THE Men'sHealth®
HOME
WORKOUT
BIBLE

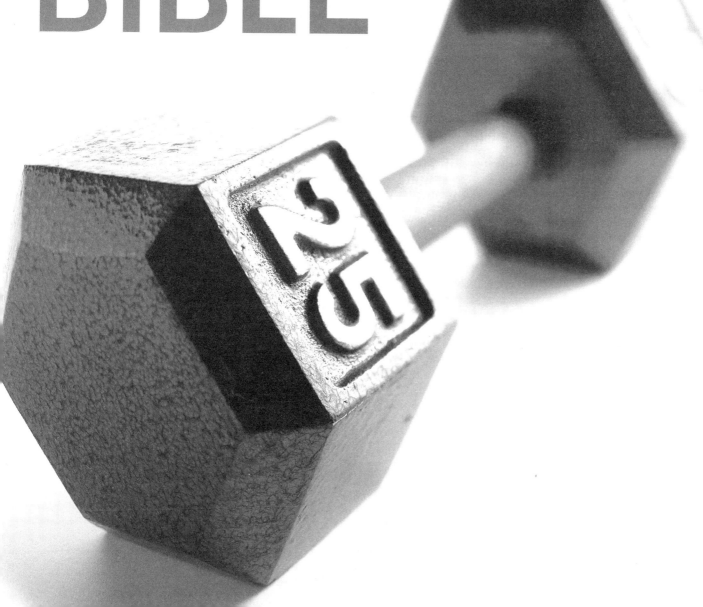

THE Men'sHealth
HOME WORKOUT BIBLE

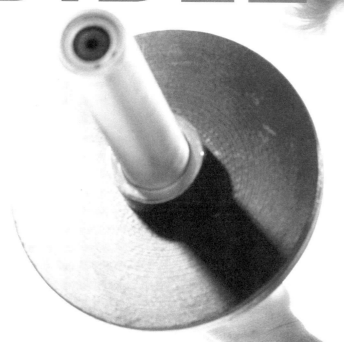

EDITED BY LOU SCHULER, Men'sHealth FITNESS DIRECTOR

WITH EXERCISE PROGRAMS BY MICHAEL MEJIA, M.S., C.S.C.S.

RODALE

© 2002 by Rodale Inc.

Illustrations © by Spencer Phippen

First published 2002
First published in hardcover 2003

Cover and Text Design by Charles Beasley
Cover Photograph by Mitch Mandel/Rodale Images
Interior photographs by John P. Hamel and Mitch Mandel/Rodale Images
Photo editing by Liz Reap
Illustrations by Spencer Phippen

Library of Congress Cataloging-in-Publication Data

The men's health home workout bible / Lou Schuler and Michael Mejia.
    p.   cm.
Includes index.
ISBN 1–57954–586–6 hardcover
ISBN 1–57954–657–9 paperback
   1. Exercise for men. 2. Bodybuilding. I. Schuler, Lou. II. Mejia, Michael.
GV482.5 .M46 2002
613.7'0449—dc21   2002008195

Distributed to the book trade by St. Martin's Press

2 4 6 8 10 9 7 5 3   hardcover
2 4 6 8 10 9 7 5 3 1   paperback

Visit us on the Web at www.menshealthbooks.com, or call us toll-free at (800) 848-4735.

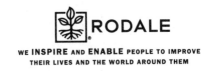

RODALE

WE **INSPIRE** AND **ENABLE** PEOPLE TO IMPROVE
THEIR LIVES AND THE WORLD AROUND THEM

CONTENTS

PART 3: HOME, SWEAT HOME

PREFACE

It's 4:30 on a cold, damp November morning. I'm stumbling downstairs to the kitchen, my eyelids still at half-mast, when I'm suddenly overcome by a feeling of impending doom. I know something isn't right, but I can't put my finger on the problem. Then, right before I take my first sip of coffee, it hits me:

It's leg day.

In a little over an hour, I'm going to have a couple hundred pounds of iron across my shoulders as I squat up and down like a Jack who can't decide whether he wants to be in or out of his box. It's not enough that I drag myself into the weight room at this unholy hour—I have to do the heaviest, ugliest exercises when I get there. Hey, maybe when I'm done I can walk barefoot over molten lava, or shave with a cheese grater.

A short while later, as the second cup of high test kicks in, the morning haze lifts from my brain and I start thinking more clearly: No one is forcing me to do this. This whole waking-up-before-dawn business is entirely self-inflicted. I could just as easily hit the snooze button a few dozen times, or not even set the alarm at all.

But I don't. Sure, I bag my workout every now and then, and go back to bed. That's usually when I'm sick or coming off a poor night's rest. Most days, I'm in my gym no matter what.

I know what you're probably thinking right now: "This guy's a trainer. It's his job to stay in shape." Fair point. There's no doubt that the shape I'm in says as much to my clients as my résumé does. A big part of my credibility is tied up in my appearance. Who's going to take fitness advice from a fat trainer?

There's more to my workouts than income enhancement, though. I could sleep in more often than not and still look like a competent trainer. What gets me up in the morning is the challenge. I like to set goals—a 300-pound bench press, a 30-inch waist, a microscopic body-fat percentage—and then achieve them through hard work, no shortcuts allowed. I like getting stronger and leaner each year while most American males are getting weaker and fatter. Most of all, I like knowing that someday I'll be able to carry my grandchildren up a flight of stairs as easily as I now carry my two young daughters.

Believe it or not, there's a reason I'm telling you all this about me: I want you to think about what motivates you—or what will motivate you if, like most North Americans, you aren't currently exercising enough to get any real benefit. Is it the fear of going up another waist size and having to buy new pants? The embarrassment of going to your high school reunion 20 pounds over your fighting weight? A doctor's order to knock your cholesterol level down a hundred points?

Maybe you're more like me, already in decent shape but having trouble pushing yourself toward the next horizon. You know that Mr. Foot remembers how to push Mr. Accelerator. You just aren't sure how hard you want to press.

In my opinion, this is a bigger dilemma for guys who work out at home than for guys who go to gyms. At the gym, there are plenty of mo-tivated lifters. Some are aiming for the biggest bench press, some for the biggest arms, some for the smallest waist. Some don't seem to have any goal other than to spend as much time as possible surrounded by iron. But a silly goal is still a goal. And when you're surrounded by guys who are working toward something, it's easier to take in their goals by osmosis, if not outright intent. Just by emulating a guy who's trying to get superior results, you'll probably make more progress than if you trained at home alone in your garage.

Trouble is, you *do* train at home alone in your garage. Where does that leave you?

Well, you have an automatic excuse for any outcome, no matter how far short of your goals you fall. It's a "Get Out of Jail Free" card for failed exercisers. Tell someone you lift weights at 5:00 A.M. while staring at your lawn mower and a couple of bags of fertilizer, and he'll understand if you never get results.

There's another way to look at this: If you succeed under those circumstances—and success probably involves finding another spot for either your weights or your fertilizer—you've achieved *more* than the guy who builds his body at the local sweat palace. While the two of you could have equal strength and physique development, in this case, the tie goes to the guy who trains at home. You know more about exercise than the gym member does, because you've had to accomplish the same results with less equipment. You know yourself better than he does, since you've tested your body and mind under adverse circumstances and know what turns your gears.

More than anything else, though, you understand what this fitness thing is really about. You know it's more than a big bench press or how you look at the beach. You know it's as much about how you feel as how you look.

I'm not downplaying the aesthetics. I want the bulging biceps and the six-pack just as much as the next guy does. Nevertheless, I think there's a point at which, to paraphrase Dennis Miller, the banal takes a back seat to the consequential. Neither you nor I walk into the weight room each morning with the idea that we're going to stave off heart disease, increase self-confidence, or sleep better at night. We just know we feel better when we exercise than when we don't. Not just better—we feel *right*. We feel strong, motivated, disciplined. After a particularly good day with the iron, maybe we even feel tough. Tougher than the guys who hit the snooze button, anyway, or the guys who put away a six-pack and a bag of Cheetos while watching *Friends* reruns. And since we accomplish all this while exercising at home, with the fridge and the TV beckoning from just a few feet away, maybe we feel tougher still.

It's not instant gratification, but it's profoundly gratifying.

—*Michael Mejia*

ACKNOWLEDGMENTS

A book of this size and scope requires a lot of people to pull together. It helps if two or three of them are sane. We got lucky and assembled a team of mostly lucid individuals, all of whom were asked to make their contributions on very short notice. Among the players:

- Writer Kelly Garrett, with whom I actually share a history in fitness journalism, although neither of us realized it until we worked together on this project. Kelly wrote the original drafts of many of the following chapters. If you see a sentence you like, he probably wrote it.

- Joan Price and Mark Anders, who contributed information and expertise to the exercise-video and exercise-equipment chapters, respectively.

- Photographers Mitch Mandel and John P. Hamel, who shot hundreds of quality photos in the time most photographers shoot dozens.

- Model Jason Cameron, who cheerfully held heavy weights and contorted body positions so Mitch and John could shoot those hundreds of pictures. Jason, besides being a model and actor, is also a personal trainer certified by the National Strength and Conditioning Association, and ended up being a full-fledged participant in the book as he helped us get the exercise images right.

- *Men's Health* assistant fitness editor Adam Campbell, who supervised the photo shoots by day and performed his writing and editing duties for the magazine on his evenings and weekends.

- Australian strength coach Ian King, C.S.C.S., our favorite trainer in the entire Southern hemisphere, whose ideas we borrowed from liberally in putting together our exercise programs.

- All the manufacturers and distributors who gave or lent us their equipment for the photo shoots. Special thanks goes to Stuart Glenn, president of Fitness Factory Outlet, who sent us tons of equipment (literally) with less than a week's notice. We also want to express our gratitude to Mike Slawinski of ProSpot Fitness, who not only lent us his prototype of the first ProSpot model designed for home use but also traveled to Emmaus, Pennsylvania, to set it up for the photo shoot.

Those are just the contributors from outside the *Men's Health* Books staff.

In-house, associate editor Deanna Portz pulled together the equipment for the photo shoots and managed the weeks-long shooting schedule.

Art director Charles Beasley designed the book and supervised almost every day of shooting, even though his wife gave birth to their second son in the middle of the project.

Research editor Deborah Pedron fact-checked all the product information and myriad other particulars.

Managing editor Kathryn C. LeSage acted as line editor as well as copy editor.

Thanks also go to executive editor Jeremy Katz, whose first days on the job were in the middle of the frantic photo shoots, and *Men's Health* vice president and editor-in-chief David Zinczenko, a believer in and champion of this project from day one.

Finally, I'd like to thank my wife, Kimberly Heinrichs—who once again found herself acting as a single parent to our three children while I disappeared on early mornings and weekends to work on this book—and Kimberly's parents, Margaret and Hugh Heinrichs, who spent many hours hosting their grandchildren so I could have more time to write and edit.

To all who contributed, thanks.

—Lou Schuler

INTRODUCTION

Welcome home.

We're glad you're ready to turn a piece of your humble abode into your personal war room. You're primed to use home exercise equipment to get your body into the shape it deserves to be in. You're not asking for much—just an awesome physique, better health, increased self-confidence, greater strength, and a longer life.

In the pages ahead, you're going to get all of that—and then some.

We assume you're not in the habit of doing things half-assed. Good. Rest assured that the information we're going to give you will be fully assed. In fact, the reason this book is more than 400 pages long is because a top-quality, beginner-friendly, long-haul home-workout program takes some time and space to explain. We're giving it 100,000 words and several hundred pictures. That doesn't cover everything, but it sure gets to most of it.

Exercise is as simple or complicated as you want to make it. It's easy (in theory) to walk for a few minutes or do some pushups or jog or stretch. When you attach performance goals to those exercises, things start getting tricky. Adding muscle, shedding fat, building strength, or improving your ability to run or jump or play a specific sport—those goals require the right exercises, the right techniques, and the right mix of hard work and recovery.

We've got all that, and more.

HOW TO USE THIS BOOK

We hope everyone who buys this book will eventually read every chapter. But we know many of you will go straight to the exercise sections and dive in. We anticipated this, because we're the same way. Our houses and garages are filled with appliances, tools, and vehicles for which we still haven't read the owner's manuals.

That's why we made the book as modular as possible. The exercise chapters are arranged according to the equipment a guy is likely to have in his home. We start with the no-equipment chapter (chapter 6, which strongly encourages you to add a chinning bar and Swiss ball to your minimalist setup), then progress to chapters on dumbbells, barbells, cable machines, and, finally, multistation home gyms. Chapter 11 shows you several routines you can do if you have all the equipment mentioned in chapters 6 through 10.

Each chapter is itself divided by muscle groups, so all the dumbbell arm exercises are in one place, all the barbell chest exercises are together, and so on. We recommend how many exercises to choose from each group, and how many sets and repetitions to do.

For the most knowledgeable and self-motivated among you, that's probably enough. But in case you don't have much experience putting together workout routines, we've taken the extra step and put some together for you.

Starting on page 357, you'll find sample routines for three skill levels (beginner, intermediate, and advanced), with six equipment options (no equipment except a chinning bar and something that can be used as a bench; dumbbells; barbell; cable; multistation; and all equipment). If you have more than one type of equipment, we've made it easy to mix and match.

If you have any questions that the book doesn't address, go to www.menshealth.com and ask it on one of our fitness message boards. This book's authors, as well as other experienced trainers and knowledgeable readers, will be happy to help you find the answer.

PART I

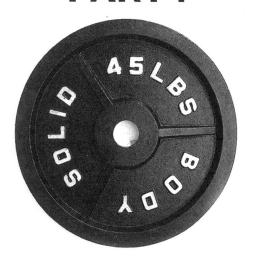

HOMEGROWN MUSCLE

CHAPTER 1

WHY WEIGHT TRAINING WORKS JUST AS WELL IN YOUR HOME

Your suspicions are correct: The home-workout experience is not quite like the commercial-gym scene.

At home, you get right to work without waiting for some unbearably bubbly employee to scan your membership card and tell you to have a nice workout.

At home, you know whose sweat is on the exercise bench.

At home, you don't have to share equipment . . . unless you have more grown kids living with you than Pa Cartwright.

Where it really counts—results—there's zero difference between a home gym and a membership gym. Regardless of venue, your muscles respond to weight training in exactly the same way: They grow. In a process called hypertrophy, your muscle cells (usually called fibers because of their elongated shape) actually get bigger so it's easier for them to hoist those barbells. This is a pretty clever strategy for what are essentially pieces of meat. Still, muscles aren't so smart that they can discern their locale. They couldn't care less whether you work out in a private residence or a crowded health club. Their only concern is adapting so that they'll be ready the next time you ask them to push around heavy weights.

PUT UP SOME RESISTANCE

An understanding of the basic physiology of muscle growth adds an important intangible to your home workouts. Instead of going through the motions like a robot, you're involved. You feel that you're working with your body's capacities instead of against its limitations. Here's the knowledge that will turn your home workouts from a chore into a labor of tough love.

Your muscles get extra, adaptation-triggering stress when they encounter resistance to their efforts. Resistance comes in many guises. It can be caused by friction or inertia or fluid or elasticity. It can be increased and decreased. It can change at different points in a movement, since your muscles are stronger in certain positions.

When you do a strength-training exercise, the resistance is usually a combination of a weighted object and gravity. In fact, **resistance training** is a common—and probably more accurate—term for what you're doing.

Not every amount of resistance will get the job done, however. After all, you use your muscles to move weight against gravity every time you lift a bottle to your lips. As far as we know, no one puts on muscle mass that way. You'll never get anywhere unless you apply enough resistance to overload the muscles you're working.

Overload sounds drastic, but all it means is giving your muscles more work than they're used to so they have a reason to make adaptations. In terms of strength training, that means lifting weights that are heavy enough to make the exercises hard to do. Obvious? Sure. But commercial-gym parking lots are paved with the expired membership cards of misguided souls who played around with piddly little poundages for a few months and wondered why nothing happened.

The overload has to be **progressive**: Your muscles must continually adapt to new challenges if they're to continue to grow. You can give them those challenges by steadily adding weight to your lifts over time. This is a factor in outfitting your home gym. A single pair of 10-pound dumbbells might be enough to overload some muscles for a while. But what happens once your muscles have successfully adapted to those weights?

Finally, your progression must be **gradual**. Your muscles adapt best when you add a little weight at a time. Jacking up weight too much or too soon is fruitless—and even dangerous.

Your training should also be gradual in the sense that **rest** is as big a factor as the actual lifting. That's because your muscles don't get stronger while they're being trained; they get stronger while they're recovering afterward. Muscle growth is a tear-it-down/build-it-up process. It's during recovery that your muscles repair the damage sustained during resistance training, coming back bigger and stronger than they were before. So you can feel good about yourself as you stare at your third *Seinfeld* rerun the day after a workout. You aren't wasting time; you're growing muscle.

Actually, you could spend that time in your home gym instead of on your couch—if you exercise different muscles than you worked the day before. For instance, you can work on your arms while your calves are recovering. That's because when you lift weights, you train only the muscles involved in the movement you're doing.

That principal, dubbed **specificity**, isn't exactly earthshattering. Most guys are already aware that their biceps won't grow in response to calf raises. But specificity is important because it means you approach muscle gain much differently than you do fat loss. Your body sheds fat from the spots where it's genetically programmed to, no matter what. There's no way you can encourage fat loss in one part of your body over another. With muscle growth, however, you can pick and choose your spots.

Specificity makes your quest for balanced, full-body muscle development a more interesting (and complex) proposition than a more general quest for fitness that is usually undertaken via walking or jogging or some other cardiovascular exercise. The specificity principal is the reason a good chunk of this book is devoted to scores of different weight-training exercises: You need a full repertoire of lifts if you're going to hit all your major muscles.

All of the exercises we'll give you emphasize one of the major muscle groups that we'll introduce in the next chapter. But only some of those exercises truly isolate the targeted muscles. The majority are **compound movements**, meaning that more than one muscle group participates in them.

The bench press is a good example of a compound exercise, since your chest muscles (in conjunction with the front parts of your shoulder muscles) move your upper arms while your triceps simultaneously straighten your arms at the elbows. Another name for compound movement is **multijoint exercise**, for the obvious reason that your muscles have to move more than one joint to complete the exercise.

Equally obvious is why movements that do involve only one muscle are called **isolation, or single-joint, exercises**. To pick the most popular example, in a biceps curl you hold your body steady while attempting to move only your elbow joint. That movement puts all the emphasis of the exercise on your biceps, the muscle responsible for bending your elbow. (Less popular isolation exercises include divorce and downsizing—they leave you lonely and cause a few elbows to bend, too.)

None of us here at *Men's Health* believe that muscles are best built one at a time. They work together in sports and other aspects of real life, so we think that's the way they should be trained most of the time. We also know that guys—ourselves included—care more about certain vanity muscles than about others. (To misquote Gordon Gekko in the movie *Wall Street*, "Vanity, for lack of a better word, is good. Vanity is right. Vanity works.") So we'll offer a collection of biceps curls and shoulder exercises to give those high-profile muscles a little isolated attention. You'll get your curls—after you've done your bench presses, squats, deadlifts, rows, and chinups.

And after you've done all of these, you'll give new meaning to the word *homebody*.

CHAPTER 2

MEET YOUR MUSCLES

Now that you understand the mechanism for building muscles, it'll help you to know a thing or two about the structure of your muscles themselves. We're not suggesting you memorize *Gray's Anatomy*. We're just asking you to put your adrenaline on hold while we give you a rundown of your main muscle groups.

As you take your muscle tour, you'll notice that we segue easily from the official Latinate names to easier-to-pronounce nicknames such as *traps*, *lats*, and *quads*. We don't do this to save ink. We just don't think you need to read *pectoralis major* or *chest muscles* at every reference where *pecs* will do just fine. (And frankly, when we were writing this book, we didn't feel like typing out all those longer terms.)

The practical payoff to demystifying your musculature is that you'll perform individual lifts better when you're familiar with the muscles that are supposed to be working. You'll put together better workouts for balanced body development. (After all, you can't write a good lineup if you don't know your players.) And you'll become accustomed to the way most of the exercises are organized throughout this book—that is, by body part (and the muscles in each body part).

Now get ready to meet your most important parts.

MIDSECTION

Sometime during the deepest, darkest days of the 1990s, ripped abs took over from bulging biceps as the dominant symbol of male virility. Even though symbols count for jack in a home training program, your abdominal muscles matter a lot. And not just because women say so.

Fitness cognoscenti like to talk about the abs and lower back as core musculature. Anything called *core musculature* has to be important, or nobody would force himself to utter such a phrase. Sure enough, these are the muscles that work nonstop to stabilize and support your torso while you do other things, such as arm or upper-torso exercises . . . or just standing around without collapsing like an empty accordion file.

So ab work delivers more than just a harder, tauter midsection and the hunk points that go with it. It also builds the core strength that helps you work the rest of your body more effectively. That's a good investment any way you look at it.

You're not going to get this result just by knocking off a set of crunches now and then (as many a guy is wont to do). You need to work *all* your core musculature; and you need to work it regularly and systematically, just like any other muscle group.

We'll show you lots of ways to do that in part 2. For now, just understand what we mean by "all" your core musculature: Like the rest of the world, we throw out the term *abs* as a catch-all for several different muscles in the abdominal area. Let's run through those, along with the major muscle group of your lower back.

Rectus Abdominis

What it is: This is the one all the fuss is about: It's the large, flat muscle wall that—assuming it's not hidden by fat—defines most of the front of your midsection from the lower chest to the pubic bone.

What it does: Besides performing the aforementioned core chores, the rectus abdominis flexes (bends) your torso by pulling your rib cage toward your hips, or vice versa. Crunches and reverse crunches do precisely those things, which is why they're the classic (but by no means exclusive) ab movements.

What you should know: The part below your navel looks, feels, and performs differently than the top part, so we'll recommend a variety of exercises to make sure you hit the whole muscle. The above-the-navel portion, incidentally, consists of three pairs of rectangular sections stacked on top of each other. The pattern is visible in many (but not all) guys with a developed rectus abdominis and little fat covering it, and is therefore to blame for the overused ab adjectives *six-pack* and *washboard*.

Obliquus Abdominis

What it is: It runs diagonally along the side of your midsection from the lower ribcage to the pubic area. You actually have a pair of muscles on each side: The *internal obliques* lie underneath the *external obliques*.

What it does: Each pair of obliques flexes your torso to its respective side. The obliques also allow you to twist at the waist and help the rectus abdominis bend your torso forward. In addition, they do their share of stabilization work.

What you should know: You'll get much better (and quicker) results if you do two kinds of movements to work your obliques. We'll show you a variety of "sideways" crunches for flexion, as well as rotational exercises for the twisting function.

Transversus Abdominis

What it is: You don't hear much about this deepest of all abdominal muscles. It's a thin

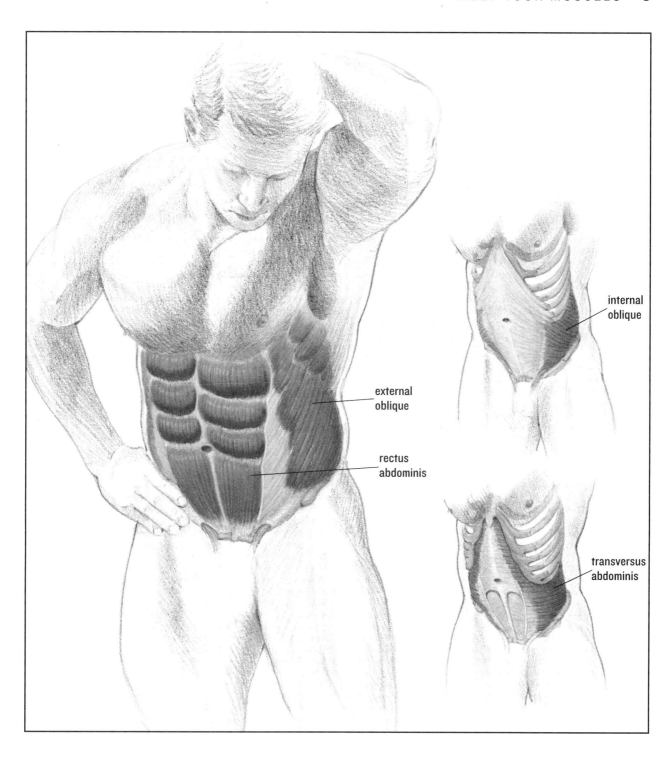

internal
oblique

external
oblique

rectus
abdominis

transversus
abdominis

strip that runs horizontally across your abdomen.

What it does: Some pretty important things such as constricting your abdomen, helping to keep your internal organs in place, forcing out your breath, and stabilizing your spine.

What you should know: A lot of exercise guides choose to ignore this one, but we figure that's not your style. Besides, the exercises you use to work the TA are interesting—almost yogalike in their emphasis on position and breathing.

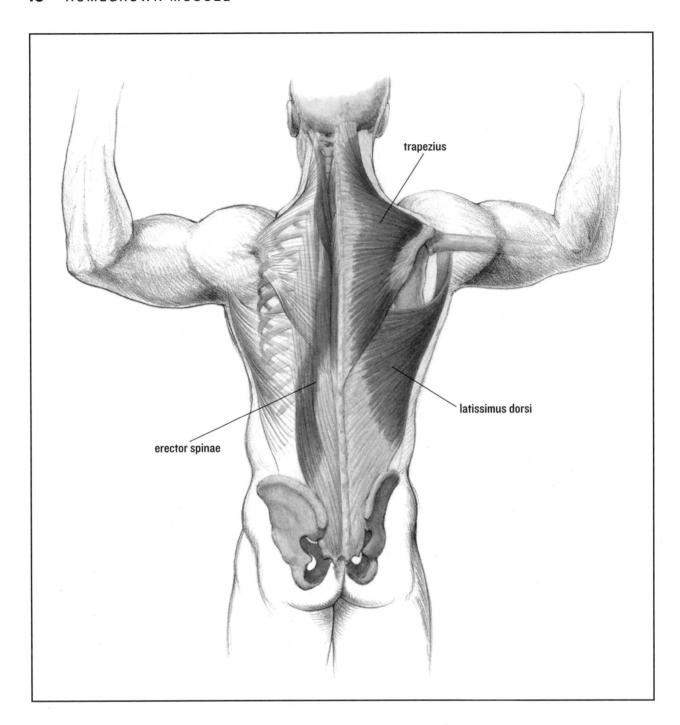

trapezius

latissimus dorsi

erector spinae

Erector Spinae

What it is: This large, powerful muscle group runs along the side of your lower spine. A pair of spinal erectors forms the main muscle group in your lower back; strengthening it reduces your chance of back pain or injury.

What it does: The name says it all: It erects your spine, straightening your torso out of a bent position. The pair also helps your obliques as you twist at the waist. And it's another key stabilizer.

What you should know: Your home is the ideal place for lower-back and all midsection work because time and convenience are your highest priority.

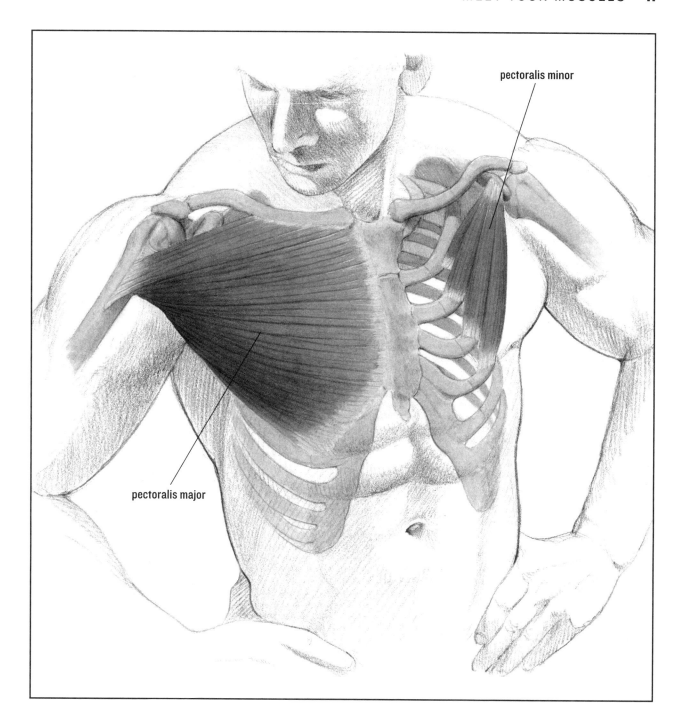

pectoralis minor

pectoralis major

CHEST AND UPPER BACK

We pair up the chest and upper back for a couple of reasons. One is that most guys are understandably gung-ho about developing an impressive, V-shaped upper torso, a worthy goal that's realized by training—guess what?—your chest and upper back.

Another is that the major muscle groups in both these body parts work to move your upper arms at the shoulder joints. (What, you thought your chest and back muscles only moved your chest and back?) Here's why that matters: When you do chest or upper-back exercises—pullups, say, or bench presses—the more-familiar arm muscles (the biceps and triceps) try to horn in and take over. That defeats your purpose. So the challenge of both chest and back work is to feel the muscles you're trying to work and then focus on them to perform the movement. That's not easy at first.

The best reason for grouping the chest with the upper back is muscular balance. As a rule, guys train their chests way too much in relation to their backs. They may be risking a postural defect, such as rounded shoulders. (We have to mention that the experts don't exactly agree on this one. Some say improper training can impair your posture; others say it's unlikely that a couple hours of exercise a week will affect your posture through all your waking hours.)

A more serious consequence of chest-heavy training is unbalanced strength. If the muscles on the front of your body are stronger than those on the back, you risk injury. Imagine that your body is a car. In any given movement, some muscles act as the engine, providing thrust and acceleration. Some act as the brakes, making sure the accelerating muscles don't pull your body apart. And some act as the chassis and suspension, keeping your body balanced during the accelerating and braking. Parity of strength from front and back and on each side ensures that all these systems work in equilibrium, rather than overwhelm each other.

You don't have to exercise your chest and back in the same workout. You just have to ensure that you work them with equal or nearly equal volume and intensity. (We'll explain what volume and intensity are later.)

Here are the specific muscles we're talking about.

Pectoralis Major

What it is: The chest muscle to the side of your breastbone. (You also have a much smaller *pectoralis minor* underneath the pectoralis major.) Your right and left pecs are like a pair of catcher's mitts: big, flat, fan-shaped, and thick. All they need is a Rawlings logo and Yogi Berra's signature.

What it does: The pectoralis's main duty is to bring your upper arm inward across your body in a motion called horizontal adduction. Your upper arms move in precisely this way when you push your hands straight out in front of you from your shoulders, as in a pushup or bench press. (Although your hands go straight up, your upper arms start outside your torso and come inward. Go ahead and see for yourself. We'll wait.).

What you should know: The upper portion of each pec runs diagonally down from your clavicle (collarbone) to your humerus (upper-arm bone). The middle part trends more horizontally from the sternum (breastbone) to the humerus. Because the intensity with which the two parts work varies at different angles, most guys use an assortment of positions and apparatuses to make sure they develop fully.

Latissimus Dorsi

What it is: It's your largest back muscle, slanting up from your lower back to your upper-arm bone. Your pair of lats pretty much defines that sought-after V-shape in the upper torso, at least from the back view.

What it does: A lot. Mainly, it pulls your upper arm toward your body—either from overhead as in a pulldown or pullup, or from in front of you as in a rowing movement. It's also a powerful internal rotator of your upper arm, so it's a big player in throwing. (An adjacent, much smaller muscle, the *teres major*, assists in these tasks.)

What you should know: The lats team with the biceps in a lot of upper-arm movements. While that's fine in real life, if you want to strengthen your lats (which you do), you have to consciously downplay the biceps' role when you do upper-back exercises in your home gym.

Trapezius

What it is: This muscle fans out from your mid-spine to your shoulder and then back in again to run up your neck. As the name implies, your pair of traps forms a trapezoid shape.

What it does: Among other things, it helps move your *scapulae* (shoulder blades) up, down, and back. Not surprisingly, shrug-mimicking exercises strengthen your upper traps, which are responsible for scapular elevation. Your lower traps do plenty of scapular depression (lowering of the shoulder blades) during pulldowns or pullups.

What you should know: Pulling back your shoulder blades is an underrated function that we'll emphasize throughout this book. Called scapular retraction, it's a group effort of the middle parts of the trapezius muscles, the back parts of the deltoids (your main shoulder muscles, which we'll get to in just a bit), and a pair of upper-back muscles called the rhomboids (technically, the rhomboidei, though if you use that term in any gym outside your home, people will think you're having a stroke). Strengthening these scapular retractors (via rowing movements, mostly) is key to upper-torso balance and pain-free shoulders.

SHOULDERS AND ARMS

Watch Pedro Martinez pitch and you'll be awed by how beautifully the human shoulder and arm can work together. As you start getting into your home workouts, you'll see that your shoulder muscles and arm muscles have significantly different responsibilities. They therefore require different exercises to make them bigger, stronger, and healthier.

Simply put, your shoulder muscles move your upper arm at the shoulder joint. Your upper-arm muscles bend or straighten your arm at the elbow. And your forearm muscles move your hand at the wrist. There are many clauses and caveats to this simple description—parts of the biceps and triceps cross the shoulder joint and help move the upper arm, and one of the forearm muscles crosses the elbow joint and works with the biceps—but it's easiest for most guys to just remember the muscles' simplest functions.

It's possible to isolate your shoulder and arm muscles, but it's not always easy. Your shoulder muscles often team with your upper-back and chest muscles to do their thing. And we've already mentioned that the muscles of your upper arm tend to butt in when you try to train other muscle groups. In fact, anytime your arms move, there's a good chance your upper-arm muscles are working. Because of that, you can actually build considerable arm size and strength without doing any biceps curls or triceps extensions.

While your shoulder joint is a complex piece of your anatomy that lets your arm move in an amazing number of directions, it's not built for heavy lifting in all of those directions. Generally speaking, you need to use lighter weights for shoulder-isolating exercises than you use for upper-arm moves.

Deltoid

What it is: It caps your shoulder and runs a few inches down your arm. But it consists of three distinct segments, each with a different job description.

What it does: The *anterior (front) deltoid* raises your arm in front of you. The *middle delt* raises your arm to the side. And the *posterior (rear) delt* draws your arm backward.

What you should know: Most guys get plenty of front-delt work with chest exercises like the bench press and pushup. Common lifts such as the front raise may constitute overkill, especially when you consider that the front delt is just a tiny strip of muscle—probably the smallest muscle on the body that a guy could specifically target.

Rotators

What they are: The small muscles of the rotator cuff, which control the turns and twists of your upper arm, lie deeper than your deltoid. The *subscapularis* is an internal rotator, meaning—ready for this?—it turns your arm inward. (This job

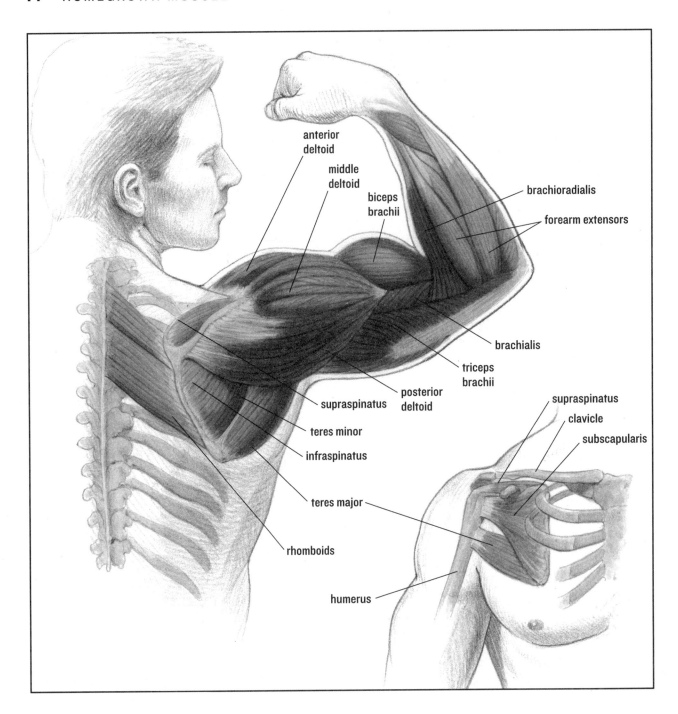

anterior
deltoid

middle
deltoid

biceps
brachii

brachioradialis

forearm extensors

brachialis

triceps
brachii

posterior
deltoid

supraspinatus

teres minor

infraspinatus

teres major

rhomboids

supraspinatus

clavicle

subscapularis

humerus

is so important that your body can't leave it to a relative peon like the subscap; the pecs, lats, and teres major also get in on the act.) The external rotators, *infraspinatus* and *teres minor*, turn your arm outward. Finally, the *supraspinatus*, which lies beneath the collarbone, helps the deltoid lift your arm out to the side.

What they do: When you cock your arm to throw a baseball, you use your external rotators. When you throw it, you use your internal rotators. When you injure your rotator cuff, you're through for the season.

What you should know: Most guys need to strengthen their external rotators, rather than their internal rotators; the latter usually get plenty of work during standard chest-and-back exercises. External-rotation exercises are usually done with cable machines (in a gym) or rubber tubing (at home or in a rehab setting). We'll show you how to do them with whatever's available—a barbell, dumbbells, or no equipment at all. The main payoff? A much-reduced risk of shoulder problems.

Biceps Brachii

What it is: Even Pee-wee Herman knows about this muscle (though he's more famous for indiscreet use of his forearm flexors). The biceps covers the front part of your upper arm. It has two sections, or "heads"—one long, one short. Though we don't normally recommend looking at pictures of bodybuilders—seeing them tends to make you forget that the aesthetic goal of weight training is to look better, not just bigger—their oversized muscles are useful when you want to see the fine lines of separation between muscles. And your arms have to get pretty huge, with your body-fat percentage in the single digits, before you can make out the separation between the two heads of each biceps.

What it does: It bends your arm at the elbow. That doesn't sound like much, but you'll be surprised at how important that flexion is to just about everything your upper body does. The long head—also called the outer head—crosses your shoulder joint and works with your front deltoid to raise your arm up in front of you. It works hardest when your hand is turned inward, when you do curls or pullups with an overhand grip, and when you do curls or chinups with a narrow grip. The short, inner head works hardest when you use a wide grip for curls, pullups, or chinups.

These are fairly trivial distinctions. For balanced strength—and to keep your workouts interesting—you'll use a variety of grips and hand positions.

What you should know: Your biceps also turns your forearm so your palm faces up—a movement called supination.

Triceps Brachii

What it is: The triceps forms a horseshoe at the back of your upper arm—or at least it will once your hard work starts paying off. As its name indicates, this is a muscle with three sections: the long head on the inside, the lateral head on the outside, and the medial head beneath the long head.

What it does: It straightens your arm at the elbow, as if you were an Atlanta Braves fan doing the tomahawk chop.

What you should know: Exercise variations can shift work from one triceps head to another (as they can for your biceps, as described earlier). Nevertheless, your entire triceps gets a workout no matter which head is emphasized.

Brachialis

What it is: Though you won't see this unless you work your way up to Arnold territory, it's right there between your arm bone and biceps.

What it does: It helps your biceps bend your elbow when your palm is facing sideways or downward instead of up.

What you should know: A simple grip change from palm-up to palm-down or palm-inward lets you work the brachialis more intensely.

Forearm Muscles

What they are: These, not surprisingly, are lots of little muscles between your elbow and your hand. Those on the palm side are collectively known as the *forearm flexors*. On the flip side are the *forearm extensors*. The biggest forearm muscle belongs to neither of those groups; it's the *brachioradialis*, up near your elbow.

What they do: The flexors bend your wrist forward; the extensors bend it back. The brachioradialis works with the brachialis on the upper arm to bend your elbow.

What you should know: Your forearm flexors also move your hand from side to side at the wrist, as in the previously alluded-to Pee-wee Pull.

LOWER BODY

From your waist down, you have some big muscles that serve you well—unless you never walk up stairs, lift, run, jump, kick, or dance. (Okay, so maybe you don't ever dance. We're pretty sure you do the other stuff at least occasionally.)

Most of the leg machines you see in health clubs isolate muscle groups to work one without involving others. At home, you'll do a lot of compound lower-body exercises, such as squats and deadlifts, to work more than one group down under. Still, a single muscle group usually does *most* of the work in any one movement, so we'll divide lower-body exercises into hip-dominant and knee-dominant categories. (We'll also have calf exercises, which compose a third category.)

Quadriceps Femoris

What it is: It's a group of four muscles on the front of your thigh that are the key to knee-dominant exercises such as squats and leg presses. For the record, the *vastus lateralis* is on the outside, the vastus medialis on the inside, the *vastus intermedius* between them, and the *rectus femoris* above them. To you, they're simply the quads.

What they do: The quadriceps extend your leg from a bent position, as in a squat or leg press.

What you should know: The rectus femoris crosses your hip joint, so it helps out in a movement called hip flexion. Since hip flexion is a part of some abdominal exercises, you'll sometimes feel the rectus femoris tighten up during your ab work.

Hamstrings

What they are: These are the main muscles at the back of your thigh, consisting of the *biceps femoris* (on the outer rear thigh) and the *semi-*

tendinosus and *semimembranosus* (both on the inner rear thigh).

What they do: You use your hamstrings to flex your knee, bringing your heel toward your buttocks. Hence, the leg curl is by far the most popular ham-building exercise.

What you should know: Your hams are also worked in hip-dominant exercises, such as deadlifts. They're big muscles designed for big jobs such as sprinting and climbing.

Gluteals

What they are: They're your butt muscles, basically. The *gluteus maximus* is the biggest, strongest muscle on your body, shaped like a construction helmet and covering the rear of your hip joint. The *gluteus medius* and *minimus* are on the outside of your hip.

What they do: The maximus works with the hamstrings on hip-dominant exercises, such as the deadlift. It also serves to move your leg straight back, in a movement that exercise physiologists call hip extension. Hip extension gives you thrusting power when you jump or sprint. The butt-blaster exercise is the purest example of isolated hip extension. We'd never tell you to do this movement, though. For one thing, it's nearly impossible to do at home with enough resistance to build serious muscle. For another . . . well, guys just look silly doing it.

The medius and minimus lift your leg out to the side. This action is called hip abduction. It's another female favorite, usually performed on that leg spreader in gyms.

What you should know: The third in the trilogy of exercises that women do to shape their thighs is hip adduction: bringing the legs together. The adductor muscles responsible for this are located on the insides of the thighs.

Hip Flexors

What they are: Opposite your glutes, on the front part of your pelvis, are the much smaller

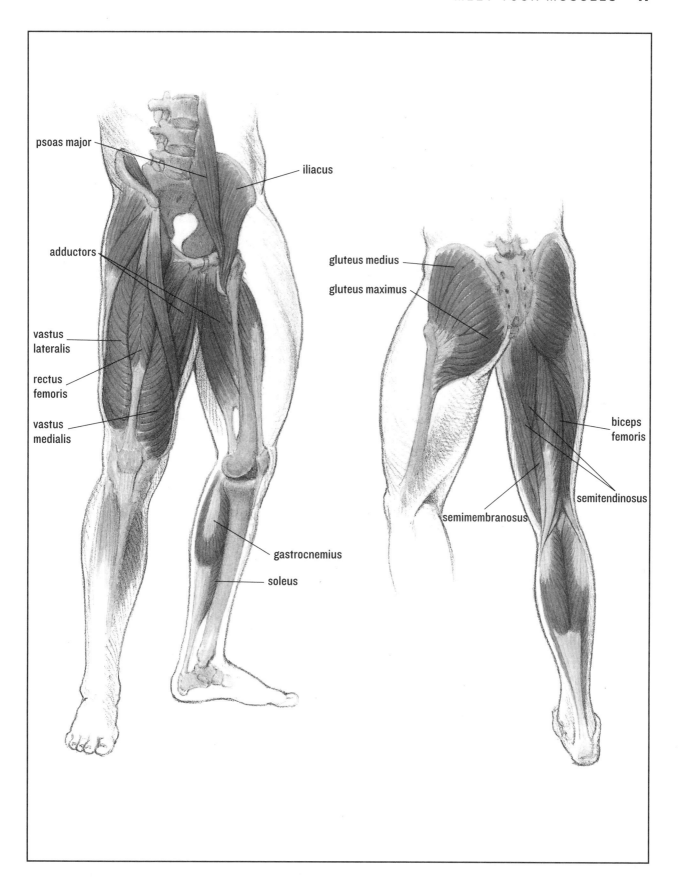

psoas major

iliacus

adductors

gluteus medius

gluteus maximus

vastus
lateralis

rectus
femoris

biceps
femoris

vastus
medialis

semitendinosus

gastrocnemius

semimembranosus

soleus

hip flexors, made up of the *psoas major* and *iliacus*.

What they do: They raise your legs in front of you. Goose-stepping soldiers are big on hip flexion.

What you should know: Your hip flexors are probably strong enough to get by without specific, targeted exercises—remember, the rectus femoris, one of the powerful quadriceps muscles, is also a hip flexor. What you need to work on is their flexibility. Tight hip flexors are the enemy of good form for all kinds of lower-body exercises and any upper-body exercises that require bending over.

Calves

What they are: These two key muscles are at the back of your lower leg. The biggest is the *gastrocnemius*, which is shaped like a butterflied salmon fillet. Under it is the *soleus*, which is more flounder-shaped.

What they do: Your calf muscles extend your foot at the ankle. They're what get you up on your toes.

What you should know: The soleus takes over from the gastroc when you do calf exercises while seated.

YOUR LOVE MUSCLE (NO, THE OTHER ONE)

Besides the skeletal muscles that move your bones, there's another muscle that's central to your fitness efforts: your heart.

As the entire civilized world knows by now, aerobic exercise trains your heart, thereby improving your cardiovascular system and your ability to use oxygen. It helps you perform aerobic tasks (such as running, swimming, and biking) for longer periods. All of this often translates into another desired benefit: fat loss.

Along with diet and strength training, aerobic (also called cardiovascular) exercise is one of the three major components of your home-fitness efforts. Like strength training, it can be undertaken with no equipment as well as with some amazingly sophisticated home equipment.

In the upcoming chapters, we'll cover the essentials of cardiovascular training and the home-equipment options for doing it. But if you've already thumbed through this book, you've probably noticed that more pages deal with strength training than with aerobics.

The main reason for this apparent imbalance is that strength work is more complex. Aerobic exercise essentially involves doing one thing for a long time. Strength training consists of lots of shorter efforts, each unique and requiring strict adherence to a precise technique. It just takes more space to explain that stuff.

Also, cardiovascular equipment is famously user-friendly. Often, the machine itself will tell you what to do and then carry on a virtual conversation with you as you do it. Weight-training equipment just sits there, waiting for you to use it. It's up to you to put it to good use—and up to us to show you how.

CHAPTER 3

YOUR HOUSE AS GYM

Your house, to the naked eye, would not be mistaken for a health club. No teal upholstery. No blaring jock rock. No chemically enhanced mutants hoisting weights that mere mortals couldn't raise without a forklift. No aspiring models working the butt blaster. In fact, there's no butt blaster, either.

That doesn't mean your digs wouldn't make a nice little fitness center. If you have a staircase, an old piano bench or a solid coffee table, some sandbags or sacks of grass seed in the garage, and (if you're already pretty damned strong) a Honda Civic to push around, you have the makings of a good-to-great workout, depending on your fitness level and ambition.

So before you spend money to fill your spare bedroom with store-bought exercise equipment, let's take a closer look at what you already have lying around.

STAIRS

Besides helping you transport yourself to and from bed each day, a staircase gives you several terrific workout options.

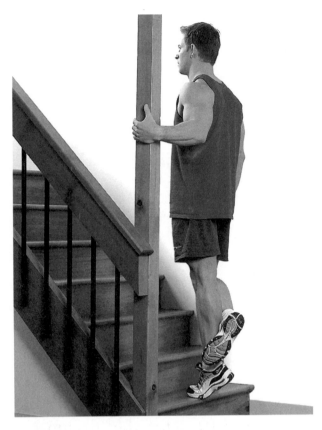

Calf raise (see page 111). A step is just the right height to stretch your calves and work them through a full range of motion.

Lunge (see page 105). When you do it on a flat surface, this is a nice exercise for your entire lower body. When you try it off a step, it becomes an even better builder of your gluteals and hamstrings.

Incline or decline pushup (see page 77). Standard pushups on a flat surface can be too challenging for a beginner or an older guy returning to exercise for the first time since his honorable discharge. If you're one of those guys, you can start out with your hands on a step and your feet on the floor.

For most exercisers, however, garden-variety pushups aren't challenging enough. You can make them tougher by putting your feet on a step.

The higher the step, the more challenging pushups become, and the more they'll work your smaller shoulder muscles and upper pectorals, instead of the meaty middle of your chest.

Stepup (see page 196). Even though you don't see many guys doing stepups in gyms, you should take advantage of these incredibly versatile lower-body exercises at home: They not only build your gluteals and hamstrings but also require strength and stability in your ankle muscles, and develop total-body balance. You can step up forward, backward, or sideways, and work different muscles each way.

Cardiovascular conditioning. Here's one for the big-city seventh-floor walk-up dwellers: A few sprints up those flights of stairs will get your heart pumping.

BENCH

Though it'd be nice to have a workout bench that inclines, declines, reclines, and reminds you to watch *SportsCenter* at 11:00, anything solid enough to hold your weight will do. Just make sure it's between 12 and 18 inches wide, and long enough to support your head, neck, and torso. If it safely gets you a few inches off the floor and allows your arms to move freely, with your elbows lower than your

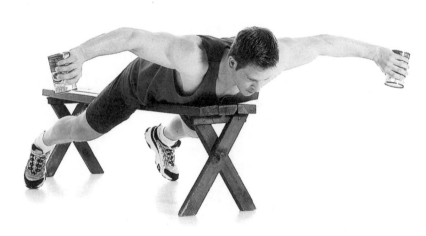

torso, that's all you need to do bench presses and flies (see pages 122 and 89).

A piano bench works well in a pinch, if you aren't lifting really heavy weights. A sturdy old coffee table is another option. Maybe you have detached picnic benches—just lay a towel on one (thus preventing splinters).

Your wife may even have one of those adjustable steps left over from the days of the aerobics junta. It'll work, too, although you may feel a temporary drop in your testosterone level the first time you use it.

Whatever your bench, add a couple of phone books or a sturdy crate to raise one end for incline and decline exercises.

SANDBAGS

In some parts of Europe, big muscles are still looked down upon; they're considered a sign that their owner is a common laborer. In America, on the other hand, every guy—whether a high school freshman or a Fortune 500 executive—wants big muscles. So, in the absence of barbells and dumbbells, it makes sense to look at how those laborers build the beef that scrawny middle-class Swedes look down upon.

A sandbag is a clumsy but effective workout tool. You can grab it by the sides to do deadlifts (see page 198), hold it against your chest to do front squats (see page 192), or pick it up off the floor and catch it on your shoulders (see the power clean on page 200).

A more unconventional use of sacks is the unbalanced deadlift, with a shovel. Put one or more sacks in the scoop of the shovel, then hold the handle and lift as you would for any type of deadlift (see page 198). The unbalanced load presents a fresh challenge to your muscles. Your back muscles, especially, have to make new adjustments to hold your spine in place while lifting. And new adjustments mean more strength and muscle mass.

You can also use sandbags for hammer curls

(see page 148), overhead triceps extensions (see page 140), and if you're in really good shape, an abdominal exercise called woodchoppers (see pages 212 and 213). You can build your grip strength and forearm size with sandbags, too. Try different grips on the bags as you lift them, and as you get stronger, squeeze harder on the bags while you work. Then see how your forearms feel afterward.

BUCKETS AND JUGS

Paint cans and water jugs come equipped with their own handles and are more versatile than you'd expect. A beginner can fill them with water for rows (see page 87) and lateral raises (see page 92).

As you get stronger, you can replace the water with sand, and perhaps even concrete. (Although we don't imagine the handle of a plastic milk jug will last long when it's lifting 15 or 20 pounds of cement.) At that point, you've got serious workout tools, so make sure you weigh them so you know what you're working with.

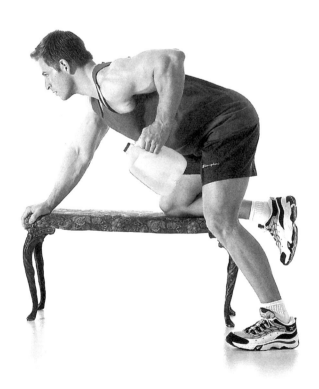

EXTERIOR WALLS

Playing wall ball with a medicine ball can help you develop strength and power for a sport (see chapter 15). Just pick a wall that's not covered in aluminum siding or Sheetrock. If you have a retaining wall, you can jump up onto it, in a type of plyometric exercise (see chapter 15 again).

JUNGLE GYM

Those kids have cost you a lot—food, orthodontist bills, the chance to be an international man of mystery. But if you bought them a jungle gym, you made an investment that will actually pay you dividends. Depending on the setup, you can use your kids' ladders and monkey bars to do pullups and chinups (see page 81), dips (see pages 95 and 96), reverse pushups (see page 86), and hanging leg raises (see page 65).

COMPACT CAR

A guy who's already strong and fit can find a hell of a workout tool in his Honda Civic or Toyota Tercel. Get it out of the driveway and push it on a flat or slightly inclined street. You need a workout partner for this one, as someone has to steer the car and be prepared to use the brake should you find yourself unable to continue pushing up that slight incline. If you're looking for an amazing lower-body muscle builder, look no further than your garage.

Note: Our lawyer insists that we include some cautionary words here. First, let us reiterate that this exercise is only for a guy who is already in very good shape. If you can do sets of 5 squats and deadlifts with 1½ times your body weight, and 10 bench presses with your body weight, you can consider yourself ready to try car pushes. No matter what shape you're in, don't try this exercise if you have lower-back problems or any type of abdominal strain.

YARD

When the weather outside isn't frightful, you can use your yard to help improve your speed, quickness, agility, and cardiovascular power.

Shuttle runs. If you have tall fences around your back yard, do short back-and-forth sprints, using some of your kids' toys as markers. We're serious about the tall fences; you'll cut your summer-barbecue invitations in half if you let anyone see you doing this.

Plyometric drills. These jumping exercises (see chapter 15 for more details) are great for improving your lower-body strength and leaping ability—if you play basketball or flag football, you'll really see the difference in your explosive power. Since the landings can be rough on your ankles, knees, and lower back, try them on the lawn, a more forgiving surface.

CHAPTER 4

THE SETUP

Though the sandbag hammer curls and jungle-gym chinups described in the previous chapter are great in a pinch, we assume you bought this book for one of two reasons:

1. You have exercise equipment, and you want to learn how to get better results with it.
2. You plan to buy equipment, and you want to make sure you get stuff that will pump up more than your Visa bill.

Regarding the first purpose, be patient—we're getting there. All of part 2 will be devoted to helping you get the most out of whatever equipment you have. Right now, we're going to help you with the second scenario by telling you about the best gear you can buy for the space you have available.

That space is, like you, unique and wonderful. Just as your parents loved you without reservation, so you'll grow to love your space, even if others have trouble seeing the charm.

However beautiful and special your home workout space is, however, you have to concede that it's limited. (Also like you—come on, admit it.)

It's great to fantasize about scoring a six-figure bonus with which to build an addition that will accommodate Body by Ed. Or, better yet, buying a McMansion in Faux Paradise, U.S.A., complete with a fully stocked workout studio.

In the real world, we all know that's going to happen for one-half of 1 percent of us. The rest of us would have to cash in our 401(k)s and the kids' college funds to come up with that kind of pump room. So we have to make smart choices.

Though prices and suppliers will change over the years, we think basic strength-training equipment will stay about the same. An Olympic barbell will still weigh 45 pounds. The bench press will still be the most popular exercise. And we'll still have to talk you into doing pullups and deadlifts.

Let's run down your equipment options.

CHINNING BARS

Chinups and pullups are the best exercises for developing your upper-back muscles while also giving your arms and shoulders a good going-over. When you can lift your own body weight 10 consecutive times, you can consider yourself a damned strong guy, pound for pound.

If you're a do-it-yourselfer, you can make your own chinning bar out of anything that will hold your weight without ripping your palms apart. Most guys just opt to spend between $10 and $37 on a simple, cheap bar that braces in a doorway. A more serious doorway bar, capable of holding up to 300 pounds, runs about $60. You could also pick up a wall-mounted bar for $145 to $180.

SWISS BALLS

Some trainers swear by these, others swear at trainers who recommend them. We like them. They make abdominal exercises different and infinitely challenging, forcing your muscles to work in new ways. Any exercise becomes more interesting when you try it on a ball instead of on the floor, a chair, or a bench. Your body must recruit more muscles to stay balanced, and if you have a strength discrepancy—if one side of your body is

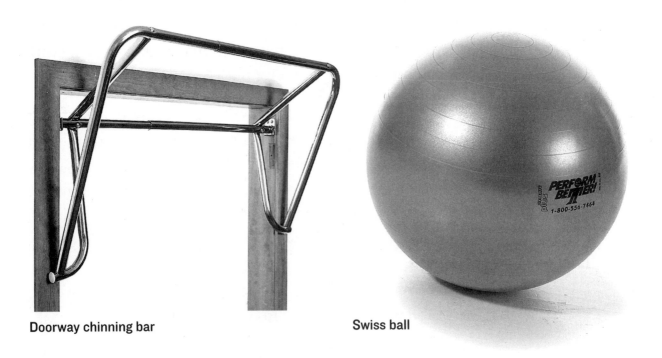

Doorway chinning bar   Swiss ball

stronger than the other—you'll quickly realize it when you use a ball for simple exercises like chest or shoulder presses.

Most catalogs and fitness-equipment stores offer balls in four sizes: 45 centimeters (for people between 4 feet 7 inches and 5 feet tall), 55 centimeters (5 foot 1 to 5 foot 6), 65 centimeters (5 foot 7 to 5 foot 11), and 75 centimeters (6 feet to 6 foot 3). You aren't completely out of luck if you're taller than 6 foot 3. You just have to go online and pay a little more for an 85-centimeter ball like the ones the guys in the NBA use.

You could pay anywhere from $15 to $45 for a ball. If you see a range of prices for balls in your size, go for one that's more expensive, and thus stronger and more durable. You may want to spend another $5 to $20 on a foot or hand pump, if you don't already own one. Trust us, you don't want to try to fill a Swiss ball with the little pump you use for your kids' rubber footballs.

Speaking of kids, they'll want to play with your Swiss ball, and there's no reason not to let them. A ball designed to support a 250-pound man doing presses with 200-plus pounds can handle some kids kicking it, throwing it, and rolling around on it. (Discourage them from using it for kickball in the street, however. The store won't take back a popped ball with Firestone tread marks.)

DUMBBELLS
Dumbbells offer enough options to confuse a financial planner. You can get a couple of handles—standard or Olympic—and load them up with the same weight plates you'd use with a barbell. You

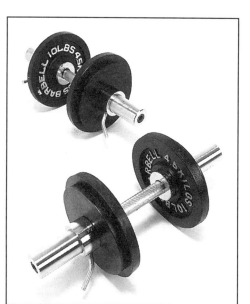

Olympic dumbbells

can get fixed dumbbells in every style—from butt-ugly hexagonal 'bells sold out of crates at your local sporting-goods store to rubber-coated, ergonomic-grip Hampton Eclipse weights that look so classy and bright you hate to call them dumb. And then there are selectorized dumbbells and quick-change systems, which are expensive but save space.

Here's a review of all the possibilities.

Adjustable dumbbells. Handles for standard weight plates can be as cheap as $7 each and can weigh anywhere from about $1\frac{1}{2}$ pounds for hollow handles to 7 pounds for solid ones. To keep the plates from sliding off the handles, you need a pair of gizmos called collars. These come in several different styles, which we'll describe in detail on page 29, in our discussion of barbells. Any of those styles are compatible with standard dumbbell handles.

Fancy threaded dumbbell handles allow you to screw on the collars as you'd screw a nut onto a bolt. Compared to the unthreaded type, these are more expensive, heavier, and in our experience, pretty useless. The collars always seem to come loose halfway through a set. You don't want to watch a collar unscrewing itself as you do an overhead triceps extension. There are better ways to crack your skull.

Olympic handles are even more expensive (about $80 a pair), heavier (11 pounds each), and kind of awkward. Each is 20 inches long, which is 6 inches longer than a standard handle. That becomes an issue on quite a few exercises. Until you get used to Olympic handles, you'll manage to make them collide during presses, smack into your legs during biceps curls, and stab you in the back during overhead triceps extensions.

Fixed dumbbells. Some guys fantasize about the girls on beer posters. We fantasize about having a complete set of fixed dumbbells. As fantasies go, ours is ambitious—the price to fulfill it would be somewhere between that of an afternoon at Fenway Park (including not only beer and peanuts but also airfare and hotel) and a 1962 Corvette.

Say you pick the cheapest weights: slag-gray hexagonal dumbbells. A set from 5 to 50 pounds (including weights in every 5-pound increment) can be had for about $230. Add a nice two-tier horizontal rack, and you're up to about $460. Those 50-pounders will seem small after a few months on one of the workout programs in this book. So you'll want to add 55- to 75-pound dumbbell pairs. That's another $300, minimum, so now

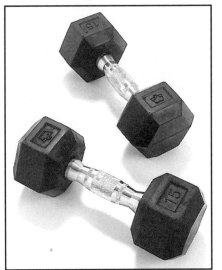

Hampton Eclipse dumbbells

you're up to at least $760. Oh, and you'll need another tier on that dumbbell rack. That takes your bill up to $800 or more.

Let's say you also follow this book's nutritional recommendations to the letter, putting on 10 pounds of extra-lean sirloin. You happily spend some money on new shirts and jackets. The downside is that your 75-pound dumbbells are no longer enough for one-arm rows and your heaviest sets of chest presses. Add five more dumbbell pairs, from 80 to 100 pounds, and you tack at least another $400 onto the price of your pump room. That puts you at about $1,200, and you still need a place to store the weights. So you move the smaller weights— the 5- to 35-pounders—to a vertical dumbbell rack, setting you back about $120.

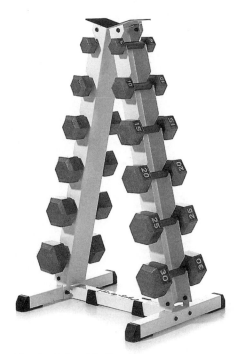

Vertical dumbbell rack

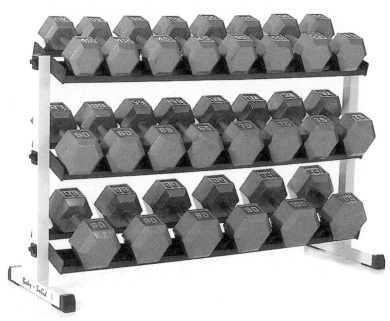

Three-tier horizontal dumbbell rack

Your total is about $1,300, not counting tax or shipping charges. And you don't have a bench yet.

Dumbbells can get a lot more expensive from there. The gorgeous Hampton Eclipse dumbbells mentioned above are more than $2,000 for a set of 5- to 50-pounders. You can find also expect to pay a lot for the rubber-coated dumbbells that are quieter and easier on your floors.

Selectorized dumbbells. The best-known are PowerBlocks. They are, literally, nested hand weights—blocks that hold thin stacks of 5 pound plates. (Other models offer differing plate weights.) To choose a weight, you adjust a selector pin. Then lift the blocks, and have at it.

You can find the Personal PowerBlock set—which allows you to select weights from 5 to 45 pounds—for around $220, and you can add a stand for about $115. The Pro Rexan set with a 40-pound add-on kit, with weights ranging from 2½ to 85 pounds, is about $550; the stand for these is $120 or so. PowerBlocks are a great space saver, and certainly cheaper than paying for a full set of dumbbells up

to 85 pounds. They're also a serious investment.

A newer, cheaper take on the same idea is Iron-Master Quick/Change dumbbells. You loosen the handles and slide on the thin plates yourself, no pins or rods required. Expect to pay $450 or so for the weights, enough plates to create 10- to 80-pound dumbbells, and a rack.

BARBELLS

The decisions you make when buying a barbell can affect your other equipment decisions. Your first choice here is between a standard and an Olympic system. A standard bar holds weight plates with a $1\frac{1}{16}$-inch hole in the middle. On Olympic plates, each hole is 2 inches across. The plates you buy for one bar aren't compatible with the other. (It's like the VHS-Betamax disparity in the early '80s, except that neither barbell system will ever become obsolete.)

So when you buy one or the other, your choice affects your adjustable dumbbells (as discussed earlier), your bench (you can use a 7-foot standard bar

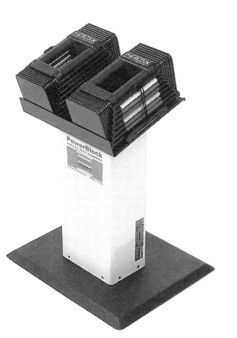
Personal PowerBlocks

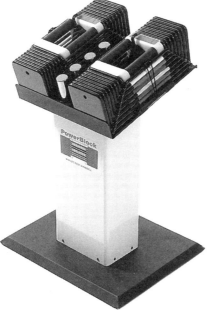
Pro Rexan PowerBlocks

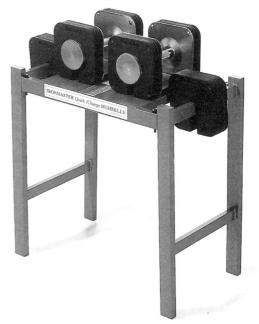
IronMaster Quick/Change dumbbells

on an Olympic bench, but not an Olympic bar on a standard bench), and any plate-loaded weight machines you buy. (We'll explain all these terms by the end of the chapter.)

Standard barbell. A 7-foot standard bar weighs 20 pounds and generally costs less than $50. Most hold up to 400 pounds of weight plates. You can also get standard combo bars and EZ-curl bars, which allow you to do arm exercises with a variety of hand positions that ease wrist strain and work your muscles differently. Each of these bars is about 4 feet long, weighs 11 to 13 pounds, and costs less than a straight barbell.

A 110-pound standard barbell set—which usually includes a 20-pound bar, 85 pounds of weight plates, two dumbbell handles, and collars (more on these later)—typically sells for $50 to $100. That's not a lot of weight for an adult male, so at some point you'll probably want to add extra weight plates to your set. We've seen standard plates for as little as 49 cents a pound.

Olympic barbell. A 7-foot Olympic bar weighs 44 pounds and holds up to 1,000 pounds' worth of weight plates. The lowest price we've seen is $75 for the bar itself. You can also get 5- or 6-foot bars, which weigh 30 and 40 pounds, respectively. Each

holds "only" 800 pounds and costs $80 to $90.

An Olympic EZ-curl bar weighs 18 pounds; combo bars are available in 18- and 20-pound versions. Any of these costs between $35 and $55.

An Olympic barbell set is about the best deal in the fitness world. We've seen a 300-pound set—including the bar, 255 pounds of weight plates, and collars—for $99. (Shipping adds more to the prices, if you buy online.) For the price of 6 weeks' dues at an average health club, you get the greatest conditioning tool ever invented.

You can get additional Olympic plates for the same price as standard plates. You can also start out with 400- or 500-pound sets for less money than you'd pay for the 300-pound set plus additional plates.

Why the extra plates? Well, for some guys, 300 pounds gets light in a hurry. For the other 99.99 percent of American males, the extra plates come in handy for convenience. Say you have an Olympic barbell, a curl bar, dumbbell handles, and a plate-loaded cable machine. Rather than move the plates from one apparatus to another each time you change exercises, it helps to have lots of plates so you can leave some near the bars, some near the cable machine, and some stacked on

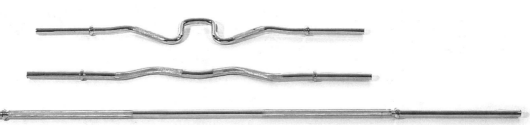

From top to bottom: standard combo, EZ-curl, and 7-foot barbells

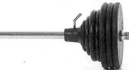

Standard 110-pound barbell set

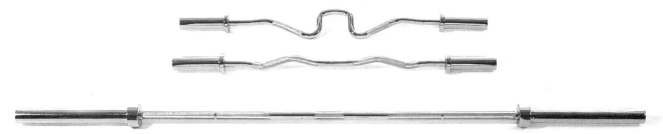

From top to bottom: Olympic combo, EZ-curl, and 7-foot barbells

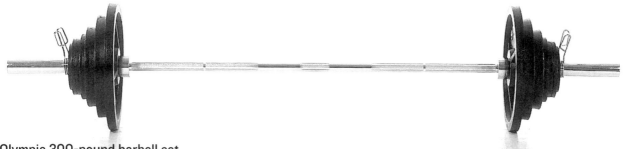

Olympic 300-pound barbell set

weight trees to impress neighbors who come over to see your home gym.

Collars. You don't need to spend a lot of time thinking about collars. Most guys just use the ones that come with the barbell set. If you buy collars separately, keep two things in mind: how fast you want to be able to change the weight plates, and how much time you want to spend calculating the extra weight the collars add.

When given a choice, we like spring collars—sort of like clothespins for barbells—because they weigh only about a pound per pair and you can get them on and off the bar faster than any other type of collar. Expect to pay at least $3 each for Olympic spring collars or $2 each for standard.

The old, standard screw-on collars we grew up with are still around, though they're no longer as popular. You're most likely to find them sold as part of a barbell set. They slow down the process of changing weight plates, and they add some weight to the bar—up to a pound on each side. If you're masochistic enough to buy them, expect to pay at least $3 each for the standard variety.

Fancier collars combine the best of both worlds—the heft of screw-on collars with the quick release and negligible weight of springs. Muscle Clamps, the best of this category, are like antilock brakes for your barbell. Expect to pay at least $35; they weigh a pound per pair.

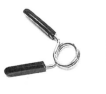

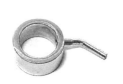

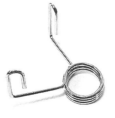

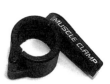

Standard spring   Standard screw-on   Olympic spring   Olympic screw-on   Muscle Clamp

BENCHES

In our experience, a guy who wouldn't think of spending less than $1,000 on a treadmill will buy the cheapest, least versatile bench he can find. It's easy to look at a piece of cardio equipment and say, "If I don't get the right one, my knees are screwed." But a mediocre bench can have a crippling effect on your workouts, too.

How can you tell whether a bench is solid? Use the rule of thumb: If you can press your thumb into the middle of the pad and touch the wooden base of the bench, the pad is too soft. Obviously, you can't do this test online or by mail-order. Still, you can always return an inadequate piece of equipment.

Perhaps the greatest challenge of owning a bench is fighting the temptation to bury it under last year's tax receipts and the kids' off-season clothing. If you start using your equipment for something other than exercise, you'll stop exercising. Lay down the law for yourself and everyone you live with: "This equipment is sacred. To clutter it up is to desecrate it—and piss me off, for which you'll suffer the consequences as soon as I add another half-inch to my arms."

Here's a closer look at your workbench options.

Dumbbell/utility bench. You can easily move this one around the room and use it for a variety of exercises. With no equipment other than a basic, $120 flat bench and some dumbbells, you can get a great workout. You're covered for any exercise that requires sitting, lying, or bracing a foot or hand against a sturdy surface. The drawback is that pushing weights week after week with no variation in angles can be tough on your joints, if not on your brain, which doesn't always warn you when you're about to pass from comfortable routine to intolerable tedium.

A good bench that inclines—adding dozens of potential exercise variations to your repertoire—costs between $130 and $270. For a bench that inclines and declines, expect to pay anywhere from $240 to $350.

The smallest sturdy bench you're going to find is about 3 feet long, 18 to 24 inches wide, and 12 inches high. So the dedicated space you need is relatively small—perhaps 10 feet by 6 feet. You also need room to stash all those dumbbell racks so your living companions don't trip over them every time they have to use the bathroom in the middle of the night. This means you have to appropriate a portion of a bedroom, a corner of a basement, or an attic.

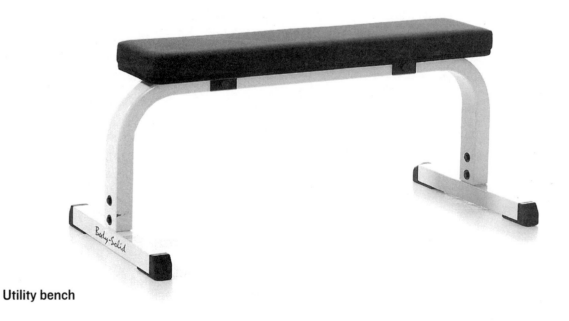

Utility bench

THE BODY YOU WANT, WITH THE MONEY YOU HAVE

One of the toughest calls a home exerciser makes is how to spend his limited funds. We're going to admit a bias that we'll show throughout this book: We think you should first invest in resistance-training equipment—whether it's a barbell, dumbbells, or weight machines—and take care of cardio equipment last. Here's why.

YOU CAN DO CARDIO EXERCISE WITHOUT EQUIPMENT. You can do any kind of cardio you want outdoors, weather permitting.

You can jump rope indoors, if you have enough headroom. (Watch out for those ceiling fans.) Rope-jumping is a fantastic cardiovascular workout that burns calories by the bucket and develops speed and hand-eye coordination at the same time. Plus, a jump rope costs $20 or less, versus $1,000 or more for a decent cardiovascular machine.

You can also get a good workout with calisthenics: pushups, jumping jacks, running or marching in place, and squat thrusts. And if you're going to do that, you may as well work out to a video. (We won't knock it if you like it, but we wouldn't do it unless we were snowed in—and maybe not even then.)

Another very cheap option, if you're a cyclist, is a stationary home trainer. It lifts your rear wheel off the ground so you can pedal away, using all your gears, in a space not much bigger than the bike itself.

YOU GET MORE WEIGHT EQUIPMENT FOR YOUR MONEY. It's hard to get a decent treadmill for less than $1,000; the best ones go for $4,000 to $5,000. You'd think stationary bikes would be cheaper, but the bottom-of-the-line Lifecycle has a sug-gested retail price of $1,499. And after spending all that money, you'd still have just one piece of equipment, allowing only one exercise.

Spend the same $1,500 on weight equipment, and you can set yourself up with a pretty good home weight room: Olympic weight set, good bench, power rack with cable attachment, Swiss ball. Right there, you have access to hundreds of exercises and every imaginable type of training program. And since most of the investment is in iron and steel, it'll last you forever.

THERE'S LESS VARIATION AMONG BRANDS OF STRENGTH EQUIPMENT. You can order a 300-pound Olympic weight set from just about any manufacturer and be assured that you're getting a worthwhile product. Some weights look cooler than others—you can spend as much as $2,450 on a set of rubber-coated chrome dumbbells from www.hamptonfit.com, for example—but the basic hexagonal dumbbells at your local sporting-goods store build the exact same muscles the exact same way.

There's more of a quality gap between the best and worst benches and weight machines, but it's nothing like the difference between a $1,000 treadmill from a warehouse shopping club and a top-of-the-line $5,000 treadmill from a company that advertises in *Runner's World* magazine.

The big caveat is that if you want or need to do aerobic exercise but can't take the ankle, knee, and lower-back pounding of outdoor running, a high-quality treadmill, stationary bike, or elliptical machine may be a good investment.

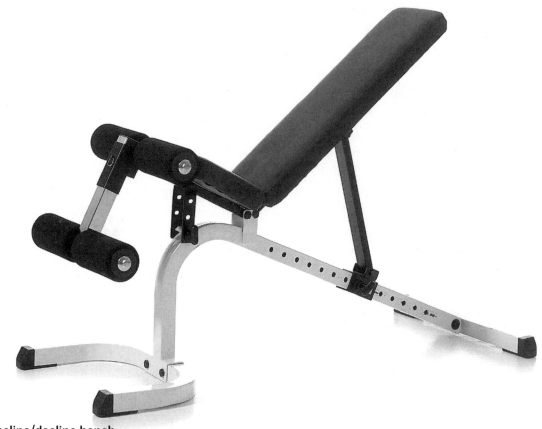

Flat/incline/decline bench

Barbell bench. This is attached to a frame with uprights that hold a barbell for bench presses. So this is not the place to go cheap: You rely on this bench to keep more than 100 pounds of iron from crashing down on your forehead. For between $150 and $300, you can get a good one that allows flat, incline, and decline presses.

The next step up is a bench that has adjustable uprights you can raise or lower to accommodate longer or shorter arms. (If your wife or kids will be using the bench, this feature will come in handy). Some in this class have uprights that rise as high as 5 feet, allowing you to rack a barbell for squats and standing shoulder presses. And some include additional attachments that let you do dips—a great exercise for your chest, shoulders, and triceps. These benches cost between $300 and $500. That seems like a lot, until you realize this one bench, along with a barbell set, gives you the ability to do almost every important strength exercise. You can do presses and dips for your chest, rows off the floor for your back, squats off the rack and deadlifts off the floor for your lower body, and a variety of arm and shoulder exercises.

The only potential downside of having your press bench and squat rack in one piece of equipment is that you need quite a bit of workout space. The bench is about 6½ feet long, and the uprights are about 4 feet wide. You need at least 4 feet in front of the bench to move around, about 4 feet behind it so you can do squats, and at least a foot on each side of the bar, depending on what size bar you have. If you use a standard 5- or 6-foot bar rather than a 7-foot Olympic bar, you can get away with less space. Still, you're looking at a space that's 11 feet square, at least. That will give you room to lift hard and heavy, with space on the periphery for your weight plates, any dumbbells you have, and any extra bars (such as an EZ-curl bar).

SQUAT RACKS AND POWER RACKS

One solution to the space problem described above is a free-standing pair of squat stands or a squat rack, which you can probably find for between $160 and $550 (with the squat stands being the less expensive). The footprint of squat

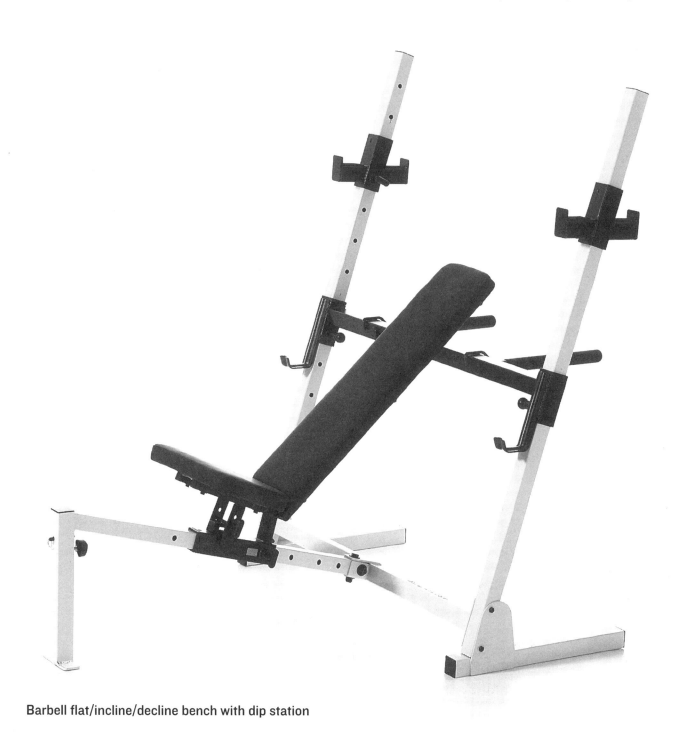

Barbell flat/incline/decline bench with dip station

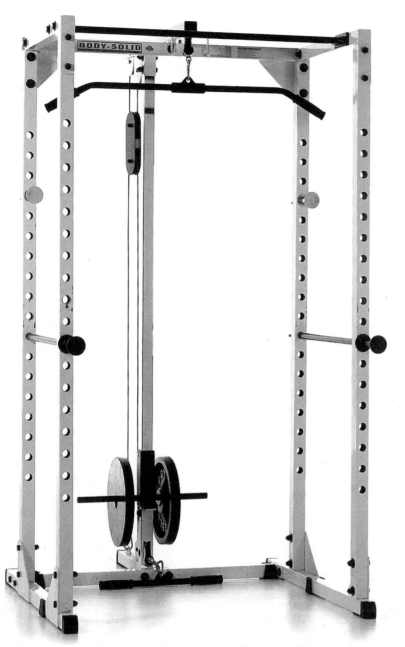

Power rack with chinning bar and plate-loaded cable attachment

bench, allows you to do heavy shrugs or biceps curls without having to load the weights onto a bar that's sitting on the floor—or to lift the bar off the floor to start the set. This is the most serious piece of strength-training equipment you can put into a room without taking over the entire room.

A power rack, on the other hand, takes over the room. This open cage of solid steel has a footprint of about 4 feet by 4 feet. If you add attachments and apparatuses to the rack's cage, it takes up even more space beyond its basic footprint. It also requires close to 7 feet of headroom (a typical height is 6 foot 8). And though the rack eliminates the need for uprights, you still need the bench itself to do chest exercises.

Nevertheless, if you're serious about weight training, the $300 to $600 you'd pay for a power rack is the best investment you could make. At some point, you'll want to test your strength in exercises like the squat and bench press. What happens if you fail on a squat? Since the weight is on your back, you can't stand up. Yes, you can let the barbell roll down your back and hit the floor. But think for a second about what 200 or 300 pounds would do to the floor. Now think about what that weight would do if it were stuck on your chest during a bench press. You might be able to roll the barbell down your torso to your lap and stand up. You might be able to tip it to one side or the other and let it crash to the floor. Or you might not be able to do anything except lie there with 300 pounds slowly crunching the life out of you.

stands is generally 1½-by-2½ feet. Squat racks are about 3 feet by 5 feet. You can position either option within a foot or two of a wall.

The name *squat rack* doesn't really do justice to this versatile tool that can be lowered for bench presses or raised for squats and standing shoulder presses. The lowest setting, minus a

A power rack provides safety bars that you can drop the bar onto if you fail at a maximum lift. You can also rest the barbell on those bars for shrugs and curls. You can easily slide a utility bench in and out of the rack for any number of exercises. For about $189 or more, you can add a plate-loaded cable-pulley system to the back of your squat rack. ("Plate-loaded" means you use your own weight plates.) This doesn't require a lot more room, and it allows you to do dozens more exercises, from lat pulldowns to cable rows to triceps pushdowns to cable biceps curls.

For $450 to $650, you can save yourself some fuss by getting a selectorized cable apparatus, which includes weight plates (the stack is usually 210 pounds) and allows you to select the weight you want by sliding in a pin.

Finally, some power racks have a crossbar on the front top that doubles as a chinning bar. (To use this you need about a foot of clearance above the top of the rack—about 8 feet from floor to ceiling.) You can also add dip bars to some power racks for about $50.

FLOOR PADS AND PLATFORMS

If you lift on a carpeted floor, you already have some padding and sound muffling in place. However, you have to consider whether you want to protect the carpet, in case you ever decide to use this room for something other than workouts.

Protection is an even bigger issue in a room with wood, tile, or linoleum floors. Sure, you can treat each weight like a sleeping infant, setting it down gently after each set. You can sing it lullabies, too. "Rock a bye, barbell, on the Mexican tile. . . ." You can't, however, baby your bar forever. Eventually, you're going to work so hard, with such heavy weights, that you'll forget to put them down softly. (The same thing might happen with the kids, but we won't joke about it.)

There are two options for quieting the clanging.

Rubber floor mats. These are usually sold as 4-feet-by-6-feet mats, in thicknesses ranging from $3/8$ to $3/4$ inch. (The heavier weights you plan to lift, the thicker the mat you'll need.) Two medium-thickness ($1/2$-inch) mats cost at least $100.

To more easily safeguard a bigger room, try interlocking 4-by-4 mats. Covering 16 square feet will set you back more than $200.

Olympic lifting platform. We mention this only because we fantasize about having such a cool fixture in our own home gyms. This 8-feet-by-6-feet, 2-inch-thick platform allows you to stand on a laminated wood center while the weight plates on the ends of your Olympic barbell sit on rubber mats. It's serious equipment, which is why you

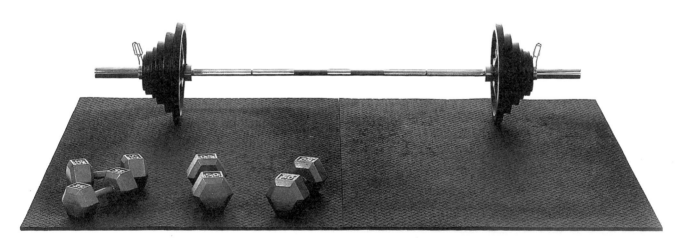

4-foot-by-4-foot rubber floor mats

usually find it only in college weight rooms, as opposed to Hank's Hypertrophy Heaven. (However, if you've gone so far as to design a logo for HHH, you can get that stamped on the wooden floor of your platform.) It's perfect for heavy lifts—deadlifts, power cleans, Olympic lifts (snatch, clean and jerk)—in which you might drop the weights at the end. You can also rest your bench and power rack on the platform. Cost? Between $550 and $750, not including your logo.

BELTS, GLOVES, STRAPS, AND WRAPS

Though we encourage you to lift without any of these accessories, we aren't going to argue if you won't lift without them.

Belts. If you've been in a gym in the past few years, you've seen lifters wearing belts for everything from bench presses to biceps curls. We once saw a guy wearing one as he walked from his car to the gym's front door. (Guess his car keys must've felt pretty heavy that day.)

The purpose of a belt is to increase intra-abdominal pressure, which provides support for your lower back on exercises such as deadlifts, squats, bent-over rows, and overhead lifts. We recommend training your own muscles to supply this pressure. The abdominal exercises in part 2 are a good way to start, and pulling in your abs on exercises like rows and deadlifts makes a belt unnecessary in most workouts. We confess we're all reformed belt-wearers. Now that we've weaned ourselves, we lift heavier weights than we ever did while wearing them.

Belts do have their place. For most guys, it's a good idea to wear one for maximum-weight lifts. Guys with back problems can use them more liberally. Our advice: Do your normal exercise belt-free, unless you have a back injury or some sort of structural anomaly (scoliosis, for example) that makes lifting more dangerous for you. If you're under a doctor's care, let him make the call.

A leather belt usually costs $20 to $30 (more for XXL). There's not much point in getting a belt that's thin in front and thick in back. You need the support in front, to increase intra-abdominal pressure, as much as you need it in back for structural integrity.

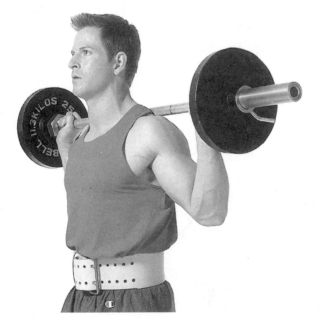

Weight belt

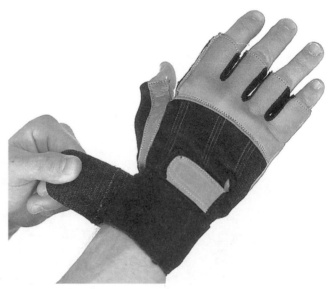

Lifting glove

Gloves. While these improve your grasp and prevent calluses, we think they also limit your grip strength. If you want to try them anyway, go for the cheapest ones that fit comfortably. Washable is good. Don't bother with more expensive gloves with leather wrap-around wrist straps. They won't give you the support you think they will. Expect to pay from $7 to $24 for lifting gloves.

Straps and wraps. Straps are $10 bands of cotton (with or without neoprene padding) or leather that help you hold on to a barbell so you can lift more weight on rows, pullups, pulldowns, and shrugs. In our view, a better way to improve your hold on the bar is to develop greater grip strength. And one of the best ways to strengthen your hands and wrists is to lift without the damned straps.

Knee wraps are a different story. Unlike gloves or wrist straps, they're allowed in powerlifting competitions, so wearing them isn't exactly cheating. More important, if you already have creaky knees that prevent you from squatting more than your body weight without support, wraps could save your joints from further damage. They cost $10 to $20 per pair.

OTHER COOL STUFF

Buying free-weight gear can be addictive. Once you have a cable setup for rows and pulldowns, for example, you'll want all the dozen or so attachments you can use with it. This reminds us of a line from comedian Steven Wright: "You can't have everything. Where would you keep it?" Here are a few things we'd force ourselves to find room for.

"Fat" bar. This 4-foot Olympic bar is 2 inches in diameter. That thickness makes it harder to hold on to, forcing you to develop more grip strength than would a thinner bar. The fat bar is great for arm exercises and makes presses and bent-over rows newly challenging. Expect to pay $70 or so.

PlateMates. You can attach one of these magnets to the outside of a dumbbell to add an extra $5/8$, $1^1/4$, $1^7/8$, or $2^1/2$ pounds of weight. Or you can put one on each end of the dumbbell to add up to 5 pounds. You'll pay $20 to $40 for a pair. For around $20, you can also get PlateMate bricks, which are specifically designed to attach to the weight stack of a cable machine.

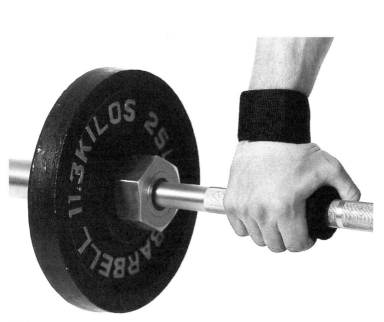

Wrist strap

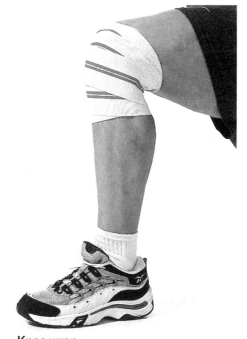

Knee wrap

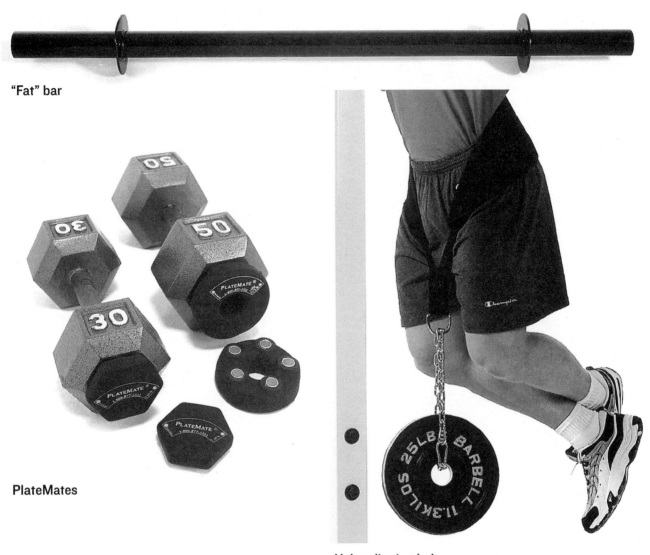

"Fat" bar

PlateMates

Nylon dipping belt

Dipping belt. As you get stronger, you'll find you can do a lot of dips before you really challenge your muscles. A dipping belt allows you to hang a weight plate or dumbbell from your waist to make an unchallenging exercise hard again. And let's face it: Having 25 to 50 pounds of iron hanging between your legs makes you feel like the biggest ape in the jungle.

It's also great for increasing your strength on pullups and chinups. Say you're stuck on 8 pullups—you've been doing that many for months, and you can't do more. Hang some weight from your waist, do sets of 4 or 5, and suddenly your body weight feels light when you do pullups without the belt. You might jump from 8 to 10 or 12 within a few weeks.

A dipping belt is also a pretty good guarantee that you'll do each exercise slowly and with perfect form. Think of what a careless mistake could do to your, uh, self-esteem.

You can pay about $30 for a nylon belt that includes the chain that holds the weight. Or for about $20, you can get a strap and chain to use with your own lifting belt.

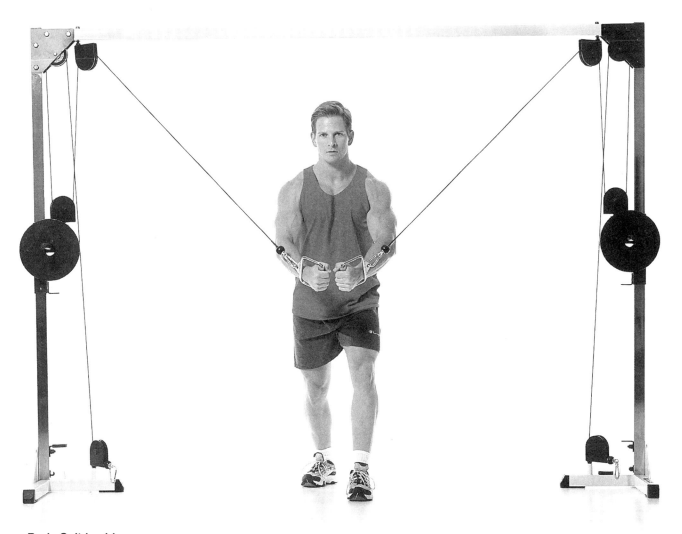

Body Solid cable crossover

CABLE STATIONS

We already mentioned that you can add a cable apparatus—plate-loaded or selectorized—to your power rack. We think that's a great choice because you should build your home workouts around free weights, with cable exercises acting as a supplement. The combined power rack/ cable apparatus takes up only slightly more space than either by itself, and it will allow you to do all the barbell exercises in chapter 8, plus most of the cable exercises in chapter 9. That's about 90 exercises right there, with dozens of possible variations.

You could, of course, buy a free-standing cable setup. These range from basic and cheap to astoundingly versatile and expensive.

The main benefit of a basic machine is that it can fit into a fairly narrow space. If you had to, you could probably squeeze it into a space 4 feet wide and still manage to do many of the exercises we'll show in chapter 9. To do the exercises safely and comfortably, however, it's best to have 5 to 6 feet between the machine and any wall. You need about 7 feet of headroom, regardless.

Unfortunately, such a machine is so basic that

it requires you to make time-sucking equipment adjustments when shifting from a high pulley (for lat pulldowns and triceps exercises) to a low pulley (for rows and biceps and shoulder exercises). It's probably made with cheap components, which means you won't have smooth, gym-quality action on lat pulldowns and seated rows. The creakier the action, the less appealing the workout becomes, and the more likely you are to let the machine turn into a $400 dustheap.

So as long as you're spending money, you may as well say to hell with simple and cheap, and spring for versatility. A cable-crossover machine allows you to do all of the exercises in chapter 9 and use the space in between the towers for free-weight exercises. (In fact, as we'll show in chapter 9, you can add free weights to some cable exercises to make them doubly challenging.) The machine is about 10 feet long, 7 feet high, and 3½ feet wide. You need even more space in two of those directions: To do exercises requiring a forward step, you need at least 6 feet in front; and to use the chinup bar that's usually attached to the top crossbar, you need about a foot more headroom.

The Body Solid cable crossover shown on the previous page costs about $500—and the prices for other models can go up considerably from there. As with any piece of exercise equipment, the closer you get to gym-quality, the more you can expect to pay.

For example, the relatively new fitness-equipment company FreeMotion Fitness sells its crossover machine for $3,750. Yes, this is serious dough. We think it's worth it, though, because the FreeMotion model allows longer ranges of motion and smoother action than any other machines we've seen, allowing you to do dozens of exercises that aren't possible with other equipment. You can work with one arm or leg at a time, and you can do moves that take your body in any path or range of motion, up to 12 feet away from the machine, which is about 6 feet farther than tradi-tional machines allow. That means you can do sport-specific exercises—simulating a golf or tennis swing, for example—that you can't do with a basic cable machine or free weights. The FreeMotion machine requires a space about 9½ feet wide, 3 feet deep (with 12 feet of clearance to do some of the exercises), and 8 feet high.

MULTISTATION HOME GYMS

These machines can't compete with free weights when it comes to helping you build muscle and strength. Worse, they restrict the functional benefit of your exercises, a topic we'll get into in chapter 19. However, they beat free weights in ease of use, safety, and attractiveness. We can't discount those attributes, because we know it's a lot easier to get into strength training with a gleaming, idiot-proof machine than with piles of iron that require a significant learning curve to use effectively.

The average multistation has apparatuses for chest and shoulder presses, leg extensions and curls, and perhaps leg presses, along with a cable station that allows a long list of high- and low-pulley exercises.

Unlike the Universal machines that sat in the middle of your high school weight room, allowing a half-dozen or more people to lift simultaneously on outward-facing stations, most home machines these days are designed to fit into corners or against walls. In some cases, they require less space than do some of the free-weight setups described previously. The simplest machines take up the space of a full-size bed. For example, the Parabody 220 is about 5½ feet long, 4 feet wide, and 7 feet high. To use it, you need a space that's about 7 feet by 6 feet.

At the more expensive end, the Parabody 777 requires a space about 8 feet by 9 feet—still less than you'd need for a good free-weight area using a 7-foot Olympic bar. You need only about 7 feet of headroom since you sit on a bench for the overhead lifts.

A higher-end machine with multiple weight stacks and all the optional workout stations could take up an entire bedroom. (Side benefit: You may finally persuade your mother-in-law to move out of your guest room if you tell her she's going to have to share it with a multistation gym and sleep on the bench.) For example, the Body Solid EXM-3000LPS requires a space about 8 feet by 6 feet. Though one side can be as close as 6 inches from a wall, you need a couple feet of clearance to each of the other two sides, and at least 4 feet of working room to the front. Now you're looking at 12 feet by 10 feet. And remember, you may want to add more equipment—free weights, treadmill, indoor climbing wall—so the 120 square feet for the machine is just a start.

You can expect your machine to come with a 200- or 210-pound weight stack, with two or three separate lifting stations connected to that stack. The more weight stacks the machine has, the more versatility you'll have—you'll spend more time lifting and less time making equipment adjustments for each exercise. Multiple weight stacks usually cost multiple thousands of dollars and require more room to accommodate them. On the positive side, you'll be able to invite your buddies

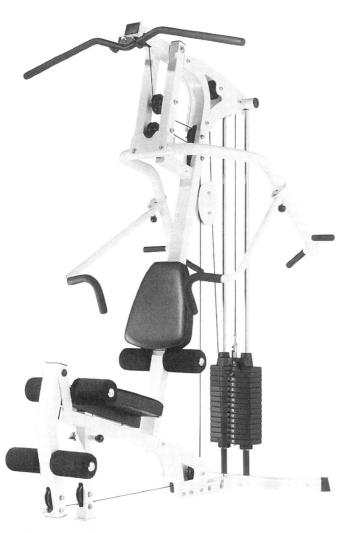

Parabody 220 multistation gym

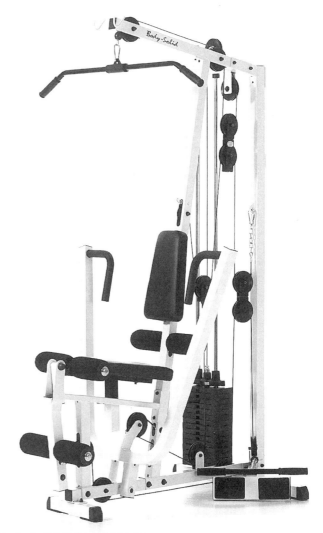

Body Solid EXM-3000LPS multistation gym

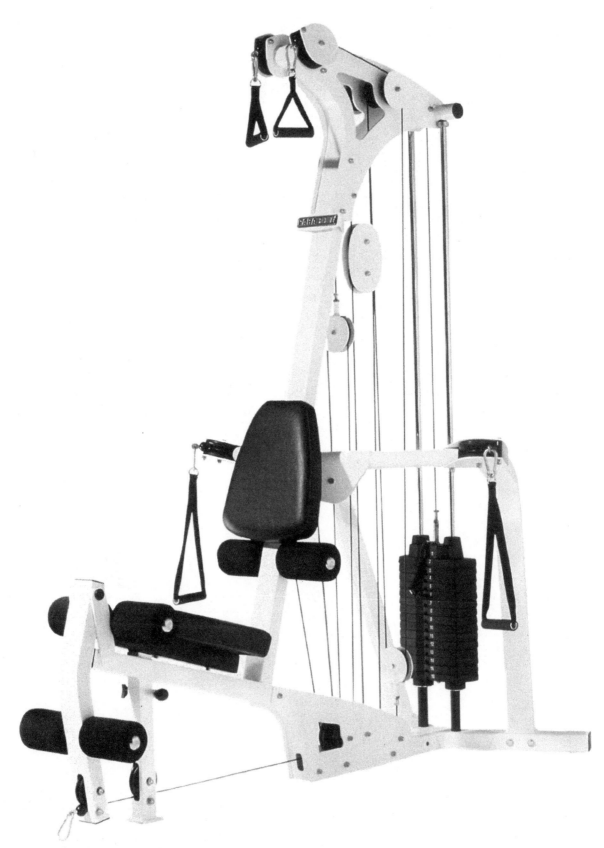

Parabody 777 multistation gym

over for a workout. Hell, you could subsidize the cost of the machine by selling home-gym memberships to your neighbors.

Some newer machines have free-floating handles that make chest and shoulder presses seem more like the dumbbell versions of those exercises. You use more muscles and develop more coordination when you have to balance two handles moving freely in space, as opposed to pushing against a single handle that balances itself. A second innovation we really like is dual cable pulleys, available on the Parabody 777 we show on the opposite page. This allows freer shoulder-joint movement on overhead cable exercises, and the ability to perform an almost unlimited variety of exercises on one machine. Its a rare case of a home machine having a cool, useful feature you won't find in gym machines. The Parabody 777 retails for just under $2,000, not including shipping and assembly.

Speaking of prices, the more you pay for a machine, the closer you'll get to health-club quality (no surprise there). Odds are a $500 machine from a big-box discount store will feel clunky and jerky. That's why we recommend buying the most expensive machine you can afford and squeeze into your space. Follow this checklist to get a machine you can grow with.

Decide what you need. Your needs are more complicated than just "heavy stuff to lift." For example, if you're going to buy or renew a gym membership even after you've purchased a machine, you don't need every possible option on your home multistation. You can, therefore, use the machine for in-home upper-body workouts, then go to your gym to work lower-body muscles. That means you don't need a leg press, which would've added a few hundred dollars to the price and taken up a lot of room. On the other hand, if you want to replicate every aspect of the gym experience without leaving your house, be prepared to pay a steep price.

Set a price range. If this were a personal-finance book, we'd tell you to base this decision on what you can afford up front, without resorting to an installment plan. Since it isn't, we'll leave financing decisions to you. We will tell you that you should decide whether a multistation is the only purchase you're going to make. If you want free weights, too, or a treadmill, you have to decide what percentage of your overall budget you can spend on the multistation.

Measure your space. Decide whether you're going to devote the whole space to the machine you're about to buy, or whether you plan to use free weights, too. We recommend keeping your space as flexible as possible and leaving enough room for a barbell bench-press station, if not a power rack. Write down the relevant dimensions, and take them with you when you shop.

Pick some stores. Start at a store that specializes in home exercise equipment. That way, you get to try out a wide range of machines and talk to salespeople who know you aren't insulting them when you ask about a dip station. Make sure you visit at least two stores. No single outlet is going to have every brand of equipment. Even if you visit two stores that have the same lines of machines, you'll be able to compare prices. It doesn't hurt to have two retailers bidding against each other for your business.

Dress for the occasion. Plan to sweat. Wear your gym shoes and loose clothing.

Take your partner. If your wife will be using the machine, too, drag her along.

Do it all. Try out the machine. Adjust everything that can be adjusted. Make sure you're challenged by the exercise options. If, for example, you can already use 90 percent of the weight stack on the chest press, you're going to outgrow one of the machine's key components in about 2 weeks. Also, give the machine a hard shake to see if it's solid.

Check the specs. The multistation should be made of 11- or 12-gauge steel. (The lower the number, the stronger the steel.) Also, make sure that the frame is welded rather than just bolted together. That's especially important for key joints on the machine. On all moving parts, it's best to have floating bushings or bearings because they'll last much longer than steel-on-steel construction. Look for aircraft-quality cable.

Pay extra for delivery and assembly. We don't care if you're a frickin' NASA engineer, pay the extra bills and have the thing delivered and put together properly.

SMITH MACHINE

We don't know who this Smith guy is, and we don't want to deprive him of his livelihood. That said, we sure don't care much for his machine. In fact, if we were the kings of the fitness universe, we'd banish these barbell-on-rails devices

ONE MAN'S TRASH . . .

Statistics show that exercise equipment is owned and used in about one-third of U.S. households. Another 18 percent of households have equipment that isn't used. That suggests that a large number of multistation home gyms are gathering dust and could probably be had for a decent offer. (That infomercial rotisserie you bought makes a fair opening bid, but expect to go up from there. You may have to throw in the breadmaker.)

A multistation doesn't have many moving parts—far fewer than a treadmill or stationary bike—so there's less that could be wrong with it. Follow most of the same steps you would when purchasing a new machine—especially the one about trying out all the exercise stations. The parts should move smoothly and adjust easily.

Check the welded parts, making sure there are no cracks. Look closely at the cables, checking for frayed wires or torn jacketing. Listen to the machine as it works. You don't want to hear crunching sounds as the cables travel. And notice where the owner keeps his machine. If it's in a damp basement or near a pool or hot tub, check for rust. Finally, contact the **U.S. Consumer Product Safety Commission (1-800-638-2772 or**

www.cpsc.gov) to make sure the manufacturer has never recalled the machine due to known defects.

Consider the size and weight of the machine. Just because you have a chance to get a $2,000 multistation for $200 doesn't mean you should cart home something so huge that you'll be doing lat pulldowns over the cat's litter box. Even if you have plenty of room to accommodate the equipment, you need a plan for moving it to your house. Our recommendation is to hire a fitness-equipment company to take the machine apart, move it to your space, and put it back together for you. An experienced crew can do in a day what it would take you at least a 3-day weekend to pull off. Professional help will cost you, so figure that into the price.

You can also buy used from secondhand and consignment stores. Finally, new-equipment retailers may take a used machine as a trade-in, spruce it up, and sell it in good condition. It's anybody's guess what you'd pay for this equipment and whether the store would be willing to help you with delivery and setup. Still, this option may be the best middle ground between brand-new gear and the crapshoot of a garage sale.

from any health club that would have us as members.

We're doubly dubious about people having these things in their homes. It's not that they're dangerous (though we do believe that, over time, they can lead to pattern-overload injuries, which we'll explain in a moment). The problem is that they're too safe.

A barbell normally travels not only up and down but also forward and back. That's the way your body naturally lifts the thing. You never move a weight straight up and down, like a piston. But that's exactly how a Smith machine forces your muscles to move—up and down, with no back and forth.

While we'll concede that a Smith machine can help you build some muscle and improve your strength, we're pretty skeptical about the usefulness of that muscle and strength. There aren't any real-life activities that require moving a counterbalanced object up and down on a pair of rails. And we have to wonder whether the unnatural movement might even inhibit your ability to move heavy objects in a three-dimensional world.

Pattern overload, mentioned above, is another concern. Say you do only one exercise for your shoulders—overhead barbell presses—and you do them only on a Smith machine. That means you work them at the exact same angle each time you enter the gym. If anything about that angle rubs them the wrong way, you're screwed.

Of course, you can say the same thing about a multistation home gym. In fact, a Smith machine may offer you some alternatives the multistation doesn't. Since you use your own bench with the Smith, you can alter angles regularly on chest presses, easing the strain on your shoulders.

The simplest Smith machines take up about as much room as a power rack: 4 feet in width and depth, with about 7 feet of headroom. You'll need about 2 extra feet to each side to accommodate the bar, and a couple of feet in front to approach it safely. Expect to pay at least $500 for this basic Smith. The machines get bigger and more expensive from there.

PART 2

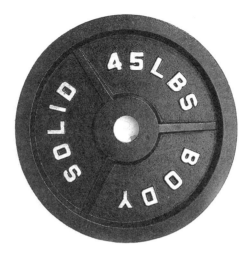

RESIDENTIAL RESISTANCE

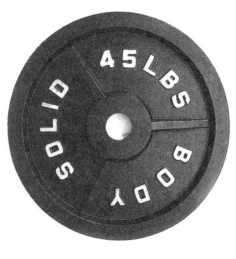

PROGRAMS

CHAPTER 5

DESIGNING A PLAN

Take a bow, homeboy. By now, you're an honorary adjunct professor of domestic body development. You know your main muscles and how to make them bigger. You have a pretty clear idea of what home strength-training equipment is all about.

There's a small matter still pending, however: What the hell are you going to do with all this knowledge?

Exercising without a plan is like hitting the road for a month-long vacation without first deciding where you're going. You may have fun for a week or two—"Hey, we're only 150 miles from Graceland!" Then you realize your vacation is already half over, and you haven't done anything really satisfying or interesting. You start thinking of all the great things you could've experienced had you done some planning. Regrets—you have a few.

Now, you may think that this analogy is stupid. Who, after all, would take a month-long vacation without picking a destination? Nobody, right? Why is it, then, that many—perhaps even most—guys start exercising with no plans, vague plans, or completely unrealistic plans?

That makes as little sense as taking a vacation to nowhere.

IF YOU DON'T KNOW WHERE YOU'RE GOING, HOW WILL YOU KNOW WHEN YOU'VE ARRIVED?

No matter what your exercise experience, we'd like you, right now, to articulate your goal. Without knowing you personally, we can guess it's similar to one of these:

- To work out three times a week.
- To get in shape.
- To build muscle.
- To lose weight.
- To play basketball without getting winded.
- To fit into size-34 khakis.
- To bench-press 200 pounds.
- To lose 13 pounds before your high school reunion, which is June 15.
- To gain 20 pounds of solid muscle, put an inch on your arms, and have six-pack abs.

Let's take a closer look at each.

To work out three times a week. This is what's called a *process goal*. You tell yourself you're going to mess around with all that exercise equipment you bought, and whatever happens, happens. This is fine for guys who have trouble getting started or staying with it—which, in a country where only about 21 percent of the population exercises at least two times a week, includes almost everybody.

We recommend that you move past your process goal as soon as you've established an exercise habit. Say you get to the point where you do some exercise every Monday, Wednesday, and Friday before work. Once you've stuck with that routine for a while, shift to an *outcome goal*, which represents a specific physiological benefit.

To get in shape. An outcome goal can be general or specific, and this particular one is about as general as you can get. Again, we aren't knocking it. We do suggest you quickly move past this vague

idea and define what you mean by "in shape." Decide whether "shape" refers to the way you look (trim waist, wide shoulders, defined muscles), the way you feel (focused, energetic, confident), or the way you perform (able to play 3 sets of tennis on a hot day, hike 10 miles with your kids, hit the weights hard for 45 minutes four times a week).

To build muscle. To lose weight. To play basketball without getting winded. Now you've gotten more specific. You know that, to reach any of these goals, you have to establish a process (exercise three or more times a week). You also have in mind an outcome that you'll be able to recognize upon reaching.

For example, you can measure your arms, neck, chest, waist, thighs, and calves right now. You can measure them again in 4 weeks. At that point, if everything but your waist is bigger, you'll know you've built some muscle.

When your specific outcome goal is weight loss, your scale tells you whether you've achieved it. You can weigh yourself first thing tomorrow morning, after you go to the bathroom but before you have anything to eat or drink. Repeat the weigh-in at regular intervals: once a week, twice a week, every day.

It may be harder to tell whether you've built up more stamina for a specific athletic performance. You may notice that you beat an opponent on a fast break when it's usually the other way around. Sometimes others may have to point this out to you. A buddy may mention that you were stronger in the second game than in the first.

To fit into size-34 khakis. To bench-press 200 pounds. To meet either of these very specific goals, you have to choose a specialized training program. A weight-loss program is different from a muscle-gain program. And a workout to improve bench-press performance is different from either a general weight-loss or muscle-gain workout.

You can't possibly miss the moment when you reach such a goal. The only way to know if you fit into those pants is to try them on. Either they fit or they don't. With the bench press, there's only one measurement, and it's concrete (well, technically, it's iron, but you get the point). Either you lift the weight or you don't.

We have a few words to add about what makes your success "official." If you have to suck in your gut or severely dehydrate yourself to fit into the pants, you haven't reached your goal. We think a fair test is whether you can fit into them after work, when you're carrying more food and water in your body than you did first thing in the morning.

The bench-press goal is even more technical. Your butt has to stay in contact with the bench throughout the lift, and your spotter cannot touch the bar during the lift. He can help you lift the bar off the uprights, but he has to let go before you begin lowering the bar to your chest. He can't touch it again until you've lowered it to your chest and then pressed it back up until your arms are straight. Of course, he has to pluck if off your chest if you fail to lift it (that's why he's there). If he touches it before you fail, you've failed anyway.

To lose 17 pounds before your high school reunion, which is June 15. In our view, this is the best type of goal you can set. You've been specific about the outcome you want, and you have a deadline. Our one suggestion for fine-tuning this goal is to measure your success in terms other than weight. Weight is an important way to keep score, but it's sort of like a batting average in baseball: It doesn't reflect how often you get on base or how far you hit the ball when you put it into play.

Say you weigh 197 pounds and wear size-38 pants. You want to get down to 180 pounds, your high school weight. You go on a comprehensive strength-training program geared toward fat loss (you'll find an example below), and you modify your diet. On June 15, you weigh 185 pounds, which means you've "failed" to reach your goal. But your shoulders are wider and your arms thicker

than they've ever been—and you wear size-34 pants, with a midsection as flat as your company's revenues. Your waist size is a better measure of your progress than your weight is.

An even better indicator is your waist-hip ratio (waist circumference at narrowest point divided by hip circumference measured at widest point). If it's under 0.9, you're in pretty good shape. (If it's over 1.0, you're in trouble.)

To gain 20 pounds of solid muscle, put an inch on the arms, and have six-pack abs. We can't knock the specifics of this goal. We can say it's pretty unrealistic. For one thing, to gain an appreciable amount of weight, you have to overeat. When you overeat, you put on fat. So while you may gain that inch of muscle on your arms, you also hide your abs under an inch of flab.

The key is to work toward this goal in stages: Put on weight for a while, then curb your diet to strip off some fat, continuing the cycle until you have the body you want.

THE MATCH GAME

Once you've perfected your goal, you have to match it to your equipment, exercise experience, and schedule.

Each of the next six exercise chapters assumes you have nothing but the equipment described therein. The body-weight chapter assumes you have nothing but your body to work with, plus a few household objects. (It helps to have a chinup bar, too, and if you're really ambitious, a Swiss ball.) The dumbbell chapter assumes you have nothing beyond dumbbells and a bench. The barbell chapter shows exercises that require a barbell and either a bench with uprights or a power rack (so you can do bench presses and squats). The cable chapter features exercises you can do with a simple apparatus that has a high and low pulley. (With apologies, we'll also show exercises with a cable-crossover machine. We know few people have these things in their homes but, damn it, we really like crossover machines.) The chapter after that shows how to maximize your multistation home gym, if you have one, and we conclude with a chapter that shows you how to make the best use of a home gym that includes everything: dumbbells, barbells, and a multistation gym with a cable apparatus.

Of course, if your goal is to build a significant amount of muscle, but the only equipment you have is your body weight and a few big bottles of laundry detergent, you don't need us to tell you that something has to give. You have to either cash in your Richie Rich comic-book collection to buy yourself a weight set, or you have to scale back your ambition. So no matter which equipment chapter applies to your current domestic arrange-

ment, we encourage you to take a look at all of them—one of them may inspire you.

Even if your equipment is a perfect match for your goals, you may pick up some new tricks from the other chapters. For instance, the body-weight exercises are useful for anybody because they can be done anywhere, anytime. And regardless of whether you have a multistation machine, that chapter could come in handy if you travel and find yourself with access to a hotel gym equipped with such a beast.

A less obvious goal-setting factor is your exercise experience. The workout chapters take this into account by categorizing each exercise as beginner, intermediate, or advanced level (or a combination thereof). They also include guide-

MIKE MEJIA'S FIVE RULES OF PROGRAM DESIGN

I. Match the routine to your goal. Fat-loss programs aren't great for adding size, and hard-core strength programs don't lend themselves to huge changes in body composition. Choose one goal and stick to it for a designated period of time. Don't try to go in two directions at once.

2. Address your weak points first. That usually means doing your least favorite exercises first. Save exercises you like and are good at until later in your workout. For instance, if your chest is strong and your back isn't, work your back before your chest.

3. Alter your routine regularly. Once you've been training consistently for 6 months or more, you'll probably get all the possible benefits of a single routine within 3 to 6 weeks. On the other hand, you have to stick with a program for 2 to 3 weeks to judge if it's doing anything for you. If you change every other workout, it's impossible to gauge your progress.

4. Work sequentially. No matter your goal, you should progress from fewer sets, lighter loads, and higher repetitions to more sets, heavier weights, and fewer reps. This ensures that you build muscular endurance and connective-tissue integrity before you increase the volume of exercise in order to add new muscle. It also increases your muscle mass before you attempt to improve your absolute strength. You reach your goal faster, with less risk of injury, when you prepare your body for a new challenge rather than just jumping into it.

5. Make compound lifts the cornerstones of your program. Exercises like squats, deadlifts, bench presses, rows, shoulder presses, and pullups build more strength and metabolism-boosting muscle than isolation exercises like chest flies, lateral raises, leg extensions, and leg curls.

lines for the appropriate number of sets and reps per exercise, depending on your experience level. This doesn't mean that grizzled, muscled veterans won't benefit from beginner- or intermediate-level lifts—trust us, those still provide plenty of work. It does mean that if you're just starting out, you're better off sticking to the beginner moves at first and then working your way up. There are no advantages to bad form, frustration, or injury.

Your skill level alone may not indicate how readily your body will adapt to the exercises. Genetics are another determinant. Some people see fast improvements in strength, muscle mass, or aerobic capacity just because they're born with that capacity. Others work diligently for months or years without seeing much difference. The more experience you have with exercise, the more you know about how your body reacts.

Finally, there's the issue of your time-and-energy commitment. The bigger your ambitions, the more time you have to set aside to reach them. If you want to make significant physiological improvements, you have to understand how much effort that's going to take.

Training time: Beginners should plan to spend 20 to 40 minutes doing resistance exercise, two or three times a week. Intermediate and advanced exercisers probably need at least 40 minutes three or four times a week. We believe the upper limit is an hour of strength training, four times a week. Beyond that, you're either wasting time—doing work at a lower intensity just to do more of it—or pushing your body past its ability to recover between one workout and the next.

Lifestyle time: Say your goal is to put on 10 pounds of muscle, and you've worked 4 hours of weight training into your schedule each week. Now you have to figure out how diligently you can follow a diet that provides enough food to build and fuel 10 extra pounds of muscle. You have to eat that food consistently, day in and day out. If you skip meals or take dietary shortcuts, you miss chances to build muscle.

You also have to get plenty of sleep. Your body releases the greatest amount of growth hormone during the deep slow-wave sleep that occurs in the first hours after you hit the sack. If your sleep patterns are irregular, your growth-hormone release will be irregular, and you may sabotage your chances of gaining muscle.

TIME PERIODS

Another vital aspect of time commitment is setting a deadline. When you decide on a date by which you want to meet your goal, you can look at a calendar and count the weeks backward from that end point, breaking down your one big goal into a series of smaller goals in a technique called periodization.

Let's say it's the end of December and you're making a New Year's resolution to reach your fitness goal by the last Friday in May—in time to look good on the beach this summer. If you plan to start your workout program on the first Monday of January, you've given yourself 21 weeks. Looking at your calendar, you see two natural breaks in your schedule: There's a week in mid-February in which you know you'll be trapped meetings at work. There's another week in early April in which you have a business trip. What you really have is a 5-week period, a week off, a 6-week period, a week off, then an 8-week period.

FIRST PERIOD: GENERAL PREPARATION

You won't reach your goal if you go all-out the first couple of weeks—you'll get hurt, burned out, discouraged, or all three. Give your body a chance to prepare for the hard work to come. Your aims in this first period are to establish a consistent workout routine, master basic exercises, and gradually increase the amount and intensity of work you do.

If your goal is fat loss: Start by performing 15-to-20 rep sets of basic, safe exercises in a circuit fashion (one exercise after another with little or no rest). Throughout the period, you work with heavier weights and do fewer repetitions per set, while also performing more sets. Though you may start the period doing one or two circuits of 10 exercises, by the end you do three circuits. And instead of doing 15 to 20 reps per set, you do 12 to 15.

If your goal is muscle gain: Start with a single 12-to-15-rep set of eight exercises. (You needn't do the same exercises each workout. You can create three different sets of exercises, and perform each once a week.) After 2 weeks, increase to 2 sets of each exercise, dropping the repetitions to 10 to 12. Add a third set by the fifth week, doing a total of 24 sets each workout.

At the end of the period, take a week off, as planned. You can do some light, enjoyable, goal-free exercise during this week, if you can squeeze it into your schedule. If you can't, don't stress out. You won't lose any of your strength or muscle size, and your body will appreciate the break.

SECOND PERIOD: MUSCLE AND STRENGTH

When you're a beginner, your body gets stronger, more muscular, and leaner simultaneously. Once you're past the beginner stage, these benefits come to you only one at a time. Sometimes you need one before you can have another.

For example, you have to get stronger before you can develop more muscle size. Your muscles need a reason to grow, and continually overloading them with heavier weights gives them a damned good reason. If you're most interested in losing fat, it helps to have bigger muscles that will speed up your metabolism.

This second period is actually a step sideways that allows you to make a huge leap forward in the final phase.

If your goal is fat loss: Throughout this 7-week period, do three workouts a week, six exercises per workout, 3 sets per exercise. Do 3 sets of 10 to 12 repetitions for 3 weeks. For the next 3 weeks, switch to a "pyramid" system in which you do sets of 12, 10, and 8 repetitions per exercise, using more weight each of the 3 sets.

If your goal is muscle gain: Create two different workouts, one for your upper body, another for your lower body. Alternate between the two. You can do a total of three or four workouts a week—depending on your schedule and how fast your body recovers—but never train more than 2 days in a row.

For the first 3 weeks, do 3 sets, with 8 repetitions each of five or six exercises per workout. Choose mostly compound or multijoint exercises (bench press, squat, deadlift, row, shoulder press, pullup or lat pulldown). If you do any isolation or single-joint exercises (biceps curl, triceps extension, lateral raise), put them at the end of the workout.

Then for the next 3 weeks, do 3 to 5 sets of 5 repetitions.

Then take your week off. Again, do some light workouts if you can and want to, but don't sweat it if you can't or don't want to.

THIRD PERIOD: THE FINAL PUSH

You have 8 weeks left to achieve your goal, and it's time to go after it head-on.

If your goal is fat loss: For 4 weeks, go to a system of giant sets and supersets. Rotate between two different workouts. In the first workout, for your lower body, do giant sets—that is, do five or six exercises in a row with no rest in between. What distinguishes these sets from the circuits you did in the first period is that giant sets involve a single muscle group, or related muscle groups. A giant set for legs might include squats, followed by leg presses, followed by leg curls or stiff-legged deadlifts, followed by wall squats or leg extensions.

Do 8 to 10 repetitions of each exercise, and do a total of 3 giant sets, resting for a minute or two in between. Follow that with 3 giant sets consisting of four or five abdominal and lower-back exercises.

In the other workout, do supersets for your upper body. That means two exercises in a row with no rest in between. One superset might be bench presses and rows; the next could be shoulder presses and lat pulldowns or pullovers; the third could be dips or chair dips and upright rows; the fourth could be pushups and reverse pushups. The point is to make sure the supersets work opposing muscle groups (chest and middle back, worked with bench presses and rows) or opposing muscle actions (vertical pushing and vertical pulling, worked with shoulder presses and lat pulldowns). Do 8 to 12 repetitions per exercise and totaling 3 supersets of each exercise pair.

The final 4 weeks, choose 18 tough exercises. Divide them up into three workouts, six exercises per workout. In each workout, do a set of 12 to 15 repetitions of an exercise, followed by 1 to 3 minutes of a cardiovascular exercise. You can do jumping jacks, use a treadmill or exercise bike, run up and down stairs, or (if you're really hard core) jump rope. You should be able to do 2 sets of six exercises per workout, and a total of 12 to 36 minutes of between-sets cardio work. Do each of the three workouts once a week.

If your goal is muscle gain: At this point, you have to make a decision: If your body has resisted muscle gain but hasn't added any fat, you need to break out the heavy muscle-building artillery. We recommend the 1-6 workout system. Pick a multijoint exercise. After a thorough warmup, do 1 repetition with a weight that's pretty damned heavy. Then do 6 reps with a lighter weight. Repeat twice, each time using more weight on the sets of 1 and 6 than you did before.

Here's an example, using barbell bench presses.

Set	Reps	Weight
1	1	185
2	6	125
3	1	195
4	6	135
5	1	205
6	6	145

By the final 2 sets, you should be at close to an all-out effort. (Observe all the precautions described in chapter 6, of course. If you don't have a spotter, a power rack with safety bars, or a ProSpot machine, use dumbbells. Multistation home gyms can also be useful for this type of workout since you don't have to worry about leaving a bar on your sternum if you fail on a repetition.)

Do two exercises per workout using this method. At the end of each workout, add a couple of supplemental exercises for your abs, lower back, arms, shoulders, or calves. Do 1 to 3 sets of 6 to 8 repetitions for these muscle groups.

Try that for 4 weeks. Then finish up with 4 weeks of compound sets. These are supersets using the same muscle group for both exercises. So, for example, you might do a set of bench presses followed by flies. Shoulder presses could be paired with lateral raises, squats with leg presses or leg extensions, deadlifts with leg curls. The idea is to completely engorge your muscles with blood on each compound set. Do higher repetitions—10 to 15—and train by instinct. Do the exercises that feel the most beneficial and produce the best pump.

If, on the other hand, you've gotten significant muscle gains but also put on a lot of fat (hey, it happens), you probably want to do an 8-week "cutting" stage. Instead of using the 1-6 system, you might do the compound sets for 4 weeks, then finish with the giant sets and supersets prescribed above for fat loss.

THE EXERCISES

Once you've finished all the mental work of setting a goal and creating a plan to reach it, you're ready to march into your home gym and start working your body. Within each workout chapter, we'll categorize the exercises by body part, using the same basic groupings we introduced in chapter 2: midsection, chest and upper back, shoulders and arms, and lower body.

Within most of those groups, the exercises are further broken down by the main muscles worked. In each shoulders-and-arms section, for example, you'll learn exercises for your main shoulder muscles (deltoids), your shoulder rotators, your triceps, your biceps, and your forearm muscles. You need this pigeonholing to put together programs that hit all your major muscle groups. We'll tell you how to select the right combination of exercises to get a balanced workout.

As you travel through these chapters, here are some other factors you'll want to keep in mind.

Weight load. You know better than we do how much weight you can handle. Still, from time to time we'll mention that a particular exercise requires a lighter-than-usual or relatively heavy weight. Take such instructions seriously—they indicate that the lift being described can't be done effectively and with good form using the weight you might instinctively choose.

Grip. The way you grab the dumbbells, barbell, or cable handles can make a big difference in the motion that follows. We'll usually advise you to use one of these grips: overhand (pronated), underhand (supinated), or neutral (palms facing each other). We'll periodically remind you which grip is which.

Unilateral versus bilateral movement. This refers to whether you work one side of your body at a time or both at once. Sometimes we give you a choice, sometimes we don't. For unilateral moves, do an equal number of reps on each side before you consider a set complete. We'll remind you of this, even though we're pretty sure you'll remember.

Lower-back posture. Your form will almost always be better when you keep your lower back in its naturally arched position. This is something we'll remind you about in many of the exercise descriptions, although it's something you should learn to do without prompting.

Sports moves. The lifts labeled SPORTS MOVES are all about speed. Good form is still essential, mind you, but you have our permission to move quickly and explosively when you do them. The whole idea is to build the kind of explosive power, quickness, coordination, and balance that will serve you on the fields of play. Fast movement is what gets you there.

Sports moves can be tricky, entailing long learning curves. That's why they're all categorized as advanced exercises. Chapter 15 will describe how best to use them. For now, we suggest that if you do them, you perform them at the beginning of your workout so your body and mind are fresh.

The well-rounded approach. Each chapter includes exercises using the main apparatus plus a Swiss ball. A ball is cheap and makes any home gym much more versatile. Here's why we're so high on inflated rubber for your home workout space.

- *Your core musculature works harder.* Working on a curved surface forces your midsection muscles to contract constantly—even when you're targeting other muscle groups.

- *The ball recruits more muscles for action.* The inherent instability of the ball puts stabilizer muscles to work. You'll often build strength in muscles you didn't even know you were working, such as the rotator cuff muscles used during dumbbell chest presses.

- *The ball does wonders for your ab workouts.* Your abs work through their full range of motion because the contour of the ball helps you start the movements in a pre-stretched position.

- *It's a bench alternative with a payoff.* When you substitute a Swiss ball for a bench, you usually need to work with lighter weights. But the strength gains you'll make in your core and stabilizing muscles mean you'll be able to work with heavier weights when you return to the bench.

- *It's the real thing.* The Swiss ball is better than a bench or chair for teaching your muscles to work in unison—as they must in sports and real life.

What's more, a ball is also one of the few exercise tools you can use more effectively at home than in a gym. Few health clubs are set up to accommodate Swiss balls. While you might find balls in the aerobics studio or the ab-crunching area, if you wanted to use one with dumbbells, a barbell, or a cable apparatus, good luck. You'd have to move equipment around to squeeze in the ball, watch that the ball didn't roll into someone's way when you were between sets, and deal with curious stares from your fellow gym users. Some people would even react with hostility if you walked into the weight room with a brightly colored rubber ball. If they weren't aware of how useful a ball can be, they'd think you were playing with children's toys in their iron sanctum.

In your home, you don't have to worry about any of that. This is probably why you're working out at home in the first place: You'd rather not deal with large-muscled, small-minded individuals who don't share your preferences in music, hygiene, or fragrances.

Variations. You'll get plenty of them. An innocuous-looking adjustment can change the effect of an exercise in a dramatic way. For example, switching from a shoulder-width spacing of your hands to a close-together grip on a bench press moves the bulk of the work from your pecs to your triceps.

Combined with the standard exercises, these variations provide literally hundreds of moves you can use to build muscle. So what are you waiting for? It's time to start your homework.

CHAPTER 6

YOUR BODY, YOUR WORKOUT

As long as gravity exists, your own body weight can provide a vigorous home workout that does all the good things any strength-training routine does—that is, build muscle mass and strength if you're a beginner, increase muscular endurance no matter your fitness level, promote fat loss, improve your health, and (to put it bluntly) make you more desirable to women of childbearing age. This chapter will show you how.

First, a slight clarification. True, most of the exercises you'll do in your no-equipment home workout require only your body weight for resistance. And you can do all of them without buying, borrowing, or stealing any of the usual tools of the trade, such as dumbbells, barbells, weight benches, or machines. Still, the no-equipment description is not absolutely literal. For example, about a half-dozen of the exercises in this chapter require a chinning bar. And, as promised in the previous chapter, we've included moves on a Swiss ball. We aren't saying you have to go out today and buy either of these things. You can make a chinning bar by hanging a hunk of PVC pipe from the crossbeams of your garage. Or as we mentioned in chapter 3, if your kids have a sturdy jungle gym, you already have a chinning bar in your yard. As for the Swiss ball, it's not necessary, just nice to have.

A few other props will come in handy: a towel, plastic jugs (fill in your own Pamela Anderson joke here), and a chair. We hope this is stuff you have sitting around. If not . . . well, we have to know: Why don't you own a chair?

There are lots of selling points for this kind of workout.

- You don't have to spend a small fortune to get fit.
- Travel is never a problem. A hotel room or friend's house is as good a venue as your own place.

SAMPLE CIRCUIT WORKOUTS

One unique benefit of no-equipment exercises is that they make it much more convenient to take advantage of a valuable workout technique called circuit training. In circuits, you do I set of each exercise in the routine before doing a second set of any exercise. Moving quickly from exercise to exercise allows you to get more work done in less time—and this is an even more efficient process when there's no weight to adjust or station to set up. Circuits also give each muscle group several minutes to recover before working again, letting you work more intensely each time you move through the circuit.

We've done the circuit planning for you with the following suggested routines—one for beginners and one for more advanced trainers. All the exercises in these circuits are described for you in this chapter.

Start with 5 to 10 minutes of continuous activity that involves large muscle groups—such as doing jumping jacks, running stairs, or skipping rope.

Then do each exercise on your circuit list in succession, pausing only long enough to get ready for the next one. Start with 12 repetitions of each exercise, eventually working your way up to 20.

When you've completed the circuit—that is, when you've done all the exercises on your list—cool down for several minutes or engage in another 3 to 5 minutes of cardio work. Then go through the circuit a second time.

BEGINNER CIRCUIT
- Pushup
- Split squat
- One-arm row, elbow out
- Towel squat
- Lateral raise
- Prone superman
- Chair dip
- Towel crunch
- Assisted chinup
- Vacuum

INTERMEDIATE/ADVANCED CIRCUIT
- Pullup
- One-leg squat
- Elevated-feet pushup
- Lunge
- Reverse pushup
- One-leg Romanian deadlift
- Triangle pushup
- Explosive calf jump
- Russian twist
- Chinup or assisted chinup
- Pulse-up
- External rotation

- Most of the best abdominal exercises use pure body weight anyway. So if you're ab-focused (who isn't?), you're set.
- Compensating for a lack of dumbbells and barbells cultivates creativity—a plus for your program.

Exercising without weights does have a few disadvantages, however. First, of course, is the problem of diminishing returns. While a beginner will certainly build muscle and strength from pushups, for example, a guy who's used to lifting weights heavier than himself won't get much out of them. Another problem is limited exercise options. Then there's the sheer difficulty (though not impossibility) of adequately working certain muscle groups, such as your upper back. (That's why we included chinning-bar exercises in this chapter—they're the best no-weight way to work your upper back.) Perhaps the biggest disadvantage is that you don't have control over how much resistance you're using. A hefty, out-of-shape guy may find his body weight too heavy to lift, while a wiry, athletic guy may be able to pop off 100 pushups without even breaking a sweat.

Still, we think this chapter offers something for everybody. Beginners may find all these exercises challenging, while intermediate and advanced exercisers will find some interesting moves to add to the workouts in later chapters. And no matter what your fitness level, something is always better than nothing. If you find yourself stranded without your regular exercise equipment, you'll still be able to do these exercises.

MIDSECTION

For a complete ab-and-lower-back workout, choose one exercise from each of the six categories. If you're a beginner, do 1 set of 10 to 15 repetitions per exercise—except while doing the vacuum, when you should do 6 to 10 repetitions.

If you're more experienced, do 2 or 3 sets of 8 to 10 repetitions of each chosen exercise. (However, if you choose the bridge or side bridge, follow the specific instructions with regard to reps.)

BEGINNER	INTERMEDIATE	ADVANCED
LOWER ABDOMINALS — Reverse crunch ------- (page 63)	**LOWER ABDOMINALS** — Pulse-up ------------- (page 64)	**LOWER ABDOMINALS** — Swiss-ball reverse crunch --------------- (page 63) — V-up ------------------ (page 64) — Hanging leg raise ------- (page 65)
UPPER ABDOMINALS — Crunch --------------- (page 66)	**UPPER ABDOMINALS** — Towel crunch ---------- (page 66)	**UPPER ABDOMINALS** — Situp ------------------ (page 66)
OBLIQUES — Oblique crunch -------- (page 67)	**OBLIQUES** — Crunch with lateral flexion -------------- (page 68)	**OBLIQUES** — Swiss-ball oblique crunch --------------- (page 67) — Oblique V-up ----------- (page 68)
ROTATIONAL MOVEMENT — Russian twist --------- (page 69)	**DEEPER ABDOMINAL AND LOWER-BACK MUSCLES** — Bridge ----------------- (page 71) — Side bridge ----------- (page 72)	**ROTATIONAL MOVEMENT** — Swiss-ball Russian twist ---------------- (page 69) — Bicycle ---------------- (page 70)
DEEPER ABDOMINAL AND LOWER-BACK MUSCLES — Vacuum --------------- (page 71)	**LOWER BACK** — Bird dog -------------- (page 73)	**DEEPER ABDOMINAL AND LOWER-BACK MUSCLES** — Jackknife ------------- (page 72)
LOWER BACK — Prone Superman ------- (page 73)		**LOWER BACK** — Back extension --------- (page 74)

EXERCISES FOR LOWER ABDOMINALS

Reverse Crunch
BEGINNER LEVEL

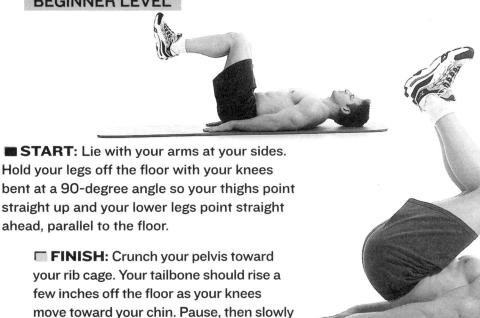

■ **START:** Lie with your arms at your sides. Hold your legs off the floor with your knees bent at a 90-degree angle so your thighs point straight up and your lower legs point straight ahead, parallel to the floor.

□ **FINISH:** Crunch your pelvis toward your rib cage. Your tailbone should rise a few inches off the floor as your knees move toward your chin. Pause, then slowly return to the starting position.

ADVANCED VARIATION
Swiss-Ball Reverse Crunch

Lie on the ball with your hips lower than your shoulders. Reach back and grab something that won't move, such as a chair weighted with sandbags. Lift and bend your legs so your thighs point up and your lower legs point ahead. (For more of a challenge, hold your legs straight out.) Do a standard reverse crunch, using your abs and hip flexors to curl your legs toward your chest.

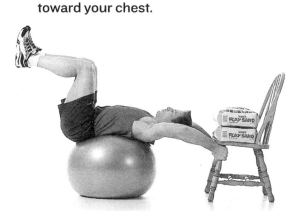

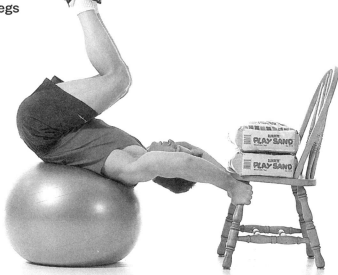

Pulse-Up
INTERMEDIATE LEVEL

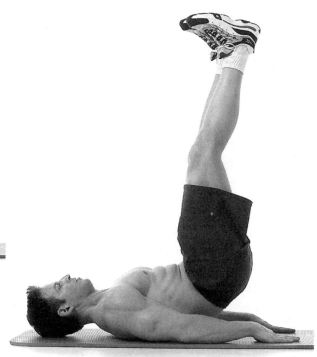

■ **START:** Lie with your hands underneath your tailbone and your legs pointed straight up toward the ceiling, perpendicular to your torso.

☐ **FINISH:** Pull your navel inward and flex your glutes as you lift your hips just a few inches off the floor. Then lower your hips.

V-Up
ADVANCED LEVEL

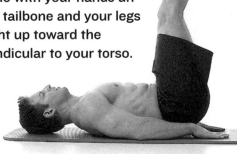

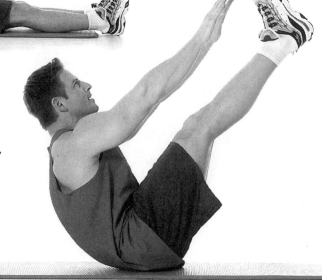

■ **START:** Lie with your legs straight out on the floor and your arms straight up in the air, fingers pointing toward the ceiling.

☐ **FINISH:** Contracting your abs, fold your body up by lifting your legs off the floor and stretching your arms toward your toes. Keep your back straight. Pause at your full extension, then return to the starting position.

Hanging Leg Raise
ADVANCED LEVEL

■ **START:** Grab a chinup bar with an overhand grip and hang with your knees slightly bent.

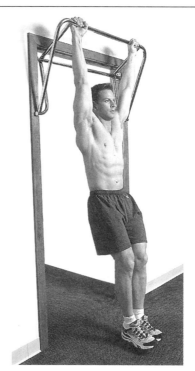

▢ **FINISH:** Use the muscles of your lower abs to pull your hips up as you curl them toward your chest. Lift your knees as close to your chest as possible, rounding your lower back at the top. Pause and feel the contraction in your lower-abdominal muscles. Then return to the starting position.

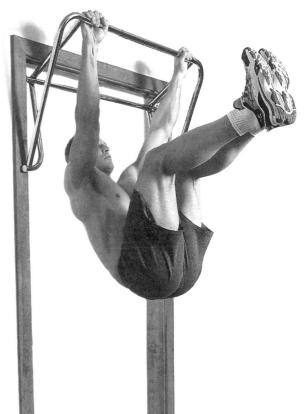

EXERCISES FOR UPPER ABDOMINALS

Crunch
BEGINNER LEVEL

■ **START:** Lie with your knees bent and your feet flat on the floor. Fold your arms across your chest or hold your hands behind your ears. (Don't interlock your fingers behind your head.)

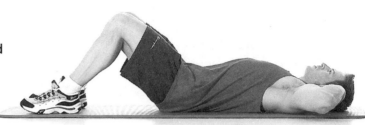

◻ **FINISH:** Use your abs to lift your head and upper torso while keeping your lower back pressed firmly against the floor. Pause with your shoulder blades a couple of inches off the floor, then slowly return to the starting position using a controlled movement.

INTERMEDIATE VARIATION
Towel Crunch

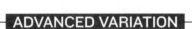

Lie with your knees bent and your feet flat on the floor. Place a rolled-up towel under your lower back. This adds to your range of motion, forcing your abs to work harder. Same movement here as the regular crunch. Pause at the top, then slowly return to the starting position, using your abs to slow your descent.

ADVANCED VARIATION
Situp

Lie with your knees bent and your feet anchored under a sturdy object such as a sofa or bed. Fold your arms across your chest or hold your hands behind your ears. Slowly lift your upper body by using your abs to flex your spine, thus bringing your chest toward your knees. Roll back down, slowly and with control.

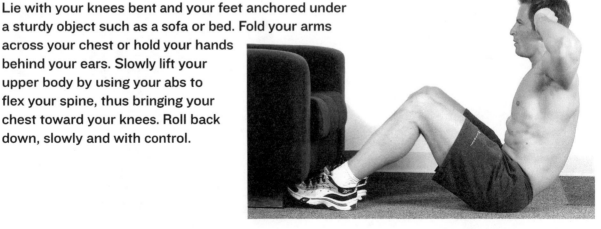

EXERCISES FOR THE OBLIQUES

Oblique Crunch
BEGINNER LEVEL

■ **START:** Lie in the crunch position, then bring your knees up and together and let them fall to one side so they're stacked on the floor. Both shoulder blades should stay on the floor. Hold your hands behind your ears.

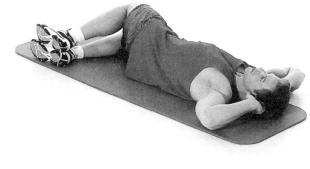

☐ **FINISH:** Lift your shoulders blades straight up off the floor, crunching your rib cage toward your pelvis, just as you would in a standard crunch. Stay in control as you lower yourself back down. Finish the set, then switch sides.

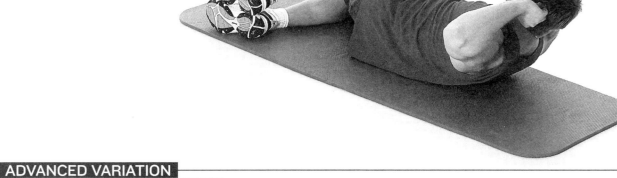

ADVANCED VARIATION
Swiss-Ball Oblique Crunch

This ball version is different from the floor exercise. Lie sideways on the ball. Keep your legs straight, brace your feet against a wall, and hold your hands behind your ears. Lift your shoulder and crunch sideways toward your hip. Hold for a second before releasing. Don't twist.

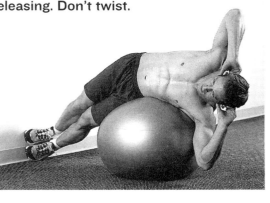

Crunch with Lateral Flexion
INTERMEDIATE LEVEL

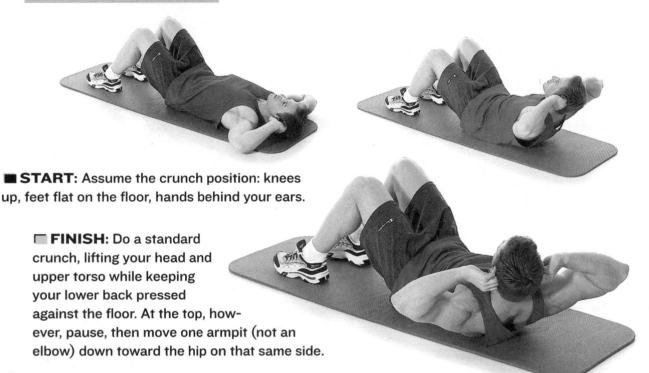

■ **START:** Assume the crunch position: knees up, feet flat on the floor, hands behind your ears.

☐ **FINISH:** Do a standard crunch, lifting your head and upper torso while keeping your lower back pressed against the floor. At the top, however, pause, then move one armpit (not an elbow) down toward the hip on that same side.

Oblique V-Up
ADVANCED LEVEL

■ **START:** Lie on your side with your body in a straight line. Fold your arms across your chest.

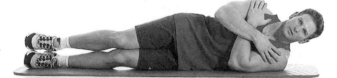

☐ **FINISH:** Keeping your legs together, lift them off the floor as you raise your top elbow toward your hip. The range of motion is short, but you should feel an intense contraction in your obliques. Pause, then slowly return to the starting position. Finish the set, then switch sides.

EXERCISES WITH ROTATIONAL MOVEMENT

Russian Twist
BEGINNER-TO-INTERMEDIATE LEVEL

■ **START:** Sit with your torso at a 45- to 60-degree angle to the floor (as if you're halfway through a situp) and your arms raised directly out in front of you. Bend your knees and keep your feet free, not anchored by anything.

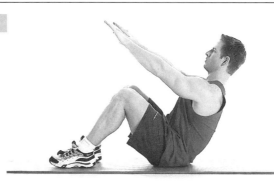

☐ **FINISH:** While maintaining this torso angle, rotate as far as possible to one side and then, without pausing, to the other.

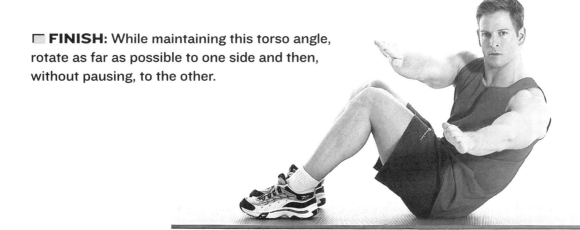

ADVANCED VARIATION
Swiss-Ball Russian Twist

Start in a regular crunch position on the ball. Lift your shoulders so that they clear the ball. With your arms extended out in front, rotate from side-to-side, as in the standard Russian twist.

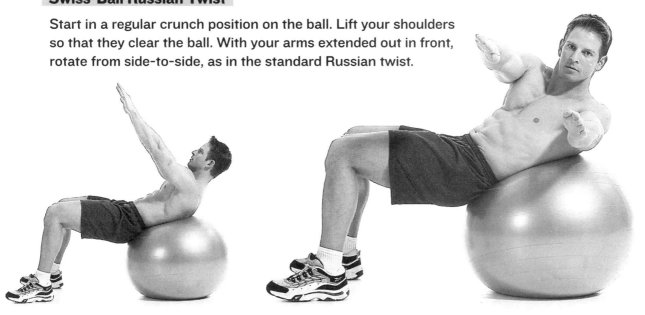

Bicycle
ADVANCED LEVEL

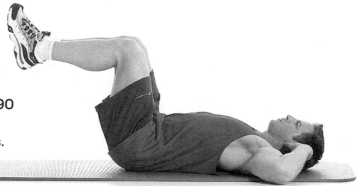

■ **START:** Lie with your knees bent at 90 degrees so your thighs point toward the ceiling. Hold your hands behind your ears.

◻ **FINISH:** Pump your legs back and forth, bicycle-style, as you simultaneously rotate your torso from side to side by moving an armpit (not an elbow) up toward the opposite knee.

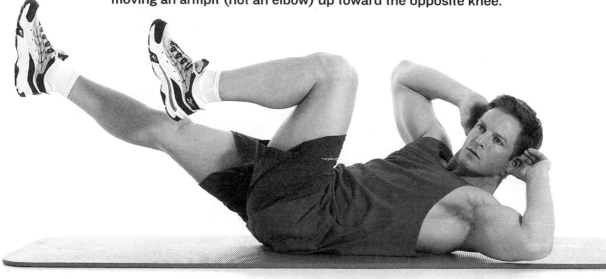

EXERCISES FOR DEEPER ABDOMINAL AND LOWER-BACK MUSCLES

Vacuum
BEGINNER LEVEL

■ **START:** Get down on your hands and knees, keeping your back flat.

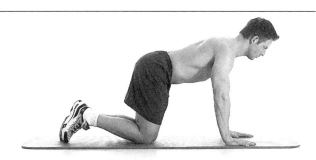

▢ **FINISH:** Take a deep breath, allowing your belly to pooch out. Then forcibly exhale and round your back like an angry cat as you lift your navel up toward your spine. When you can exhale no more, keep your back rounded and your navel in as you purse your lips and take shallow breaths through your nose for several seconds. That's I repetition; it should take 20 to 30 seconds. Inhale as you flatten your back to the starting position.

Bridge
INTERMEDIATE LEVEL

■ **START:** Get into a modified pushup position with your weight on your forearms and toes. Your body should form a straight line from head to heels (don't let your back sag).

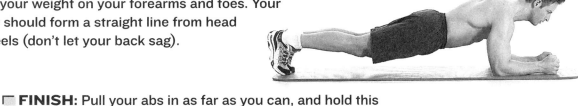

▢ **FINISH:** Pull your abs in as far as you can, and hold this position for 20 to 60 seconds, breathing steadily. Relax. If you can do the entire 60 seconds, I rep is enough. If not, try for any combination of reps that gets you up to 60 seconds.

Side Bridge
INTERMEDIATE-TO-ADVANCED LEVEL

■ **START:** Lie on your nondominant side (if you're right-handed, that would be your left side). Support your weight with that forearm and the outside edge of that foot. Your body should form a straight line from head to ankles.

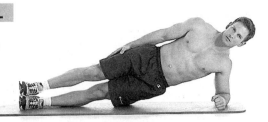

☐ **FINISH:** Pull your abs in as far as you can, and hold this position for 10 to 30 seconds, breathing steadily. Relax. If you can do the entire 30 seconds, 1 rep is enough. If not, try for any combination of reps that gets you up to 30 seconds. Then repeat on your other side.

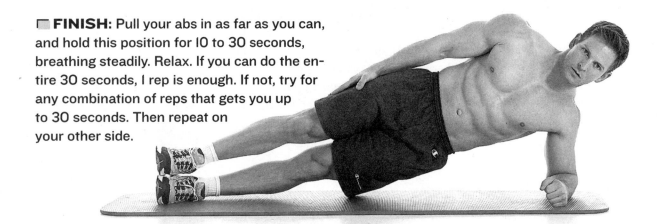

Jackknife
ADVANCED LEVEL

■ **START:** Get into a pushup position with the tops of your feet and your shins on the ball and your hands on the floor.

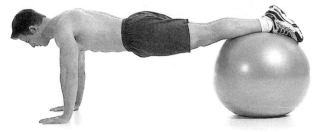

☐ **FINISH:** Pull your knees close to your chest, letting the ball roll slightly forward. Keep your arms straight, and squeeze your abs hard at the top.

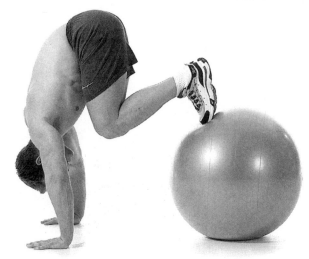

EXERCISES FOR THE LOWER BACK

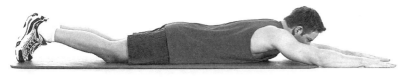

Prone Superman
BEGINNER LEVEL

■ **START:** Lie facedown with your legs straight and your arms stretched straight in front of you, with your hands on the floor.

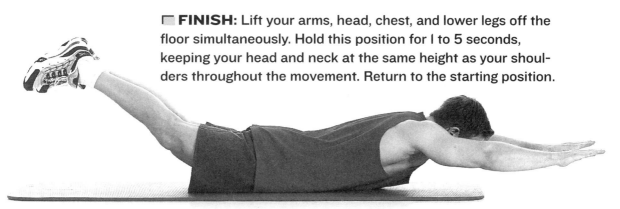

☐ **FINISH:** Lift your arms, head, chest, and lower legs off the floor simultaneously. Hold this position for I to 5 seconds, keeping your head and neck at the same height as your shoulders throughout the movement. Return to the starting position.

Bird Dog
INTERMEDIATE LEVEL

■ **START:** Start on all fours, with your knees and toes on the floor and your palms facedown in front of you.

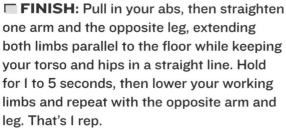

☐ **FINISH:** Pull in your abs, then straighten one arm and the opposite leg, extending both limbs parallel to the floor while keeping your torso and hips in a straight line. Hold for I to 5 seconds, then lower your working limbs and repeat with the opposite arm and leg. That's I rep.

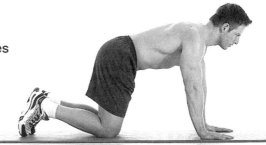

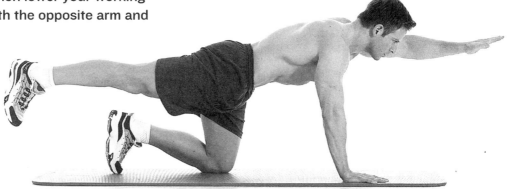

Back Extension
ADVANCED LEVEL

■ **START:** Lie with your abs and chest on the ball, your back rounded, and your legs straight behind you, braced against the base of a wall. Fold your arms across the ball (or stretch them out in front of you for more of a challenge).

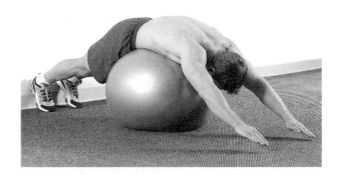

▢ **FINISH:** Uncoil your torso and lift your chest a couple of inches off the ball.

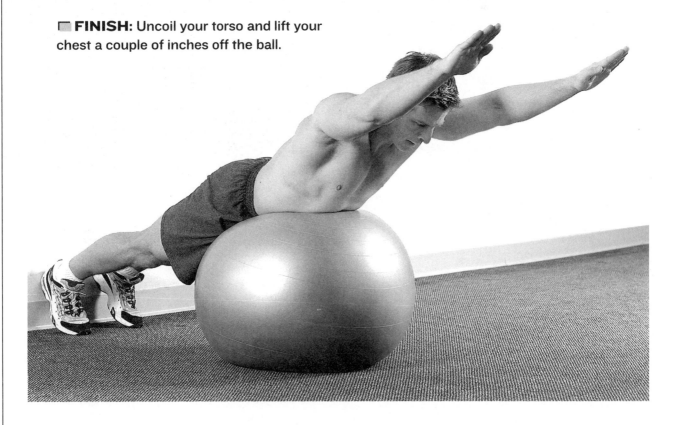

CHEST AND UPPER BACK

Beginners should choose any one chest exercise and do 2 sets of 10 to 15 reps. Also choose two upper-back exercises, making sure at least one of them focuses on scapular retraction—in other words, pulling your shoulder blades closer together in back, as in rows and reverse flies. Do 2 sets of 10 to 15 reps of each.

Intermediate and advanced lifters should choose two chest exercises and do 2 to 3 sets, with 8 to 10 reps of each (except for the box pushup—see the specific instructions for that one). Then choose three back exercises (at least one of which should include scapular retraction) and do 2 or 3 sets of 8 to 10 reps per exercise.

BEGINNER

CHEST
- Pushup --------------- (page 76)

UPPER BACK
- Assisted chinup --------(page 81)
- Supinated reverse pushup --------------(page 85)
- One-arm row, elbow in --------------------(page 87)
- One-arm row, elbow out --------------------(page 87)
- Bent-over row --------(page 88)
- Seated reverse fly -----(page 88)

INTERMEDIATE

CHEST
- Slow pushup ----------(page 76)
- Stop-and-go pushup ---(page 76)
- Stacked-feet pushup ---(page 76)
- Elevated-feet pushup --(page 77)
- Lifted-feet pushup -----(page 77)
- Swiss-ball pushup -----(page 77)
- Towel fly -------------(page 79)

UPPER BACK
- Chinup----------------(page 81)
- Pullup ----------------(page 81)
- Wide-grip pullup -------(page 82)
- Reverse pushup -------(page 85)
- Prone reverse fly ------(page 89)
- Swiss-ball prone reverse fly -----------(page 89)

ADVANCED

CHEST
- Staggered-hands pushup --------------(page 78)
- Walking pushup -------(page 78)
- Towel fly -------------(page 79)
- Plyometric pushup -----(page 80)
- Box pushup -----------(page 80)

UPPER BACK
- One-arm chinup -------(page 82)
- Weighted chinup or pullup -------------(page 83)
- Sternum chinup -------(page 83)
- Swiss-ball pullup ------(page 84)
- Towel pullup ----------(page 84)
- Elevated-feet reverse pushup --------------(page 86)
- Swiss-ball reverse pushup --------------(page 86)

EXERCISES FOR THE CHEST

Pushup
BEGINNER LEVEL

■ **START:** Support your body with the balls of your feet and with your hands, positioning the latter slightly wider than shoulder-width apart, palms flat on the floor. Straighten your arms without locking your elbows.

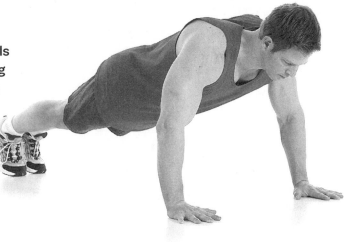

□ **FINISH:** Lower your torso until your chest is just a fraction of an inch off the floor. Push yourself back to the starting position.

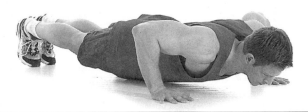

INTERMEDIATE VARIATIONS
Slow Pushup

Lower your body in an exaggeratedly slow movement to keep your chest and arm muscles under tension longer.

Stop-and-Go Pushup

From the top position, go down one-third of the way and stop for 2 or 3 seconds. Lower yourself another third and stop again. When you reach the bottom position, stop a third time before pressing back up quickly.

Stacked-Feet Pushup

Put one foot on top of the other so only the lower one supports your body. Then do a standard pushup.

Elevated-Feet Pushup

To increase the demand on your upper chest, put both feet up on a step or piano bench and do standard pushups. (You get extra style points for using a bench as dainty as ours.)

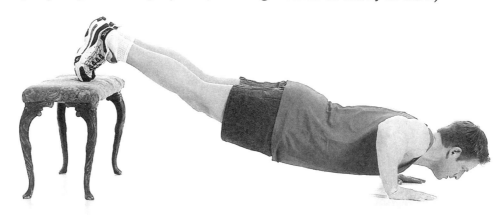

Lifted-Feet Pushup

From the elevated-feet starting position, straighten and lift one leg a few inches off the support surface as you lower and raise your torso. This is tough, since you're moving more body weight against gravity *and* increasing the work your muscles have to do to keep you stabilized.

Swiss-Ball Pushup

Get into pushup position with your knees, shins, and feet—or, to make it harder, just your shins and feet—on the ball. Then do standard pushups.

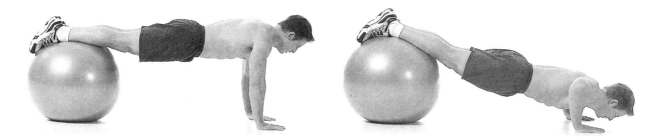

Pushup

ADVANCED VARIATIONS

Staggered-Hands Pushup

Add a greater challenge to your abdominal and shoulder muscles by placing one hand a few inches farther forward than the other. Alternate hands on each set.

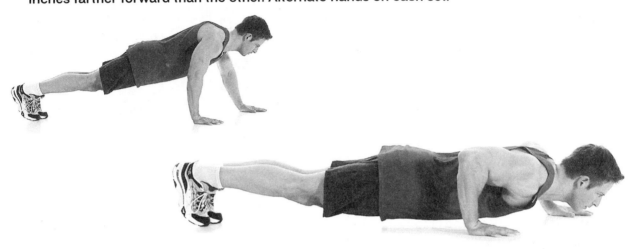

Walking Pushup

If you have a smooth surface that gives you 15 to 20 feet of clearance—such as a linoleum basement floor or a hardwood hallway—try this gut-ripper: Get into pushup position with your toes resting on a medium-size towel (or each foot resting on a smaller towel). Then "walk" your hands forward, dragging your toes behind you. Keep your back straight and your elbows bent slightly.

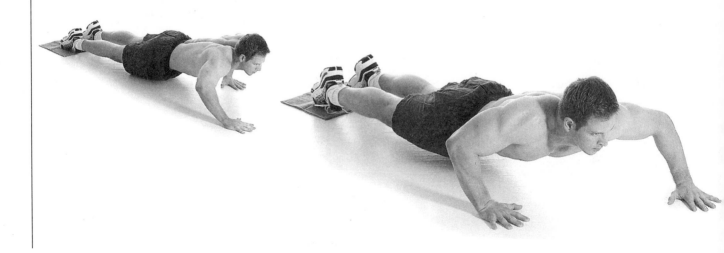

Towel Fly

INTERMEDIATE-TO-ADVANCED LEVEL

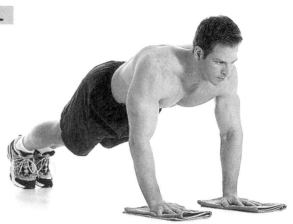

■ **START:** Assume the pushup position on a hardwood or tile floor—a rug or mat won't work for this one. Place a small, thick towel under each hand.

▢ **FINISH:** Keeping a slight bend in your elbows, move your arms up and out to your sides atop the sliding towels so your hands are in line with your ears. Then use your chest to move the towels back in, simulating a dumbbell fly.

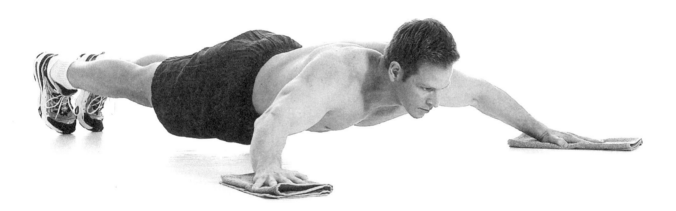

Plyometric Pushup
ADVANCED LEVEL

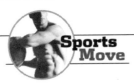

Sports
Move

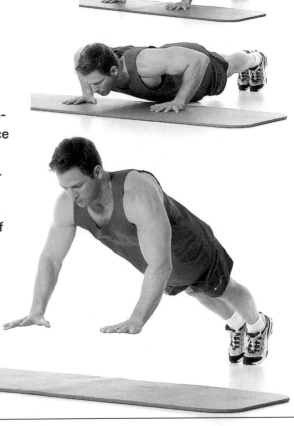

■ **START:** Assume the basic pushup position on a thick, well-padded carpet or an exercise mat. (Or better yet, use both: Put your wife's yoga mat on a well-padded surface.)

☐ **FINISH:** Lower yourself to the bottom position, then quickly push up with enough force so that your hands come off the floor. (You may have seen guys do this with a hand clap. Don't bother—it's just for show, and it increases your injury risk.) Catch yourself with your elbows slightly bent, then lower yourself with a controlled movement.

VARIATION
Box Pushup

Set up two low, sturdy boxes or steps about 3 feet apart. Get into pushup position so that the boxes are just outside your hands, and lower yourself. Then push up so hard that you land with a hand on each box. Immediately begin another pushup, lowering yourself and pushing up again. Land with your hands on the floor, between the boxes. That's I repetition; keep your sets to 5 or fewer reps.

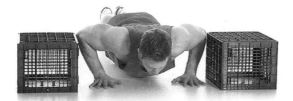

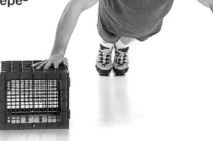

EXERCISES FOR THE UPPER BACK

Chinup
INTERMEDIATE LEVEL

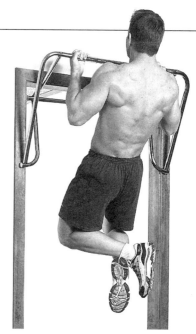

■ **START:** Grab a chinning bar with an underhand, shoulder-width grip, and hang with your elbows slightly bent.

☐ **FINISH:** Pull your chin above the bar, hold for a second or two, and lower your body with control.

BEGINNER VARIATION
Assisted Chinup

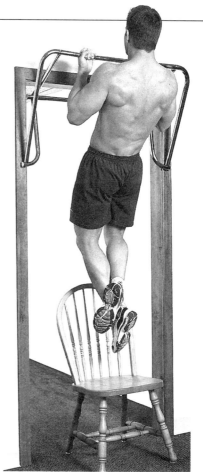

If you find it hard to do even one chinup from the hanging position (which is far from unusual among beginning and even intermediate exercisers), stand on a chair and push off a bit with your legs.

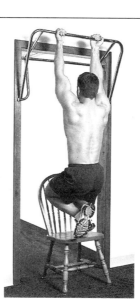

INTERMEDIATE VARIATIONS
Pullup

Same as a chinup, but with an overhand, slightly wider grip. This puts your biceps in a weaker position, forcing your upper-back muscles to do more of the work.

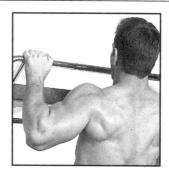

Chinup

INTERMEDIATE VARIATIONS
Wide-Grip Pullup

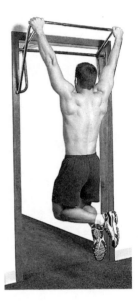
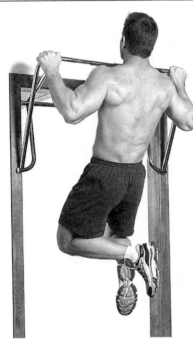

Place your hands well outside your shoulders, putting your biceps in a still-weaker position and further increasing the demand on your lats as you pull yourself up. This shortens your range of motion, decreasing your overall back-muscle stimulation; and yet it's more difficult than the previous two variations.

ADVANCED VARIATIONS
One-Arm Chinup

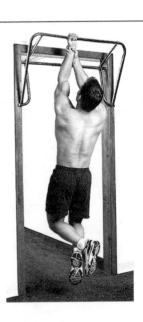
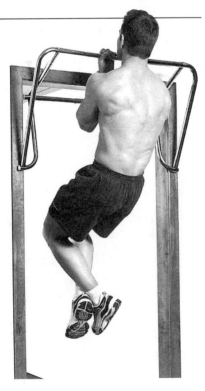

Grab the bar with one hand, using an underhand grip. Grab your wrist with the other hand. Pull yourself up.

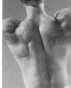

Weighted Chinup or Pullup

Wear a full backpack or fanny pack and do a regular chinup or pullup.

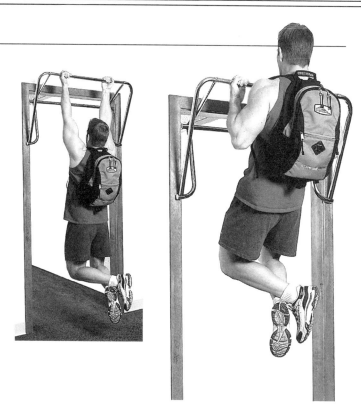

Sternum Chinup

If you have a few extra feet of clearance above your chinning bar, pull your chest up to the bar and lean back. This works your middle-back muscles a little harder.

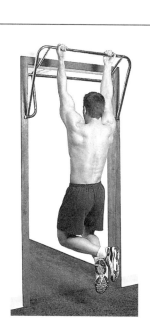
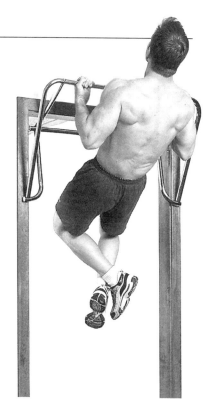

Chinup

ADVANCED VARIATIONS
Swiss-Ball Pullup

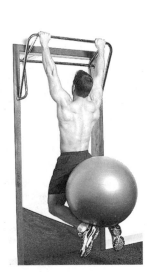

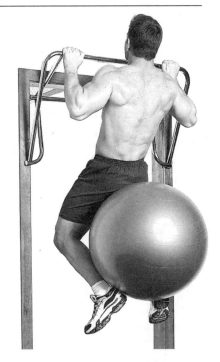

Ask a buddy to position a Swiss ball behind you so you can hold it between your hamstrings and calves as you perform any kind of pullup or chinup. This will help you minimize swinging and maintain a good chest-out position.

Towel Pullup

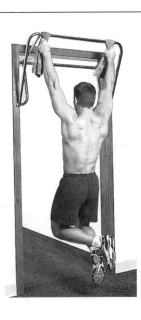

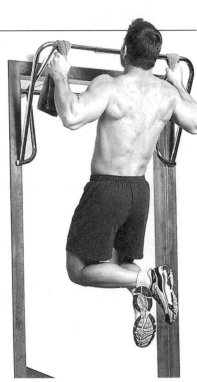

Probably the toughest variation of all: Place two hand towels over the chinning bar and grab each by its ends. Then go ahead and perform any of the pullup variations. Note that you won't be able to get your chin above the bar; pull yourself to the level of your hands or slightly higher.

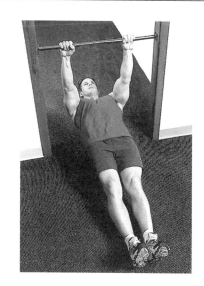

Reverse Pushup
INTERMEDIATE LEVEL

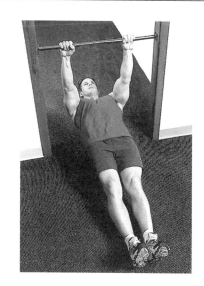

■ **START:** Affix your chinning bar in a doorway, about 3 feet above the floor. Lie down so the bar is directly over your chest. Grab the bar with an overhand grip that's slightly wider than shoulder-width. Lift your torso and legs off the floor so that only the backs of your heels remain planted. Pull in your abs and hold your body in a straight line from head to heels.

◻ **FINISH:** Pinch your shoulder blades together as you pull your chest up as close as possible to the bar.

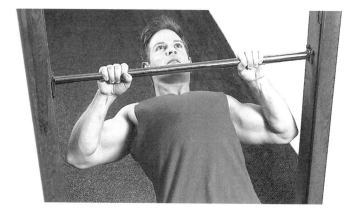

BEGINNER VARIATION
Supinated Reverse Pushup

Use an underhand grip that's slightly narrower than shoulder-width, to shift more work to your biceps and lats and away from your scapular retractors (middle traps and rhomboids).

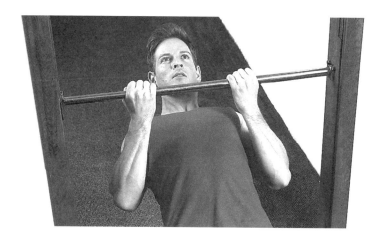

Reverse Pushup

ADVANCED VARIATIONS
Elevated-Feet Reverse Pushup

Rest your feet on a footstool or small bench, then do a standard reverse pushup.

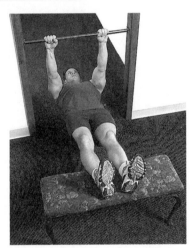

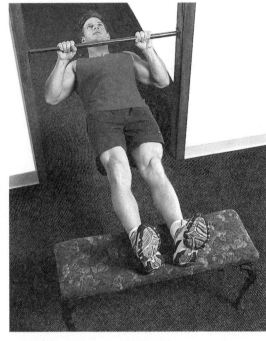

Swiss-Ball Reverse Pushup

Keep the backs of your heels and calves on the ball as you perform standard reverse pushups. It's even harder with just your feet touching the ball.

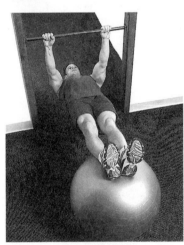

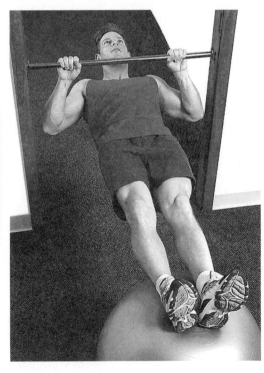

One-Arm Row, Elbow In
BEGINNER LEVEL

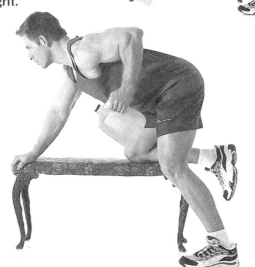

■ **START:** Grab a full plastic water or detergent bottle with your non-dominant hand, and place your other hand and knee on a sturdy bench (a piano bench works great). Plant your dominant foot flat on the floor, and let your working arm hang down slightly ahead of your shoulder, with your palm facing the bench. Keep your back straight.

▢ **FINISH:** Pull your working elbow up and back, past your torso. Pause for 2 full seconds, then slowly return to the starting position. Finish the set with that arm, then switch to the other.

One-Arm Row, Elbow Out
BEGINNER-TO-INTERMEDIATE LEVEL

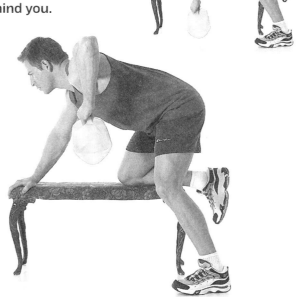

■ **START:** Same as the elbow-in version, but with your working arm out away from your body and your palm facing behind you.

▢ **FINISH:** Pull the weight straight up (not back) until your elbow is slightly higher than your back. Pause, then slowly return to the starting position.

Bent-Over Row
BEGINNER-TO-INTERMEDIATE LEVEL

■ **START:** Lay a full suitcase in front of you. (As discussed in chapter 3, you can use anything for a weight—luggage, a sandbag, a couple of cinder blocks, a railroad tie, whatever.) Stand with your legs comfortably apart, then bend over at your hips with your knees bent and your back flat, and grab the sides of the bag.

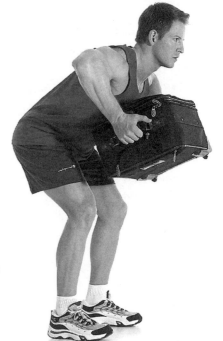

▢ **FINISH:** Use your back and biceps to pull the suitcase up to your chest, keeping it close to your body. Pause, then slowly return to the starting position.

Seated Reverse Fly
BEGINNER-TO-INTERMEDIATE LEVEL

■ **START:** Sit on the edge of a chair with your legs together and an un-opened soup can (or some other light object) in each hand. Lean forward at the waist until your chest is as close to your thighs as you can get it without rounding your back. Let your arms hang down in line with your calves, with your elbows bent slightly (5 to 10 degrees) and your palms facing behind you.

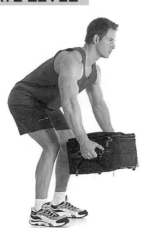

▢ **FINISH:** Raise the cans to either side in an arcing motion until your arms are parallel to the floor and your wrists are in line with your ears. Pause at the top, then slowly return to the starting position, keeping the same small bend in your elbows throughout the movement.

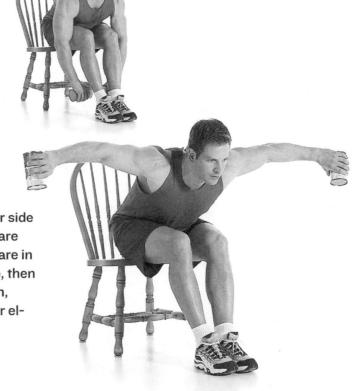

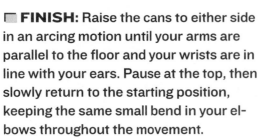

Prone Reverse Fly
INTERMEDIATE LEVEL

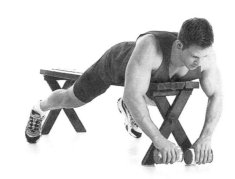

■ **START:** Lie facedown on a sturdy bench or table. Hold a pair of soup cans (or other light objects) in an overhand grip about an inch off the floor, with your elbows slightly bent and your upper arms as close as possible to perpendicular to your torso.

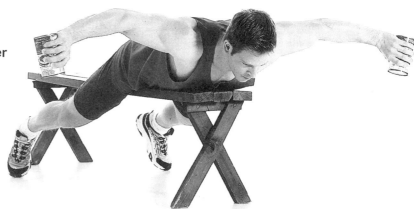

▢ **FINISH:** Pinch your shoulder blades together as you raise your arms in a wide, arcing motion to either side until they're parallel to the floor. Hold for a second or two at the top, then slowly return to the starting position. You should feel constant tension in your rear deltoids and upper back throughout the movement.

VARIATION
Swiss-Ball Prone Reverse Fly

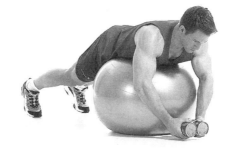

Do reverse flies with your chest on a Swiss ball instead of a bench. The more limited range of motion actually helps keep maximum tension on your back muscles.

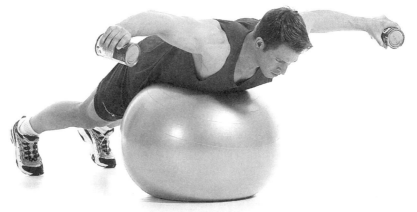

SHOULDERS AND ARMS

Beginners should do 1 or 2 sets of 10 to 15 reps of the external rotation and the lateral raise. Also, choose two triceps exercises, doing 1 or 2 sets of 10 to 15 reps of each. For your biceps, do 1 set of 10 to 15 reps (each arm) of the self-resisted biceps curl, plus 1 or 2 sets of 10 to 12 reps of the towel curl.

At the intermediate and advanced levels, do 2 or 3 sets of 8 to 10 reps of the external rotation and two other shoulder exercises. Do 2 or 3 sets of 8 to 10 reps of the triangle pushup and one-arm triceps extension. Do 2 or 3 sets of 6 to 10 reps of the towel curl and supinated close-grip chinup.

BEGINNER	INTERMEDIATE	ADVANCED
SHOULDER MUSCLES	**SHOULDER MUSCLES**	**SHOULDER MUSCLES**
External rotation -------(page 91)	Alternating lateral raise ---------------------(page 92)	External rotation with lean ------------------(page 91)
Lateral raise ----------(page 92)	Upright row -----------(page 93)	Pike pushup------------(page 93)
TRICEPS	**TRICEPS**	Slow negative pike pushup --------------(page 93)
Double triceps kickback ------------(page 95)	Triangle pushup --------(page 97)	Swiss-ball shoulder press ---------------------(page 94)
Chair dip --------------(page 95)	One-arm triceps extension ------------(page 97)	**TRICEPS**
BICEPS	**BICEPS**	Full-elevation chair dip -------------(page 96)
Self-resisted biceps curl ------------------(page 99)	Supinated close-grip chinup --------------(page 100)	Swiss-ball chair dip ----(page 96)
Towel curl------------(page 99)		Stabilizing pushup -----(page 98)

EXERCISES FOR THE SHOULDER MUSCLES

External Rotation
BEGINNER-TO-INTERMEDIATE LEVEL

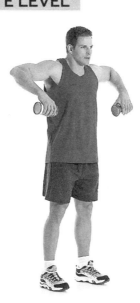

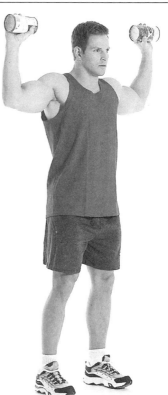

■ **START:** With a soup can or other light object in each hand, hold your arms out to your sides with your elbows bent 90 degrees so your upper arms are just an inch or two below your shoulders and almost parallel to the floor, and your forearms are pointed in toward your torso.

▢ **FINISH:** Keep your upper arms still and use your elbows to rotate your forearms up until they are as close to perpendicular to the floor as possible. Return to the starting position.

ADVANCED VARIATION
External Rotation with Lean

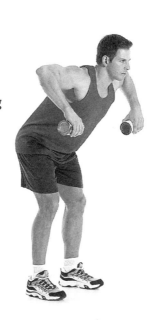

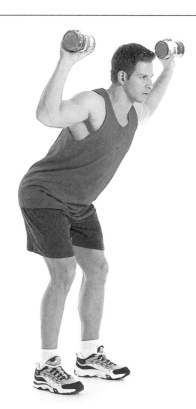

Increase the challenge by leaning forward 30 to 45 degrees at the waist.

Lateral Raise
BEGINNER LEVEL

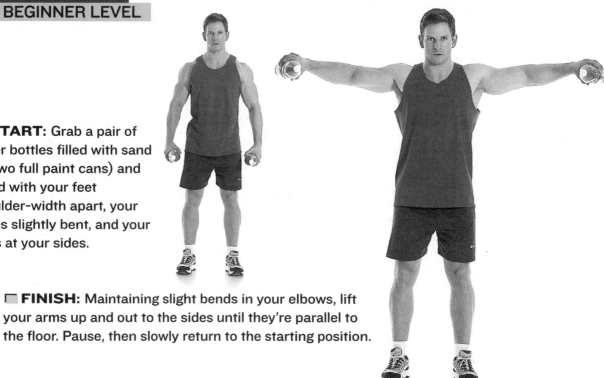

■ **START:** Grab a pair of water bottles filled with sand (or two full paint cans) and stand with your feet shoulder-width apart, your knees slightly bent, and your arms at your sides.

☐ **FINISH:** Maintaining slight bends in your elbows, lift your arms up and out to the sides until they're parallel to the floor. Pause, then slowly return to the starting position.

INTERMEDIATE VARIATION
Alternating Lateral Raise

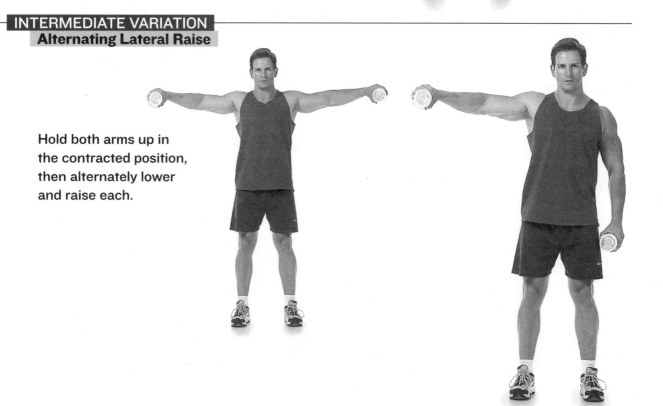

Hold both arms up in the contracted position, then alternately lower and raise each.

Upright Row
INTERMEDIATE LEVEL

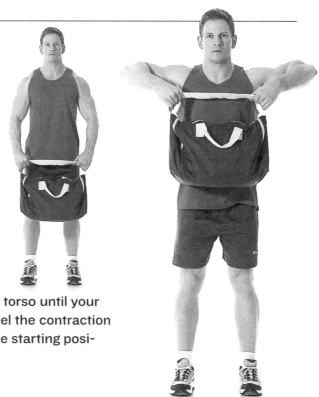

■ **START:** Fill your gym bag or carry-on suit-case with books or something else heavy enough to create a challenging weight. Hold the bag by its straps with both hands. Let your arms hang straight down, with your hands 12 to 24 inches apart. (The farther you place them apart, the easier and more natural the exercise is for your shoulders.)

◰ **FINISH:** Lift the bag straight up along your torso until your upper arms are parallel to the floor. Pause to feel the contraction in your delts and traps, then slowly return to the starting posi-tion, staying in control.

Pike Pushup
ADVANCED LEVEL

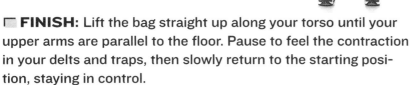

■ **START:** Get into the standard pushup position with your hands about shoulder-width apart. Walk your feet forward until they're 2½ to 3 feet behind your hands and your hips stick way up.

◰ **FINISH:** Keep your legs straight as you execute a pushup, feeling the work in your shoulders and triceps.

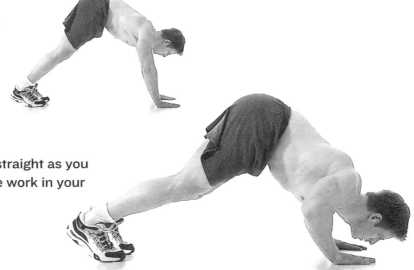

VARIATION
Slow Negative Pike Pushup

For even more of a challenge, go extremely slowly during the lowering phase.

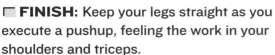

Swiss-Ball Shoulder Press
ADVANCED LEVEL

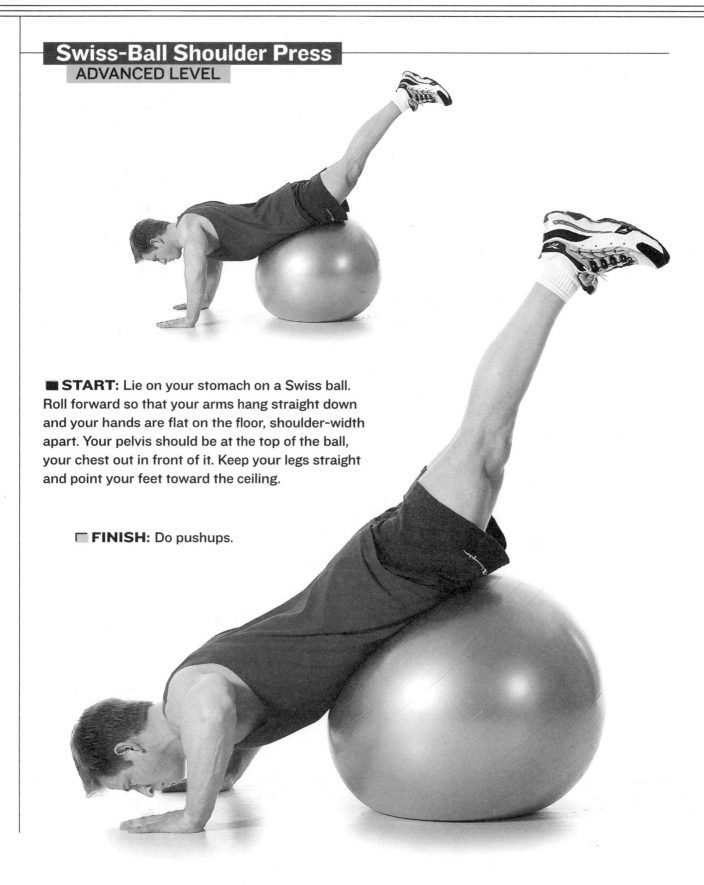

■ **START:** Lie on your stomach on a Swiss ball. Roll forward so that your arms hang straight down and your hands are flat on the floor, shoulder-width apart. Your pelvis should be at the top of the ball, your chest out in front of it. Keep your legs straight and point your feet toward the ceiling.

▢ **FINISH:** Do pushups.

EXERCISES FOR THE TRICEPS

Double Triceps Kickback
BEGINNER-TO-INTERMEDIATE LEVEL

■ **START:** Holding a household object (can, water bottle, brick) in each hand, bend at the hips until your torso is nearly parallel to the floor. Keep your knees slightly bent and your back slightly arched. Fix your upper arms against your sides, also parallel to the floor. Let your forearms hang straight down, perpendicular to the floor.

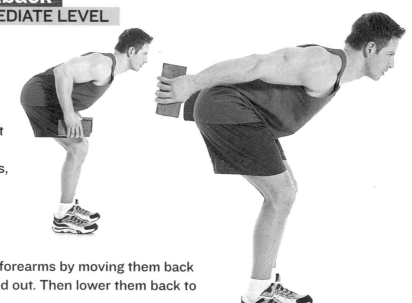

▢ **FINISH:** Straighten your forearms by moving them back until they're completely locked out. Then lower them back to the starting position.

Chair Dip
BEGINNER-TO-INTERMEDIATE LEVEL

■ **START:** Hold on to the seat of a sturdy chair behind you, with your knees bent and your feet flat on the floor—as if you were seated in another, invisible chair.

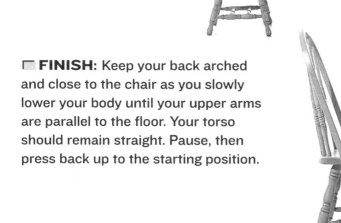

▢ **FINISH:** Keep your back arched and close to the chair as you slowly lower your body until your upper arms are parallel to the floor. Your torso should remain straight. Pause, then press back up to the starting position.

Chair Dip

ADVANCED VARIATIONS
Full-Elevation Chair Dip

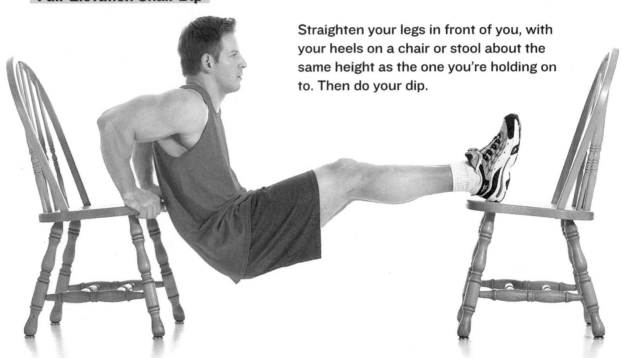

Straighten your legs in front of you, with your heels on a chair or stool about the same height as the one you're holding on to. Then do your dip.

Swiss-Ball Chair Dip

Do chair dips with your heels on a Swiss ball. The chair or bench should be against a wall so it doesn't move.

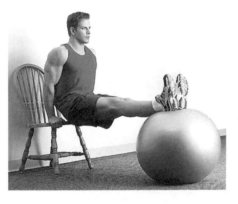

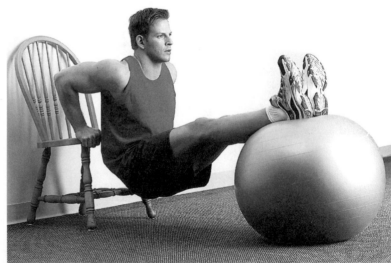

Triangle Pushup
INTERMEDIATE-TO-ADVANCED LEVEL

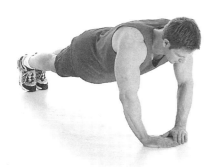

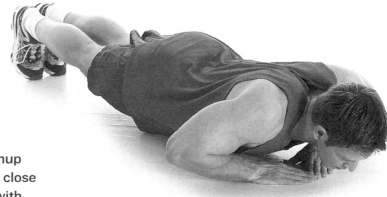

■ **START:** Start in the regular pushup position, but with your hands placed close enough together to make a triangle with your thumbs and forefingers.

▢ **FINISH:** Keeping your elbows in so your upper arms form a 45-degree angle with your torso, lower your chest as close to the triangle as possible. Then return to the starting position.

One-Arm Triceps Extension
INTERMEDIATE-TO-ADVANCED LEVEL

■ **START:** Lie on your side with your legs, hips, and shoulders stacked over each other. Reach your bottom arm across your body and grab your opposite shoulder. Place your free hand on the floor, in front of your chest.

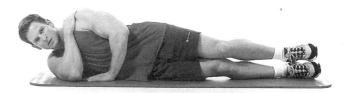

▢ **FINISH:** Use your upper triceps to push your entire upper torso off the floor so that only your hips and legs remain in contact with the floor. Return to the starting position. Finish the set with that arm, then switch sides.

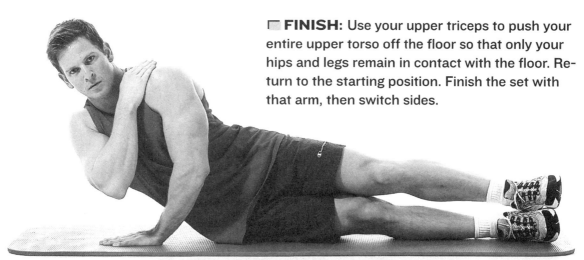

Stabilizing Pushup
ADVANCED LEVEL

■ **START/FINISH.** Stand with your feet shoulder-width apart, bend forward at your waist, and place your arms 8 to 10 inches apart on a Swiss ball that's a few feet in front of you. (The farther away from the ball you are, the harder the exercise is.) Your weight should be on the balls of your feet. Pull your abs in toward your spine. (It's important to tense your abs and lower back to stabilize your body as you do this.) Do pushups.

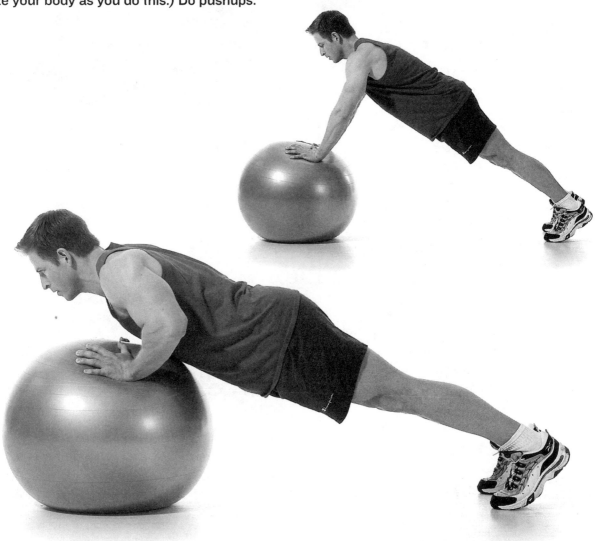

EXERCISES FOR THE BICEPS

Self-Resisted Biceps Curl
BEGINNER LEVEL

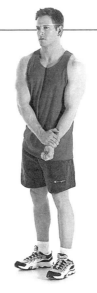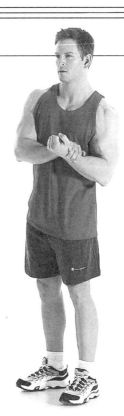

■ **START:** Stand with your knees slightly bent and your abs tucked in, your nondominant arm down at your side with your palm facing forward. Put your opposite palm over your wrist.

☐ **FINISH:** Make a fist with your working hand and execute a biceps curl with that arm while resisting it with the other. Shift the resistance on the way so your palm pushes the working arm down. Return to the starting position. Finish your set, then repeat, with the other arm doing the work.

Towel Curl
BEGINNER LEVEL

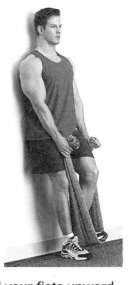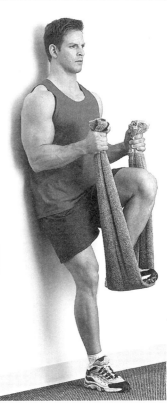

■ **START:** Fold a large bath towel lengthwise a few times and hold it at either end, your palms facing each other, as you stand with your back against a wall. Move your feet out about a foot in front of you, and place one of them in the middle of the towel (at the bottom of the U that the towel makes as you hold it). Start with both knees slightly bent.

☐ **FINISH:** With your arms straight down, curl your fists upward toward your shoulders while using your foot to resist the movement. Keep your upper arms still and against your body so all the pulling power comes from your elbow joints. Pause at the top, using your arms to resist your leg's attempt to push the towel back down to the floor. Return to the starting position.

Supinated Close-Grip Chinup
INTERMEDIATE-TO-ADVANCED LEVEL

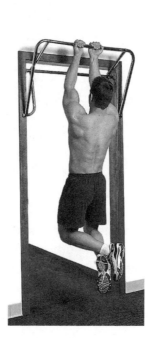

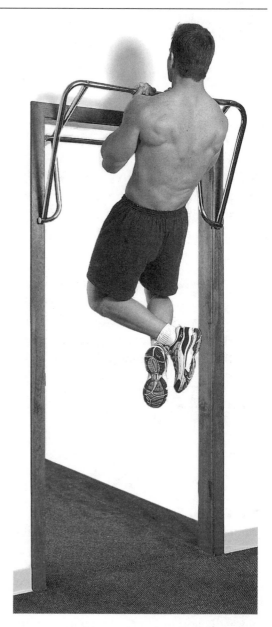

■ **START:** Hold on to a chinning bar with an underhand grip that's less than shoulder width (the close grip emphasizes the biceps). Bend your elbows slightly so you're not quite at a full dead-hang.

■ **FINISH:** Pull yourself up until you get your chin over the bar. Pause, then lower to the starting position.

LOWER BODY

We've divided the exercises for the thighs and gluteals into two categories. In *knee-dominant exercises*, the hardest-working muscles are the ones that straighten the knee joint—the quadriceps (we could also have called these *quad-dominant exercises*). *Hip-dominant exercises* straighten the hip joint—they raise your torso back up when it's bent forward at the hips. These work hamstring and gluteal muscles. We also provide a set of exercises for the calves, which do some work with knee- and hip-dominant exercises but not through a full range of motion.

Beginners should choose two knee-dominant and two hip-dominant exercises, and one for the calves. Do 1 or 2 sets of 12 to 15 reps of each.

Advanced and intermediate lifters should select three knee-dominant and three hip-dominant exercises, and two for the calves. Do 2 or 3 sets of each. The recommended rep count is 12 to 15 for the calf raises (but not the calf jumps), and 6 to 8 for the rest. If you do split jumps, 4 to 6 reps on each leg per set is enough.

BEGINNER

KNEE-DOMINANT
- Towel squat ----------(page 102)
- Split squat ----------(page 103)
- 10-second-stop ski squat --------------(page 104)

HIP-DOMINANT
- Lying hip extension ---(page 107)
- Reverse hyperextension --------------------(page 110)

CALVES
- One-leg calf raise ------(page 111)
- Seated calf raise -------(page 111)

INTERMEDIATE

KNEE-DOMINANT
- Swiss-ball wall squat ---------------(page 102)
- Bulgarian split squat ---------------(page 103)
- Ski squat ------------(page 104)
- Lunge ----------------(page 105)

ADVANCED

KNEE-DOMINANT
- Swiss-ball Bulgarian split squat ----------(page 104)
- Split jump ------------(page 105)
- One-leg squat --------(page 106)

HIP-DOMINANT
- Elevated-leg lying hip extension -----------(page 107)
- Swiss-ball lying hip extension -----------(page 108)
- Swiss-ball lying hip extension/leg curl ---(page 108)
- One-leg Romanian deadlift -------------(page 109)
- King deadlift ----------(page 109)
- Swiss-ball reverse hyperextension ------(page 110)

CALVES
- Explosive calf jump ----(page 112)

KNEE-DOMINANT EXERCISES

Towel Squat
BEGINNER LEVEL

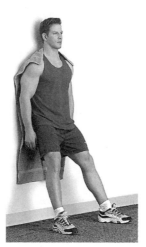

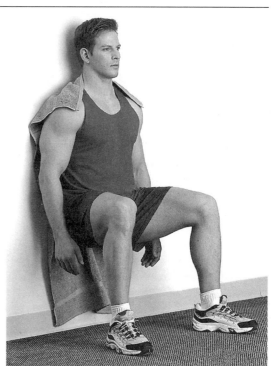

■ **START:** Stand leaning against a wall with your feet slightly wider than shoulder-width apart and about 2 feet in front of you. Put an unfolded towel behind you so that your back presses against it rather than directly on the wall.

☐ **FINISH:** Bend your knees and let your back slide down the wall along with the towel until your upper thighs are parallel to the floor. Pause, then push yourself back up.

INTERMEDIATE VARIATION
Swiss-Ball Wall Squat

Get into position as for the towel squat, but put a Swiss ball, not a towel, between you and the wall. The ball will press against your middle or lower back in the up position, and against your upper back in the down position.

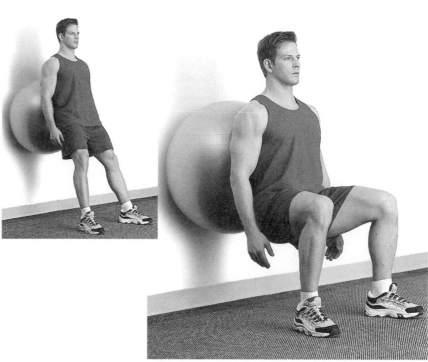

Split Squat
BEGINNER LEVEL

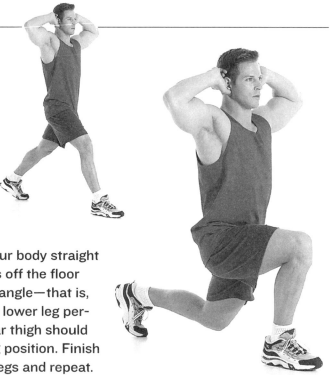

■ **START:** Stand with one leg 3 to 4 feet in front of the other, with your toes pointed forward. Your front foot should be flat on the floor, but only the ball of your back foot should be planted. To help yourself balance, line up each foot with its corresponding buttock, not with the other foot. Keep your torso erect. Rest your hands behind your head.

☐ **FINISH:** Bend both knees to lower your body straight down until your back knee is a few inches off the floor and your front leg is bent at a 90-degree angle—that is, with the thigh parallel to the floor and the lower leg perpendicular to the floor. Your torso and rear thigh should form a straight line. Return to the starting position. Finish the set, then switch your front and back legs and repeat.

Bulgarian Split Squat
INTERMEDIATE LEVEL

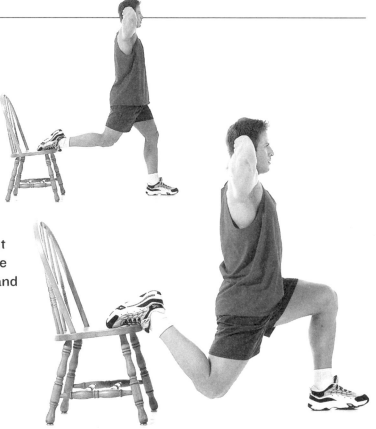

■ **START:** Place one foot on the floor 2 to 3 feet in front of you and rest the instep of the other on the surface of a chair, bench, or bed 2 feet behind you. Hold your hands behind your ears.

☐ **FINISH:** Balancing on your front foot, execute a split squat. Finish the set, then switch your leg positions and repeat.

Bulgarian Split Squat

ADVANCED VARIATION
Swiss-Ball Bulgarian Split Squat

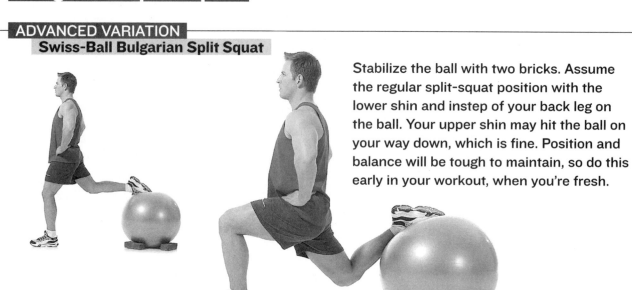

Stabilize the ball with two bricks. Assume the regular split-squat position with the lower shin and instep of your back leg on the ball. Your upper shin may hit the ball on your way down, which is fine. Position and balance will be tough to maintain, so do this early in your workout, when you're fresh.

Ski Squat
INTERMEDIATE LEVEL

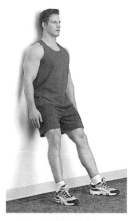

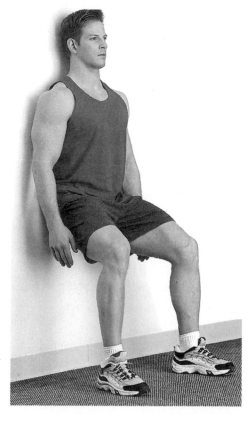

■ **START:** Lean back against a wall with your feet 2 feet in front of you as in the towel squat—but without the towel.

☐ **FINISH:** Bend your knees to descend just a few inches, and freeze there for 30 seconds. Slide down another few inches and stop again for another 30 seconds. Stop two or three more times as you work your way down until your butt is almost touching the floor. That's the end of the first set.

BEGINNER VARIATION
10-Second-Stop Ski Squat

Same exercise, with 10-second stops.

Lunge
INTERMEDIATE LEVEL

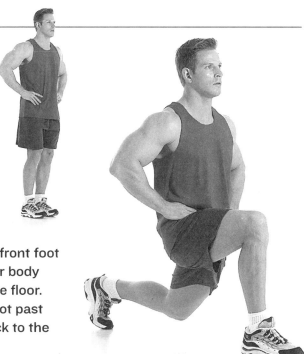

■ **START:** Stand with both feet together and your hands on your hips.

□ **FINISH:** Take a long step forward so your front foot lands 2 to 3 feet in front of you, and lower your body until the top of your front thigh is parallel to the floor. Your forward knee should be over your toes, not past them. Quickly and forcefully push yourself back to the starting position.

Split Jump
ADVANCED LEVEL

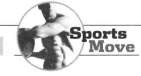

Sports Move

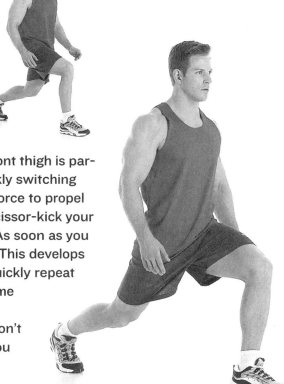

■ **START:** Start in the split-squat position— one foot 2 feet ahead of you and the other 2 feet behind.

□ **FINISH:** Instead of descending until your front thigh is parallel to the floor, stop halfway down. Then, quickly switching directions, push yourself back up with enough force to propel your entire body off the floor. While in the air, scissor-kick your legs so you land with the opposite leg forward. As soon as you land, lower yourself and jump into the next rep. This develops quickness, explosive power, and the ability to quickly repeat explosive movements (useful in a basketball game when a rebound is tipped several times and you have to jump again and again to pull it down). Don't pause between reps—pop them off as fast as you can without sacrificing good form.

One-Leg Squat
ADVANCED LEVEL

■ **START:** Stand between two objects sturdy enough to hold on to for balance—a chair and banister, for example, or a doorway. Place your dominant leg about a foot in front of your other leg and lift the forward leg a few inches off the floor.

☐ **FINISH:** Squat down with your planted leg while holding your forward leg off the floor. Lower yourself until your lifted leg is as close to parallel to the floor as possible, then push yourself back up. Keep your torso as erect as you can. Finish the set, then switch leg positions and repeat.

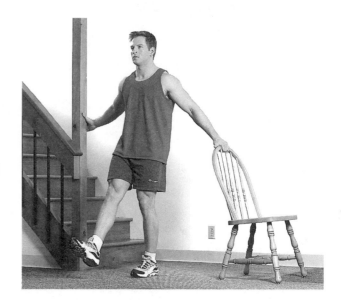

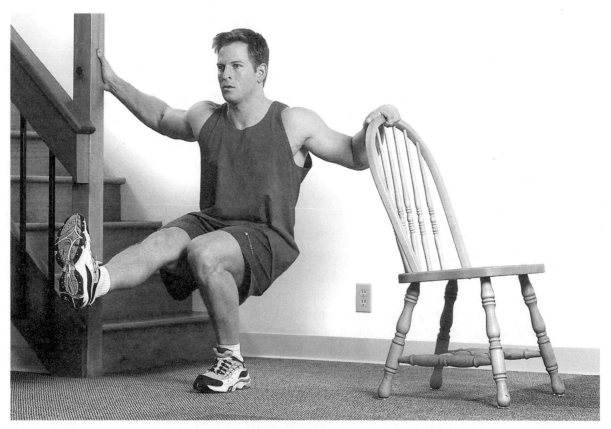

HIP-DOMINANT EXERCISES

Lying Hip Extension
BEGINNER-TO-INTERMEDIATE LEVEL

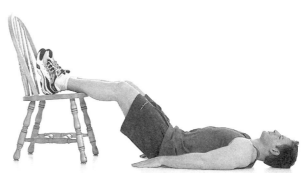

■ **START:** Lie on the floor with your arms at your sides and both heels up on a chair or bench, with your knees bent.

□ **FINISH:** Pushing with your gluteals and hamstrings, dig your heels down into the seat of the chair and lift your hips until your body forms a ramp that descends from your knees to your shoulders. Pause, then return to the starting position.

ADVANCED VARIATIONS
Elevated-Leg Lying Hip Extension

For a greater challenge, straighten one leg and hold it directly over its hip before you lift up. The elevated leg should stay perpendicular to the floor throughout the exercise.

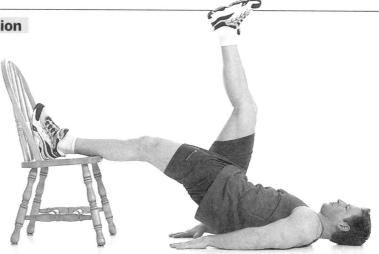

Lying Hip Extension

ADVANCED VARIATIONS
Swiss-Ball Lying Hip Extension

To go spherical with this movement, put your heels and calves on a Swiss ball (rather than just your heels on a bench) and spread your arms on the floor for added stability. Everything else is the same.

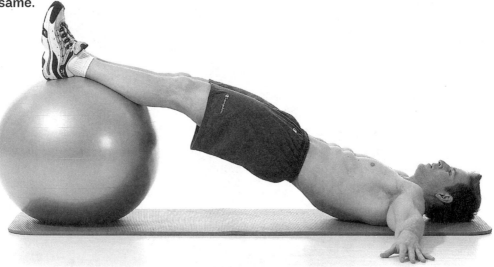

Swiss-Ball Lying Hip Extension/Leg Curl

Set up on the Swiss ball exactly as you would for the lying hip extension described above. Perform the same movement, but don't go back down just yet. Instead, at the top, execute a leg curl by using your hamstrings to roll the ball toward your butt. Hold at the point of greatest contraction, straighten your legs, and then lower your body to the starting position.

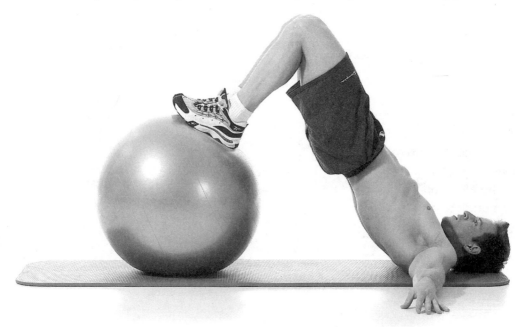

One-Leg Romanian Deadlift
ADVANCED LEVEL

■ **START:** Stand with your feet shoulder-
width apart, your knees slightly bent, your abs
tucked in, your shoulders pulled back, and your
arms at your sides. Lift one foot an inch or two
off the floor and shift it over next to (but not
touching) the other leg.

▢ **FINISH:** Bending at the hips, lower your
torso until it's as close to parallel to the floor as
you can get it without rounding your back.
Pause, then push with your heel to rise back up.

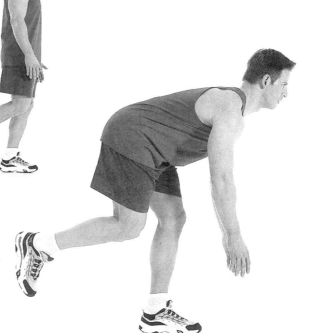

King Deadlift
ADVANCED LEVEL

■ **START:** Lift one foot behind you so that
your shin is parallel to the floor, flamingo-
style.

▢ **FINISH:** Allow your torso to lean slightly forward
(but do not bend at the hips as in the one-leg
Romanian deadlift) as you lower your body straight
down, until your hanging leg is almost touching the
floor. Pause, then push back up to the starting
position.

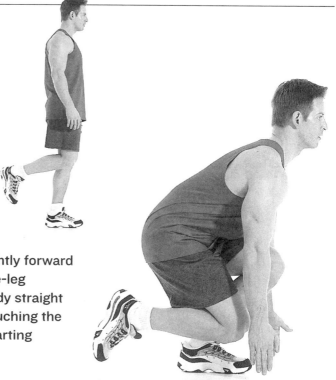

Reverse Hyperextension
BEGINNER-TO-INTERMEDIATE LEVEL

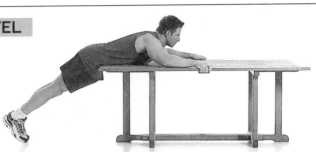

■ **START:** Lie facedown, with your torso on a piano bench or sturdy table from the navel up, and your legs hanging off behind you so they nearly touch the floor.

□ **FINISH:** Holding on to the sides of the bench, use your gluteals and hamstrings to lift your legs straight up into the air until they're just above parallel to the floor and your body forms a straight line. Hold that position for a few beats, then return to the starting position.

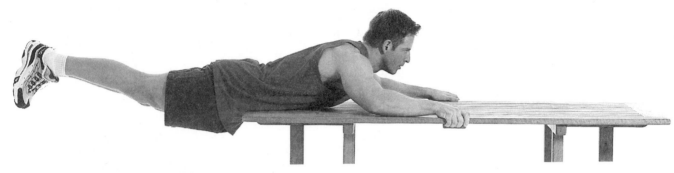

ADVANCED VARIATION
Swiss-Ball Reverse Hyperextension

Set a Swiss ball in front of something sturdy you can grab on to, like a chair weighted with heavy objects such as sandbags. Lie on your chest on the ball, and raise your straight legs off the floor. Hold for a few seconds. For more range of motion, place the ball on top of a bench or box and then lie on it. Make sure the ball can't roll off the surface you've set it on, or wear a football helmet and mouth guard.

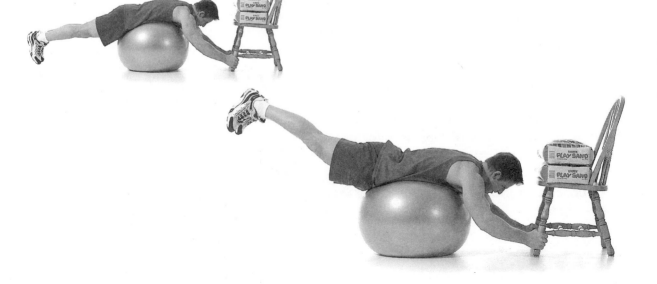

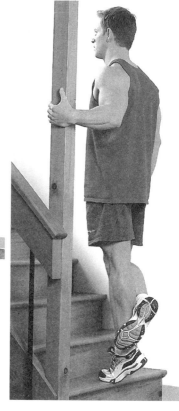

EXERCISES FOR THE CALVES

One-Leg Calf Raise
BEGINNER LEVEL

■ **START:** Stand with the ball of your non-dominant foot on the edge of a step or wooden block that's several inches high. Hook your other foot around the back of your non-dominant heel. Hold on to a banister or anything sturdy to stay balanced.

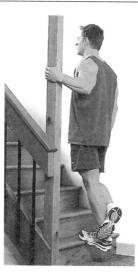

▢ **FINISH:** Let your nondominant heel drop as low as it'll go off the step. Then change direction and push off the ball of that foot until the heel is a couple of inches above the step.

Seated Calf Raise
BEGINNER LEVEL

■ **START:** Sit at the end of a chair or bench with your legs bent 90 degrees at the knees. Place the balls of your feet on a wooden block or a couple of phone books. Hold some weight—a couple of I-gallon water bottles or a sack of sand or fertilizer, for example—on top of your knees.

▢ **FINISH:** Lower your heels as far as they'll go, then slowly raise them as high as you can.

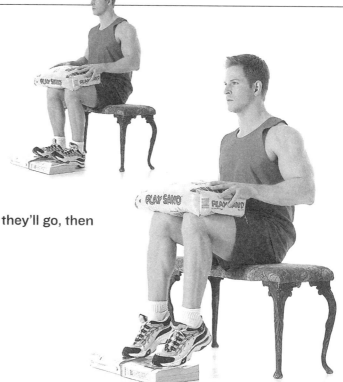

Explosive Calf Jump
ADVANCED LEVEL

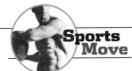

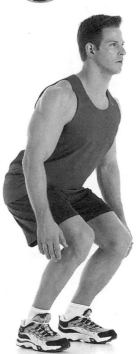

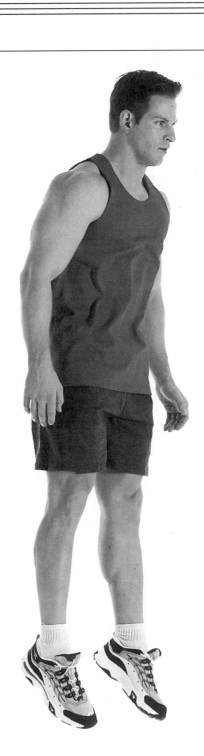

■ **START:** Bend your knees and squat straight down until your thighs are halfway to parallel to the floor (in a quarter-squat).

☐ **FINISH:** Quickly and explosively jump into the air as high as possible, concentrating on pushing off with your calves rather than with the larger hamstrings or quadriceps. As you land, immediately descend into a quarter-squat and jump again.

CHAPTER 7

DUMBBELLS: THE SMART CHOICE

What's so great about a home dumbbell workout? It's simply the purest partnership of man and iron. The necessary equipment is basic and compact: Besides an assortment of the dumbbells themselves, the only other thing you need is a sturdy workout bench (preferably one that inclines and declines).

Dumbbells give you more room to maneuver not only by taking up minimum space but also by allowing you a greater range of motion. You can move them higher, lower, farther back, and closer together than you can any barbell or machine weight. For example, while you hold a dumbbell, your shoulder and upper-back muscles can fully rotate your arm in every anatomically feasible direction. Try that with a barbell and at some point you're going to get clocked with the bar. The freedom of movement permitted by dumbbells can increase your strength, muscle mass, and flexibility—all at the same time.

The ability to work each side of your body independently of the other is another advantage afforded by 'bells. Most guys are stronger on one side than on the other, and there's no better way to discover that than by having each arm hold a separate weight. Dumbbells let you even things up by working your weaker side first or assigning it a few more reps.

Last but certainly not least, dumbbell exercises more readily recruit your smaller, "hidden" muscles to help the big boys do the work. They're able to do this thanks to the greater range of motion you usually use with dumbbells, and because it takes more individual muscles to stabilize your body when you move two limbs independently, rather than together. The stronger these small stabilizing muscles get, the more weight you'll be able to use.

MIDSECTION

Not many guys use dumbbells for abdominal and lower-back exercises. A lot of them believe using free weights during midsection work is unsafe for the lower back. Of course, any exercise is dangerous if you do it wrong. That's why you've got us to tell you how to do things right.

Another common worry is that, because you do ab exercises with higher numbers of repetitions, adding weight will make your muscles "bulky" rather than "cut" or "defined." While your midsection muscles can get bigger, they can't become huge. They just aren't designed for significant hypertrophy.

Having said that, we have to point out that these ab and lower-back exercises are for intermediate and advanced lifters. If you're a beginner, use the no-weight midsection exercises in chapter 6, doing 1 or 2 sets of 10 to 15 reps of two ab exercises and one lower-back exercise. Move up to these dumbbell exercises once you're ready for a new challenge.

If you're intermediate or advanced, go ahead with 2 or 3 sets, 8 to 12 reps each, for two of the following ab exercises and one lower-back exercise.

INTERMEDIATE

ABS
- Reverse woodchopper - (page 116)
- Weighted crunch ------ (page 116)
- Swiss-ball weighted crunch -------------- (page 117)
- Long-arm weighted crunch -------------- (page 117)
- Weighted Russian twist --------------------- (page 118)

LOWER BACK
- Back extension -------- (page 119)
- Good morning --------- (page 119)

ADVANCED

ABS
- Swiss-ball weighted Russian twist ------- (page 118)

LOWER BACK
- Prone cobra ---------- (page 120)

EXERCISES FOR THE ABS

Reverse Woodchopper
INTERMEDIATE LEVEL

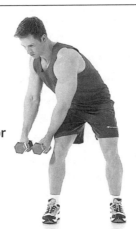

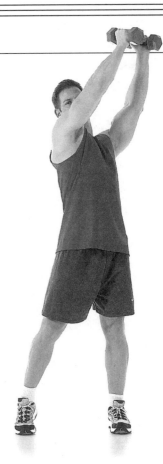

■ **START:** Stand with your feet flat on the floor and your knees bent. Hold a pair of light dumbbells to one side of your body so that both weights are just outside your knee. Your arms are straight.

□ **FINISH:** Keeping your arms straight and your eyes forward, lift the dumbbells up and across your body in an arcing motion as you straighten your legs. Finish with both arms stretched over your shoulder and your opposite heel off the floor as if you were about to begin chopping wood. Slowly lower the dumbbells to the starting position—remember to work your abs on the way down. Finish the set on that side, then repeat on the other side.

Weighted Crunch
INTERMEDIATE LEVEL

■ **START:** Lie on the floor in the crunch position—knees bent, feet flat on the floor. With both hands, hold the sides of a dumbbell on your upper chest, just below your chin.

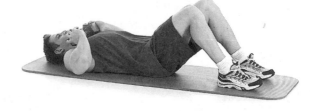

□ **FINISH:** Keep your lower back pressed against the floor as you use your abs to crunch your rib cage toward your pelvis. Your shoulder blades should rise a few inches off the floor. Pause, then slowly return to the starting position.

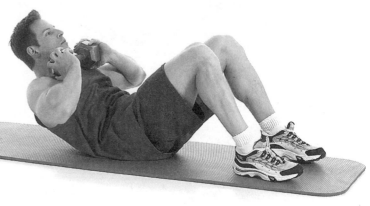

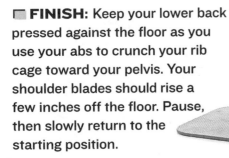

Swiss-Ball Weighted Crunch

Lie on a Swiss ball with your head slightly below your chest. Hold a dumbbell by its sides at your upper chest. Your shoulders should move a few inches off the ball as you perform your crunch.

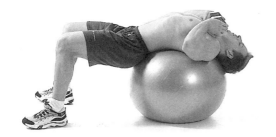

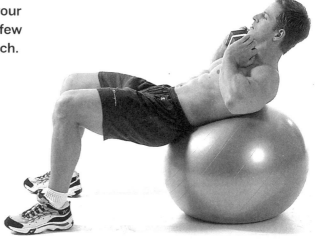

Long-Arm Weighted Crunch
INTERMEDIATE-TO-ADVANCED LEVEL

■ **START:** Lie on the floor with your knees up and your feet flat. Hold a light dumbbell in each hand and stretch your arms straight back behind you.

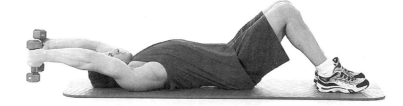

□ **FINISH:** Crunch your rib cage toward your pelvis. Don't generate momentum with your arms—make your abs do all the work. Pause, then slowly return to the starting position.

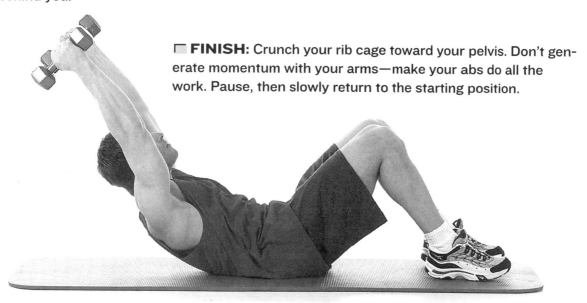

Weighted Russian Twist
INTERMEDIATE-TO-ADVANCED LEVEL

■ START: Sitting on the floor with your knees bent and your feet flat, hold a light dumbbell at the ends with your arms extended straight out in front of you. Lean back until your torso is at a 60- to 75-degree angle from the floor. Pull your belly in.

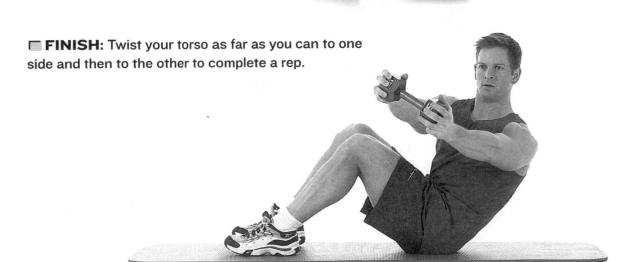

▢ FINISH: Twist your torso as far as you can to one side and then to the other to complete a rep.

ADVANCED VARIATION
Swiss-Ball Weighted Russian Twist

Do the exercise while sitting on a Swiss ball instead of on the floor. Your hips and legs may shift a bit because of the ball's instability, and you won't be able to lean back as you did on the floor.

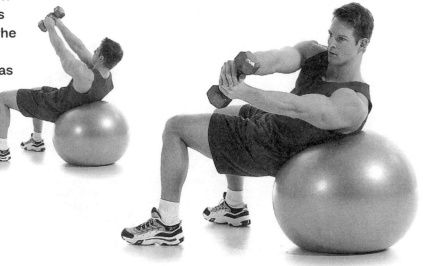

EXERCISES FOR THE LOWER BACK

Back Extension
INTERMEDIATE LEVEL

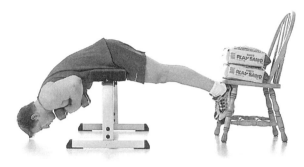

■ **START:** Place a sturdy bench some 3 feet in front of a solid piece of furniture. Make sure that you can get your feet under it at about the same height as the bench. Lie facedown on the bench so that your hips are on it but your upper body, starting at the navel, hangs off it. Hook the backs of your heels underneath the piece of furniture behind you. Grab two dumbbells.

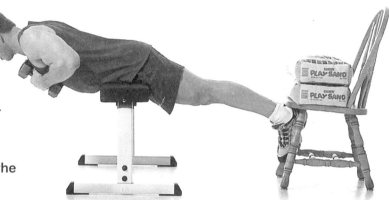

☐ **FINISH:** With your back rounded (not straight) and the dumbbells clutched to your upper chest, uncoil your back to raise your upper body. When your torso is parallel to the floor and your back is straight, hold. Then slowly lower to the starting, rounded-back position.

Good Morning
INTERMEDIATE-TO-ADVANCED LEVEL

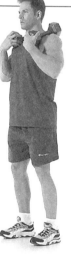

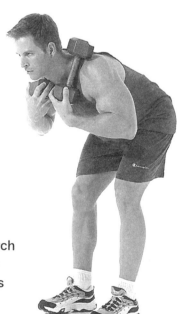

■ **START:** Stand with your feet shoulder-width apart and your knees slightly bent. Rest a light dumbbell on each shoulder with the weighted ends facing forward and backward and the bars sitting on your traps. Hold the front ends of the dumbbells.

☐ **FINISH:** Keeping a slight bend in your knees and the natural arch in your lower back, bend forward at the waist until your chest is almost parallel to the floor. Pause, then push down with your heels as you raise yourself back to the starting position.

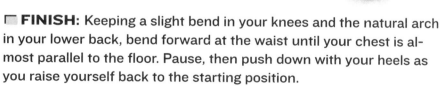

Prone Cobra
ADVANCED LEVEL

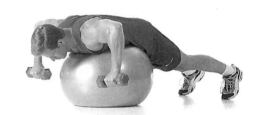

■ **START:** Grab a pair of light dumbbells with an overhand grip and lie facedown with your torso rounded over a ball and your legs straight behind you (or you can brace your feet against a wall, if necessary). Hold the dumbbells up near your chest, with your elbows out.

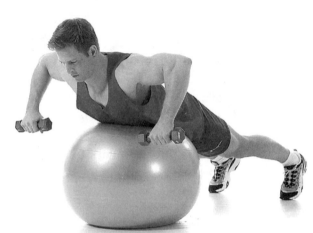

▢ **FINISH:** Do a back extension by un-curling your spine and lifting your chest several inches off the ball. Then, holding this torso position, perform an external rotation by pivoting your upper arms and lifting the weights up toward your ears. Keep your elbows at the same angle throughout, and keep your upper arms roughly parallel to the floor and perpendicular to your torso. Lower the weights to chest level, then lower your torso to the starting position.

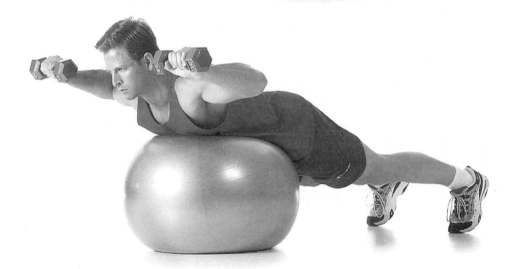

CHEST AND UPPER BACK

Using the following flexible guidelines, you can create excellent upper-torso home workouts.

If you're a beginner, select one type of chest press and one type of fly, and do 1 or 2 sets of 10 to 15 reps. For your back, select two rowing movements, or one row and the pullover. Do 2 or 3 sets of 10 to 15 reps each.

If you're intermediate or advanced, select two chest presses and one fly, doing two to three sets of 6 to 10 reps of each of the three exercises. For your back, select two rows, one pullover, and one reverse fly. Do one to two sets of 10 to 12 reps of each of the four exercises.

You can adjust these guidelines for posture reasons, based on the relative development of your chest and back. Go back and have another look at chapter 5 for information on how to do that—and why you might need to.

BEGINNER

CHEST
- Bench press ---------- (page 122)
- Elbows-in bench press -------------------- (page 122)
- Alternating or piston-style bench press -------- (page 122)
- Fly ------------------- (page 125)

UPPER BACK
- Prone reverse fly ------ (page 127)
- Seated reverse fly ----- (page 128)
- Bent-over row --------- (page 129)
- Elbow-in one-arm row ------------------ (page 130)
- Pullover -------------- (page 131)

INTERMEDIATE

CHEST
- Swiss-ball press --------- (page 122)
- Incline bench press ------- (page 123)
- Swiss-ball incline chest press ------------------ (page 123)
- Decline bench press ------ (page 123)
- Swiss-ball decline chest press ------------------ (page 123)
- Rotating-grip bench press -- (page 123)
- Swiss-ball fly ------------ (page 125)
- Incline or decline fly ------ (page 125)
- Swiss-ball incline or decline fly -------------- (page 125)

UPPER BACK
- Swiss-ball prone reverse fly ---------------------- (page 127)
- Supinated seated reverse fly ---------------------- (page 128)
- Pronated seated reverse fly ---------------------- (page 128)
- Neutral-grip bent-over row -------------------- (page 129)
- Pronated bent-over row ---(page 129)
- Alternating or piston-style bent-over row ----------- (page 129)
- Elbow-out one-arm row ----(page 130)
- Two-hand pullover -------- (page 131)
- Swiss-ball pullover ------- (page 131)

ADVANCED

CHEST
- Straight unilateral bench press --------------- (page 124)
- Swiss-ball multiangle chest press --------- (page 124)
- T-pushup ------------- (page 126)

UPPER BACK
- One-leg bent-over row ----------------- (page 129)
- Alternating pullover ---- (page 131)

EXERCISES FOR THE CHEST

Bench Press
BEGINNER LEVEL

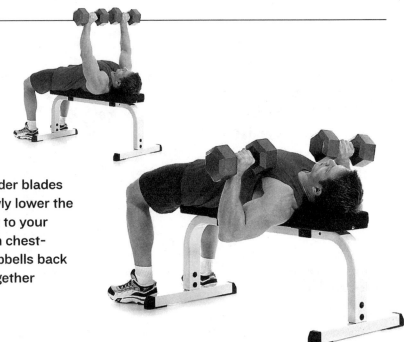

■ **START:** Lie on a flat bench holding two dumbbells up over your middle chest with an overhand grip and straight arms.

▢ **FINISH:** Pinching your shoulder blades back, bend your elbows and slowly lower the dumbbells until they're right next to your armpits, a few inches higher than chest-level. Pause, then press the dumbbells back up, bringing your hands close together without clanking the weights.

BEGINNER-TO-ADVANCED VARIATIONS
Elbows-In Bench Press

If you have chronic shoulder problems (a lot of guys do), switch to a neutral grip—palms facing each other—and move your elbows in closer to each other, keeping them that way as you lower the dumbbells. This shifts more of the work from your pecs to your triceps, but it will help you do flat, incline, or decline presses without pain.

Alternating or Piston-Style Bench Press

Work each side independently by holding your arms, front delts, and pecs taut in the bottom position, then pressing up and bringing down one dumbbell before doing a complete repetition with the other (alternating). Or increase stabilizer strength and improve upper body coordination by pressing up with one arm while the other is coming down (piston-style).

INTERMEDIATE VARIATION
Swiss-Ball Press

Grab a pair of dumbbells that are lighter than those you'd use for the standard bench version. Lie so that only your head, neck, and shoulder blades are in contact with the ball—your lower back should be off it. With your feet shoulder-width apart, push to lift your hips until they're parallel to the floor and your knees are bent at a 90-degree angle. Then simply press the weights up over your chest as in the standard bench press.

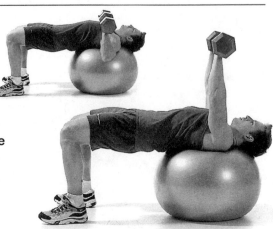

INTERMEDIATE-TO-ADVANCED VARIATIONS
Incline Bench Press

To work your upper pecs more, incline the bench 10 to 30 degrees and start the movement with the weights over your collarbone or chin. Perform the exercise as you would a flat-bench press, noticing a slight arc in the movement as you lower the dumbbells toward your armpits.

Swiss-Ball Incline Chest Press

Lie with your head, neck, and upper back completely in contact with a Swiss ball. Keep your feet flat on the floor, and bend your knees as you lower your hips until your hips are lower than your chest. Hold the dumbbells within an inch or two of your upper chest, then press them up over your collarbone.

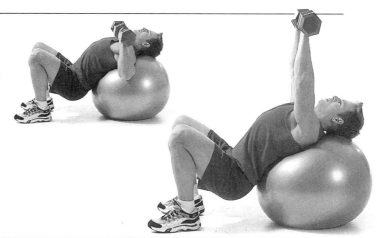

Decline Bench Press

Declining the bench about 45 degrees will target your pecs. Start the movement with the dumbbells over your lower chest, then lower and raise them as you would in a flat-bench press. You'll notice that the range of motion is shorter and that you're surprisingly strong in this position.

Swiss-Ball Decline Chest Press

Set up a pair of your heaviest dumbbells in front of the ball and hook your insteps beneath them as you lie back on the ball far enough that your chest is slightly lower than your hips. From that position, execute your dumbbell presses.

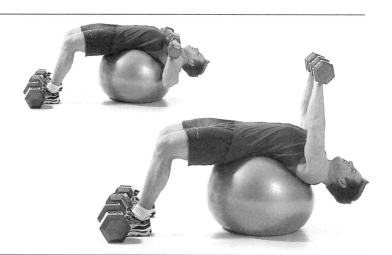

Rotating-Grip Bench Press

Work your pecs harder by starting with a neutral grip and then rotating the dumbbells inward as you press up so you finish in the standard palms-out position. This adds internal rotation of your upper arms, making your pecs do more work.

Bench Press

ADVANCED VARIATIONS

Straight Unilateral Bench Press

Work with just one dumbbell by pressing with one arm while holding on to the side of the bench with the opposite hand. Switch sides and do the same number of reps, or address a strength imbalance by doing an extra set or two with your weaker side.

Swiss-Ball Multiangle Chest Press

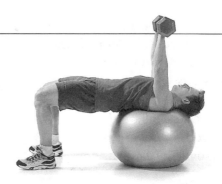

This variation gets you working harder on the down phase of the lift. Start by executing a chest press from the flat Swiss-ball position. Holding the dumbbells over your chest in the top position, slowly lower your hips to the incline pressing position. Once there, stay in control as you lower the dumbbells back down to within an inch or two of your chest. Then use your legs to push yourself back up to the flat-press position before you start the next repetition.

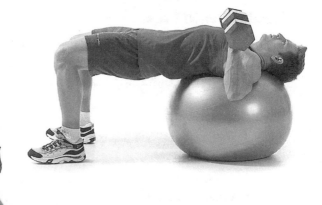

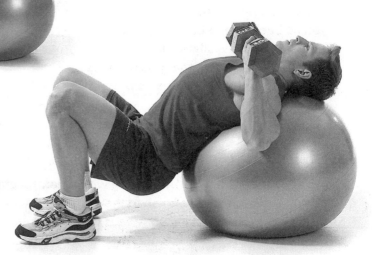

Fly
BEGINNER LEVEL

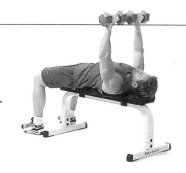

■ **START:** Grab a pair of dumbbells that are lighter than those you'd use for bench presses. Lie on the bench, holding the dumbbells in an overhand grip over your mid-pec region, arms straight up.

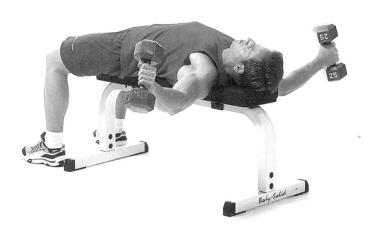

☐ **FINISH:** Maintaining a slight bend in your elbows, lower the dumbbells down and back until your upper arms are parallel to the floor and in line with your ears. Then use your chest to pull the weights back up to the starting position, retracing the same route in reverse. Keep your shoulder blades pinched back toward each other throughout, and flex your pecs at the top of the movement.

INTERMEDIATE VARIATION
Swiss-Ball Fly

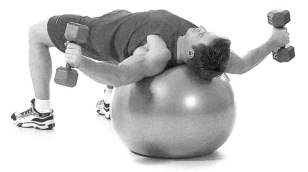

Set up on a ball exactly as you would for a flat chest press, with only your head, neck, and shoulder blades in contact with the ball. Then do a standard fly, making sure you can see your upper arms at the bottom of the range of motion. (It's tempting to go lower—but dangerous to your shoulders.)

INTERMEDIATE-TO-ADVANCED VARIATIONS
Incline or Decline Fly

As with presses, you move more of the workload to your upper pecs if you incline the bench 45 to 60 degrees and start with the dumbbells over your collarbone. Or decline the bench 10 to 30 degrees to concentrate on your lower pecs, and start the movement with the dumbbells over your lower chest.

Swiss-Ball Incline or Decline Fly

Set up with your head, neck, and back completely in contact with a ball, and do the incline fly as described above. Or set up on a ball with your feet anchored by heavy dumbbells and your head lower than your hips. Then do the standard fly.

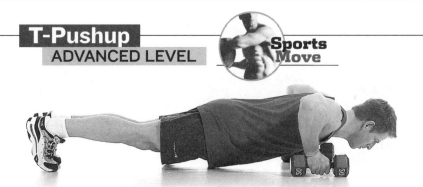

T-Pushup
ADVANCED LEVEL

Sports Move

■ **START:** Hold a pair of light dumbbells with a neutral grip, and get into the down position of a standard pushup, with your hands directly below your shoulders.

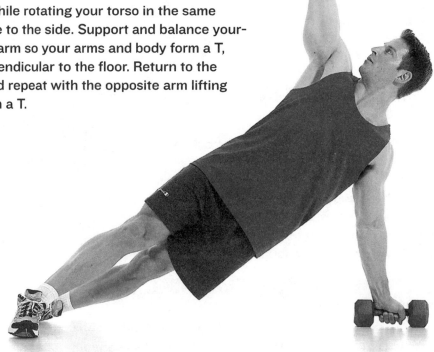

▢ **FINISH:** Execute a basic pushup. Then hold the top position and lift the dumbbell in your nondominant hand toward the ceiling while rotating your torso in the same direction so you face to the side. Support and balance yourself with your other arm so your arms and body form a T, with your arms perpendicular to the floor. Return to the starting position, and repeat with the opposite arm lifting the dumbbell to form a T.

EXERCISES FOR THE UPPER BACK

Prone Reverse Fly
BEGINNER LEVEL

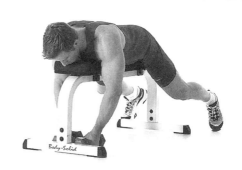

■ **START:** Grab a pair of light dumbbells and lie facedown on a bench, letting your arms hang off the sides. Hold the dumbbells with a neutral grip.

▢ **FINISH:** Pinch your shoulder blades together as you use your rear delts and upper-back muscles to raise your arms in a wide, arcing motion out to the sides. Hold for a second or two at the top, then stay in control as you lower the weights. Don't rest the weights on the floor.

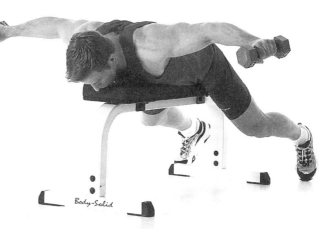

INTERMEDIATE VARIATION
Swiss-Ball Prone Reverse Fly

Lie with your chest on a ball instead of a bench. Execute a standard prone reverse fly, keeping your legs as straight as possible.

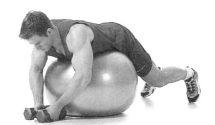

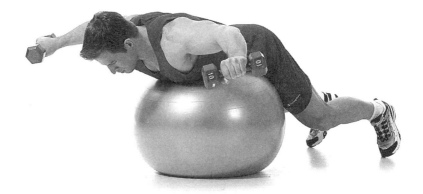

Seated Reverse Fly
BEGINNER LEVEL

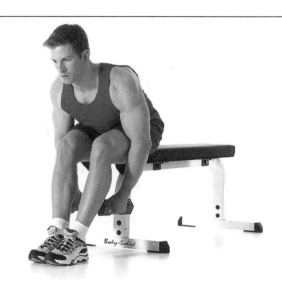

■ **START:** Grab a pair of light dumbbells and sit with your legs together on the front edge of a bench. Lean forward at the hips to get your chest as close to your thighs as you can without rounding your back (keep it slightly arched, in other words). Let your arms hang down from your sides in line with your calves as you hold the dumbbells with a neutral grip.

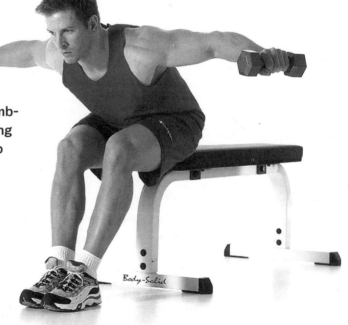

□ **FINISH:** Use your rear delts and upper-back muscles to raise the dumbbells up to either side in a wide, arcing motion until your arms are parallel to the floor, your elbows just below shoulder level and your wrists in the same plane as your ears.

INTERMEDIATE-TO-ADVANCED VARIATIONS
Supinated Seated Reverse Fly

While the neutral grip spreads the stress fairly evenly over your entire upper back, this under-hand-grip variation puts more stress on your external rotators.

Pronated Seated Reverse Fly

Switching to an overhand grip shifts more work to your rear delts.

Bent-Over Row
BEGINNER LEVEL

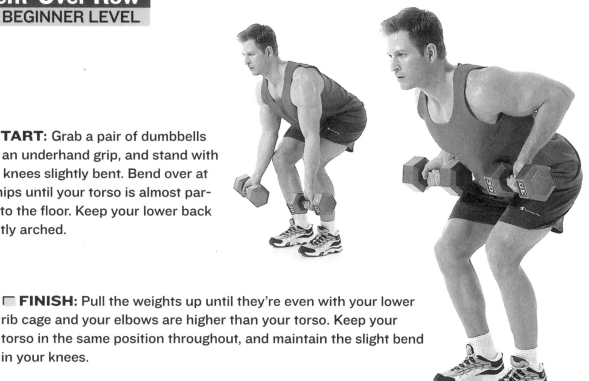

■ **START:** Grab a pair of dumbbells with an underhand grip, and stand with your knees slightly bent. Bend over at the hips until your torso is almost parallel to the floor. Keep your lower back slightly arched.

☐ **FINISH:** Pull the weights up until they're even with your lower rib cage and your elbows are higher than your torso. Keep your torso in the same position throughout, and maintain the slight bend in your knees.

INTERMEDIATE-TO-ADVANCED VARIATIONS
Neutral-Grip Bent-Over Row

With a neutral grip, you're essentially doing two simultaneous elbow-in one-arm rows (see page 130). Start with the dumbbells hanging slightly in front of your shoulders and arc them back toward your hips as you lift them.

Pronated Bent-Over Row

A pronated (overhand) grip gives you the two-arm equivalent of the elbows-out one-arm row.

Alternating or Piston-Style Bent-Over Row

When you're ready, try bent-over rows one arm at a time, using any grip. Do a complete repetition with one arm before repeating with the opposite arm (alternating), or raise one dumbbell while lowering the other (piston-style).

ADVANCED VARIATION
One-Leg Bent-Over Row

Work on your balance and coordination by doing this exercise while standing on one leg. Use any grip or style of repetitions (two-arm, alternating, or piston-style).

Elbow-In One-Arm Row
BEGINNER LEVEL

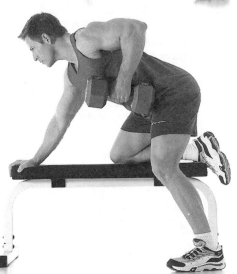

■ **START:** Holding a dumbbell in your nondominant hand, place your opposite hand and knee on a bench. Keep your back flat as you let the dumbbell hang down to your side so your arm lines up just in front of your shoulder.

◰ **FINISH:** Concentrate on using your upper-back muscles as you pull the dumbbell up and back toward your hip, keeping your elbow close to your body. Pause, then slowly return to the starting position.

Elbow-Out One-Arm Row
INTERMEDIATE-TO-ADVANCED LEVEL

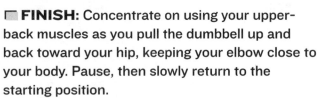

■ **START:** Start as you would for the elbow-in version, but hold a lighter dumbbell with an overhand grip. Your arm should hang directly below your shoulder rather than in front of it. This position shifts work from your lats to the rear delts, rhomboids, and mid-traps.

◰ **FINISH:** Keeping your forearm perpendicular to the floor, pull your elbow straight up until the dumbbell is as high as you can get it without altering your torso position.

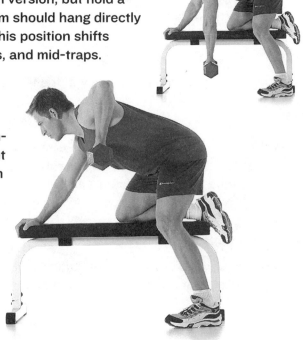

Pullover

BEGINNER-TO-INTERMEDIATE LEVEL

■ **START:** Lie lengthwise on a bench—not perpendicular to it, as you often see in gyms (if you frequent such places). Press your head, torso, lower back, and glutes firmly against the surface. Your feet should be flat on the floor (or, if you prefer, flat on the end of the bench). Place one hand around the handle of a dumbbell and wrap the other one over the gripping hand. Extend your arms directly above your collarbone, holding the dumbbell bar perpendicular to the floor.

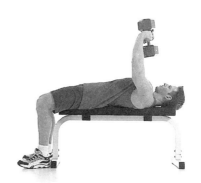

☐ **FINISH:** Keeping your back flat against the bench to elongate your lats, slowly lower the weight behind your head until your arms are in line with your ears. Pause, then pull the weight back up. Slightly bend your elbows throughout.

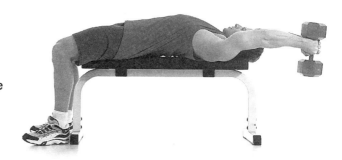

INTERMEDIATE VARIATIONS
Two-Hand Pullover

Use two dumbbells—one in each hand with a neutral grip—to increase the involvement of your smaller muscles.

Swiss-Ball Pullover

Hold a dumbbell with a hand-over-hand grip as you lie with your head, neck, and upper back in contact with a ball. Bridge your hips up so your thighs are parallel to the floor and your knees are bent 90 degrees. Lift your arms directly over your chest, lower them behind your head, and do a standard pullover.

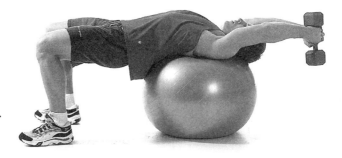

ADVANCED VARIATION
Alternating Pullover

Make the two-dumbbell version even harder by alternating arms—keeping one up while lowering the other back.

ARMS AND SHOULDERS

To get an excellent all-dumbbell workout for arms and shoulders, beginners should select one shoulder press, one shrug or upright row, the side-lying external rotation, one triceps movement, and one biceps curl. Do 1 or 2 sets of 10 to 15 repetitions per exercise.

Intermediate and advanced lifters should do 2 or 3 sets of 6 to 10 reps of the following exercises: one lateral raise; one shoulder press; one shrug, upright row, or hang clean; one scarecrow; two triceps movements; and two different biceps curls.

BEGINNER

SHOULDERS
- Lateral raise --------(page 133)
- Shoulder press ------(page 134)
- Neutral-grip shoulder press --------------(page 134)
- Upright row ---------(page 135)
- Neutral-grip shrug --(page 135)
- Side-lying external rotation ------------------(page 136)

TRICEPS
- Lying triceps extension ----------(page 139)
- Unilateral triceps kickback ---------(page 142)

BICEPS
- Seated curl ---------(page 144)
- Standing curl -------(page 144)
- Seated concentration curl ---------------(page 146)

FOREARMS
- Wrist curl -----------(page 150)
- Unilateral wrist curl ---------------(page 150)
- Wrist extension -----(page 150)
- Unilateral wrist extension ----------(page 150)

INTERMEDIATE

SHOULDERS
- Alternating lateral raise ----(page 133)
- Rotation press -------------(page 134)
- Alternating upright row ----(page 135)
- Piston-style upright row ---(page 135)
- Standing scarecrow -------(page 137)

TRICEPS
- Rotation lying triceps extension ----------------(page 139)
- Alternating or piston-style lying triceps extension ---(page 139)
- Swiss-ball lying triceps extension ----------------(page 139)
- Cross-body unilateral extension ----------------(page 140)
- Overhead triceps extension ----------------(page 140)
- Unilateral overhead triceps extension with lean -------(page 141)
- Bilateral triceps kickback --(page 142)
- Close-grip bench press ------(page 143)

BICEPS
- Supinated seated curl ------(page 144)
- Incline curl ----------------(page 144)
- Swiss-ball curl ------------(page 145)
- Alternating curl -----------(page 145)
- Piston-style curl -----------(page 145)
- Multiangle dumbbell curl ---(page 146)
- Swiss-ball preacher curl ----(page 147)
- Standing concentration curl ----------------------(page 147)
- Hammer curl --------------(page 148)
- Hammer curl variations ----(page 148)

ADVANCED

SHOULDERS
- Alternating press --------(page 134)
- Piston-style press -------(page 134)
- Swiss-ball alternating or piston-style shoulder press ---------(page 134)
- Overhead shrug ---------(page 136)
- Prone scarecrow -------(page 137)
- Hang clean -------------(page 138)

TRICEPS
- Two-dumbbell overhead triceps extension -------(page 141)
- Piston-style overhead triceps extension -------(page 141)
- Alternating overhead triceps extension ------(page 141)
- Swiss-ball overhead triceps extension -------(page 141)

BICEPS
- Seated curl with static hold --------------------(page 145)
- Strict curl --------------(page 145)
- 45-degree prone curl ---(page 148)
- 45-degree prone curl variations -------------(page 148)
- Zottman curl -----------(page 149)

EXERCISES FOR THE SHOULDERS

Lateral Raise
BEGINNER LEVEL

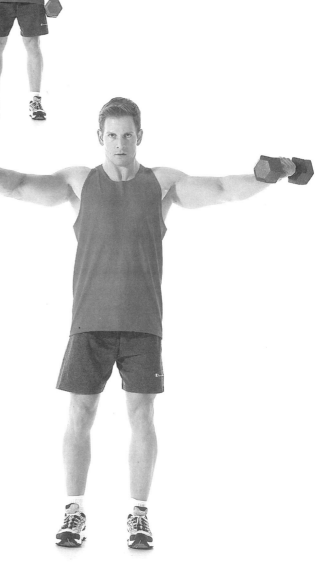

■ **START:** Stand holding a pair of dumbbells at your sides with an overhand grip, your elbows slightly bent. Bend slightly forward at the hips, keeping your lower back in its naturally arched position.

▢ **FINISH:** Raise your arms up and out to the sides until they're parallel to the floor, keeping the same bend in your elbows. Pause, then slowly return to the starting position.

INTERMEDIATE-TO-ADVANCED VARIATION
Alternating Lateral Raise

Start with the dumbbells up, your arms parallel to the floor. Slowly lower and then raise one arm. Repeat with the opposite arm.

Shoulder Press
BEGINNER LEVEL

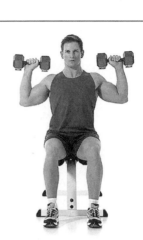

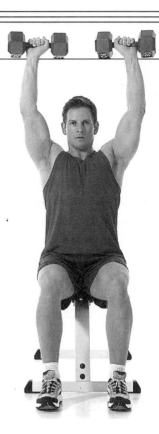

■ **START:** Grab two dumbbells and sit on the edge of a bench (or stay standing, if you prefer). Hold the weights with an overhand grip above each shoulder, in line with your jaws.

▢ **FINISH:** Press the dumbbells straight up, but not up and in (no clanking—it takes tension off your shoulder muscles and annoys the hell out of whoever else is home). Pause, then slowly return to the starting position without letting the weights rest on your shoulders.

BEGINNER VARIATION
Neutral-Grip Shoulder Press

This is less effective but more joint-friendly, especially if you have shoulder problems.

INTERMEDIATE VARIATION
Rotation Press

Start with an underhand grip. As you lift, rotate outward from your shoulders (not your wrists) so your palms face forward at the top position.

ADVANCED VARIATIONS
Alternating Press

Do either the shoulder or rotation press one arm at a time: raise one dumbbell, lower it, then raise and lower the other.

Piston-Style Press

On either version of the press, push one dumbbell up as the other comes down.

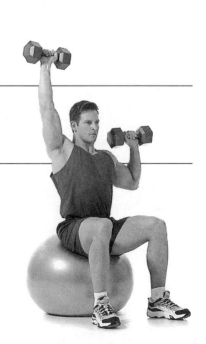

Swiss-Ball Alternating or Piston-Style Shoulder Press

The Swiss-ball version of a standard shoulder press is simply a matter of doing the exercise while sitting on a ball. However, if you switch to alternating or piston-style movements, your round perch adds a noticeable challenge.

Upright Row
BEGINNER LEVEL

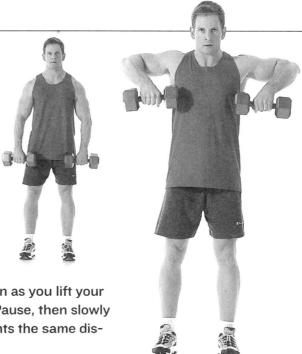

■ **START:** Stand with your feet hip-to-shoulder-width apart and your knees slightly bent. With an overhand grip, hold a pair of dumbbells in front of your thighs, at arm's length and shoulder-width apart.

☐ **FINISH:** Keep your forearms pointed down as you lift your upper arms until they're parallel to the floor. Pause, then slowly return to the starting position. Keep the weights the same distance apart throughout the exercise.

INTERMEDIATE-TO-ADVANCED VARIATIONS
Alternating Upright Row

Pull one elbow up and lower it, keeping the other dumbbell down.

Piston-Style Upright Row

Pull one elbow up as you lower the other.

Neutral-Grip Shrug
BEGINNER-TO-INTERMEDIATE LEVEL

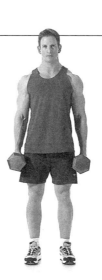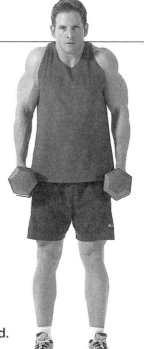

■ **START:** Stand holding two moderately heavy dumbbells at your sides, with a neutral grip. Keep your shoulders relaxed and in line with your ears.

☐ **FINISH:** Shrug your shoulders up as if you were trying to touch them to your ears. Hold at the top position, then slowly return to the starting position. Don't bend your elbows or let your head move forward.

Overhead Shrug
ADVANCED LEVEL

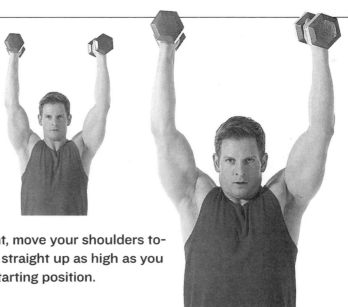

■ **START:** Hold a pair of light dumbbells over your head with a neutral, shoulder-width grip.

☐ **FINISH:** Keeping your arms straight, move your shoulders toward your ears to shrug the dumbbells straight up as high as you can. Pause, then slowly return to the starting position.

Side-Lying External Rotation
BEGINNER LEVEL

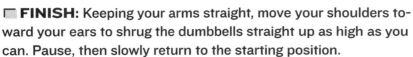

■ **START:** Grab a very light dumbbell with your nondominant hand and lie on opposite side with a rolled-up towel on your top hip. Bend your top elbow 90 degrees and rest it on the towel so upper arm is parallel to your torso and your forearm hangs down in front of your abs. Turn your palm toward your midsection.

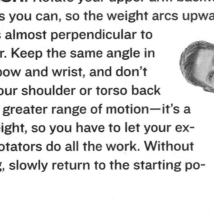

☐ **FINISH:** Rotate your upper arm backward as far as you can, so the weight arcs upward until it's almost perpendicular to the floor. Keep the same angle in your elbow and wrist, and don't move your shoulder or torso back to get a greater range of motion—it's a light weight, so you have to let your external rotators do all the work. Without pausing, slowly return to the starting position.

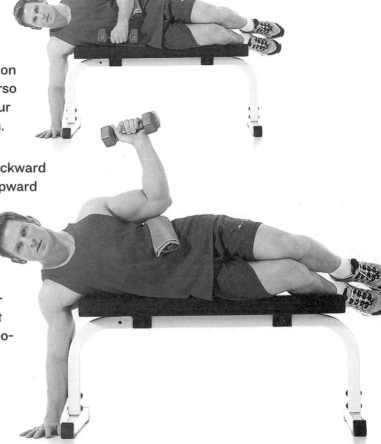

Standing Scarecrow
INTERMEDIATE LEVEL

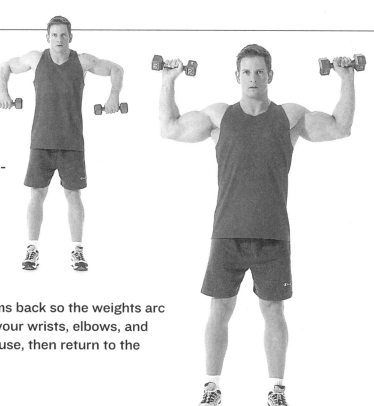

■ **START:** Stand holding a light dumbbell on either side of your lower chest, with your forearms pointing straight down and your upper arms out to the sides yet slightly lower than parallel to the floor.

▢ **FINISH:** Rotate your upper arms back so the weights arc upward as high as possible. Keep your wrists, elbows, and shoulders in the same position. Pause, then return to the starting position.

Prone Scarecrow
ADVANCED LEVEL

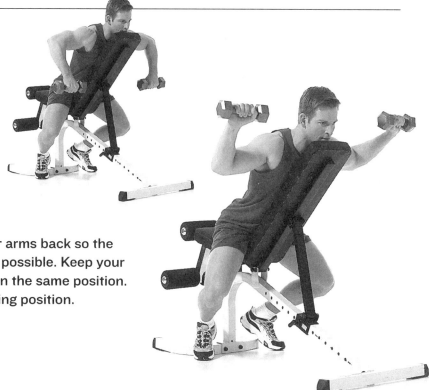

■ **START:** Grab a pair of dumbbells and lie facedown on a bench that's inclined about 45 degrees. Hold the weights overhand with your forearms pointing straight down and your upper arms slightly lower than parallel to the floor.

▢ **FINISH:** Rotate your upper arms back so the weights arc upward as high as possible. Keep your wrists, elbows, and shoulders in the same position. Pause, then return to the starting position.

Hang Clean
ADVANCED LEVEL

Sports Move

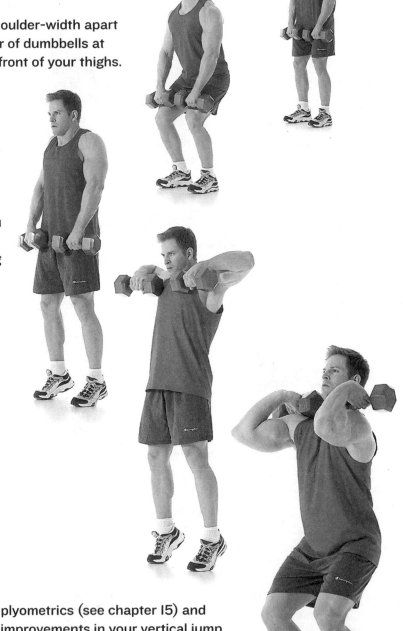

■ **START:** Standing with your feet shoulder-width apart and your knees slightly bent, hold a pair of dumbbells at arm's length, with an overhand grip, in front of your thighs. Bend forward a bit at the waist.

▢ **FINISH:** This is a multipart sequence that you execute quickly and powerfully. Dip your knees, as if you were about to jump. Then quickly reverse the motion as if you were jumping, rise up on the balls of your feet, and immediately shrug the weights upward. As that momentum moves the weights up, continue in a wavelike manner by pulling them up in the air. Finally, dip down with your knees and hips to "catch" the weights on your shoulders. The weights will roll to the ends of your fingers, your wrists will bend back, and your upper arms should end up parallel to the floor, in front of your torso. Quickly return to the starting position—this is one exercise where there's no benefit to pausing and slowly lowering the dumbbells.

This exercise, combined with plyometrics (see chapter 15) and squats, will produce amazing improvements in your vertical jump and lead to better performance in every sport this side of chess. The key is to make the move as much like a jump as possible. Work on your form with light weights for weeks before attempting this with heavier loads. You'll know you've hit it when the weights snap into place on your shoulders on each repetition.

EXERCISES FOR THE TRICEPS

Lying Triceps Extension
BEGINNER LEVEL

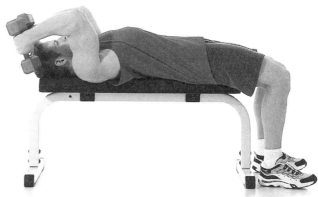

■ **START:** Grab a pair of dumbbells and lie on a bench. With a neutral, shoulder-width grip and straight arms, hold the dumbbells up over your forehead.

▢ **FINISH:** Bend at the elbows as you lower the weights down to the sides of your forehead. Keep your upper arms in the same position, and pause when your elbows are bent just past 90 degrees. Return to the starting position.

INTERMEDIATE VARIATIONS
Rotation Lying Triceps Extension

Start with an overhand grip. Rotate your arms inward as you lower them, so your palms face the sides of your head at the bottom position. Then rotate them back outward as you return to the starting position.

Alternating or Piston-Style Lying Triceps Extension

Keep one dumbbell in the top position while the other arm performs the movement, then switch to complete the repetition (alternating). Or raise one dumbbell at the same time that you're lowering the other.

Swiss-Ball Lying Triceps Extension

Lie with only your head, neck, and shoulder blades in contact with a ball—your lower back should be off of it. Then with your feet shoulder-width apart, push to lift your hips until they're parallel to the floor and your knees are bent at a 90-degree angle. Do standard lying triceps extensions, angling your arms back slightly as you hold the dumbbells overhead, to ensure more work for the long head of your triceps.

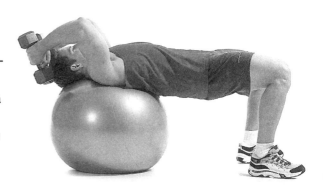

Cross-Body Unilateral Extension
INTERMEDIATE LEVEL

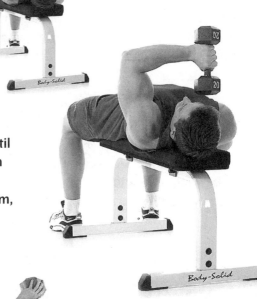

■ **START:** Sit on a bench and lean toward your dominant side, grabbing the side of the bench to steady yourself. With an overhand grip, hold a dumbbell in your nondominant hand and raise it at arm's length above your shoulder so your arm and torso are at the same angle.

▢ **FINISH:** Bend your elbow to lower the weight until it's an inch or two above your jaw. Pause, then return to the starting position. Keep your upper arm in the same position throughout. Finish the set with that arm, then repeat with the other.

Overhead Triceps Extension
INTERMEDIATE LEVEL

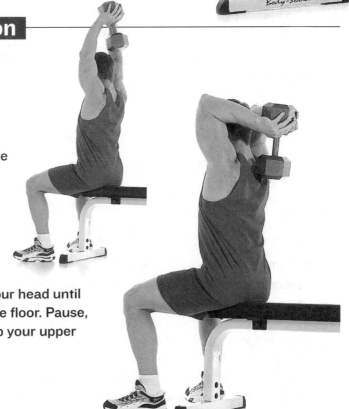

■ **START:** Grab the end of a moderately heavy dumbbell with both hands, and sit at the end of a bench. With your palms around the bar and pressing up on the inside of the upper weight plate, lift the weight over your head, and hold it there with your elbows close to your head.

▢ **FINISH:** Lower the weight behind your head until your forearms are just past parallel to the floor. Pause, then return to the starting position. Keep your upper arms in the same position throughout.

ADVANCED VARIATIONS

Two-Dumbbell Overhead Triceps Extension

Perform the same movement while holding a dumbbell in each hand with a neutral grip, taking special care to keep your elbows close to your head.

Piston-Style Overhead Triceps Extension

With two dumbbells, lower one as you raise the other.

Alternating Overhead Triceps Extension

Do the two-dumbbell version one arm at a time.

Swiss-Ball Overhead Triceps Extension

This is basically the same as the standard overhead triceps extension, except that the ball requires you to balance, making the exercise more challenging.

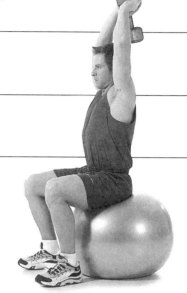

Unilateral Overhead Triceps Extension with Lean
INTERMEDIATE-TO-ADVANCED LEVEL

■ **START:** Grab one light dumbbell in your nondominant hand with an overhand grip, and sit sideways on a bench. Lean so your torso is at about a 75-degree angle to the bench. (You don't have to break out the protractor here; you just want to be somewhere between 45 and 90 degrees.) Support your body with your other hand on the bench. Hold the dumbbell straight up over your head, following along the same angle as the rest of your body.

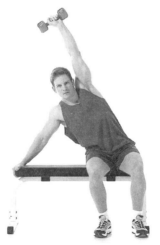

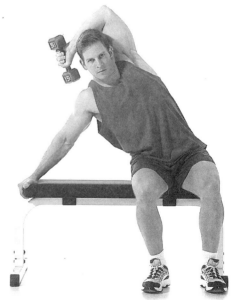

☐ **FINISH:** Lower the weight at an angle behind your head, toward the opposite ear. Pause, then return to the starting position. Keep your upper arm at the same angle throughout. Finish the set with that arm before repeating with the other.

Unilateral Triceps Kickback
BEGINNER LEVEL

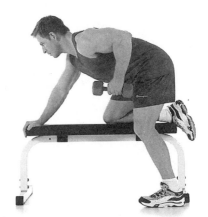

■ **START:** Grab a light dumbbell in your nondominant hand and place your opposite hand and knee on a bench. (This is the same basic starting position as the one-arm row.) Plant your nondominant foot flat on the floor. Bend forward at the hips so your torso is parallel to the floor. Hold the dumbbell at the side of your abdomen with a neutral grip, elbow pointed toward the ceiling.

☐ **FINISH:** Lift the weight up and back until your arm is straight. Keep your elbow pointed toward the ceiling and the rest of your body steady. Pause for 2 full seconds, then slowly return to the starting position. Finish the set on that side before repeating on the other.

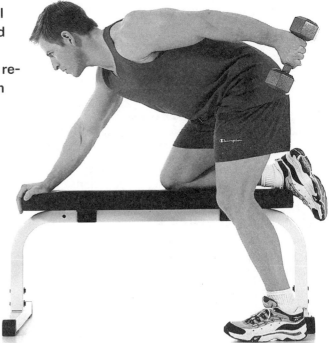

INTERMEDIATE-TO-ADVANCED VARIATION
Bilateral Triceps Kickback

Do this version standing in the bent-over-row position: slightly bent knees, slightly arched back, leaning forward at the hips with your torso almost parallel to the floor. With a dumbbell in each hand, hold your upper arms next to your torso as you extend both forearms straight back, pause, and then slowly return to the starting position.

Close-Grip Bench Press
INTERMEDIATE-TO-ADVANCED LEVEL

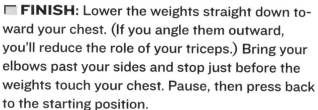

■ **START:** Grab a pair of dumbbells with a neutral grip, to maximize your triceps workload. Lie on a bench and extend both arms directly over your chest.

▢ **FINISH:** Lower the weights straight down toward your chest. (If you angle them outward, you'll reduce the role of your triceps.) Bring your elbows past your sides and stop just before the weights touch your chest. Pause, then press back to the starting position.

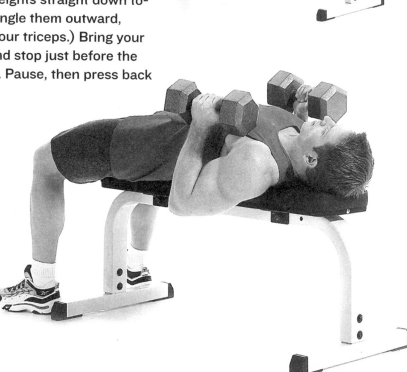

EXERCISES FOR THE BICEPS

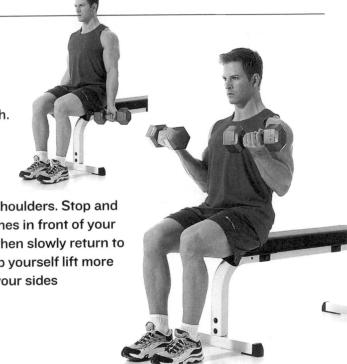

Seated Curl
BEGINNER LEVEL

■ **START:** Sit up straight at the end of a bench. With an underhand grip, hold two dumbbells straight down, at arm's length.

□ **FINISH:** Curl the weights toward your shoulders. Stop and squeeze when the dumbbells are 6 to 8 inches in front of your shoulders. Hold the contraction for a beat, then slowly return to the starting position. Don't lean back to help yourself lift more weight, and keep your upper arms against your sides throughout the exercise.

BEGINNER-TO-ADVANCED VARIATION
Standing Curl

You can do the curl and the first two variations that follow (supinated and static-hold seated curls) standing up as well.

INTERMEDIATE VARIATIONS
Supinated Seated Curl

For a more forceful contraction that combines the biceps' two major functions (elbow flexion and wrist supination), start with your palms facing each other in the down position and rotate them as you curl so they face your shoulders at the top. Rotate them back on the way down.

Incline Curl

To shift more of the focus to the outer head of your biceps (the part that produces a peak), do the curls while sitting back on an inclined bench. Start with the bench at about 75 degrees, and work your way down slowly. The more dramatic the incline, the tougher it will be on your shoulders.

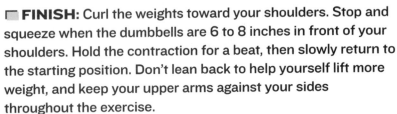

Swiss-Ball Curl

Sit on a ball as you perform a seated curl or any variation of it.

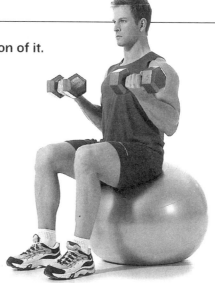

INTERMEDIATE-TO-ADVANCED VARIATIONS
Alternating Curl

You can vary almost any curl by curling one arm at a time. Do the complete curl with one arm before starting the movement with the other arm.

Piston-Style Curl

Curl one arm up as the other comes down.

ADVANCED VARIATIONS
Seated Curl with Static Hold

Curl one dumbbell halfway up and leave it there as you do the entire set with your other arm. Then switch arms and do the same thing. The isometric hold in one biceps makes this one a killer.

Strict Curl

Stand with your back against a wall while you perform the curls.

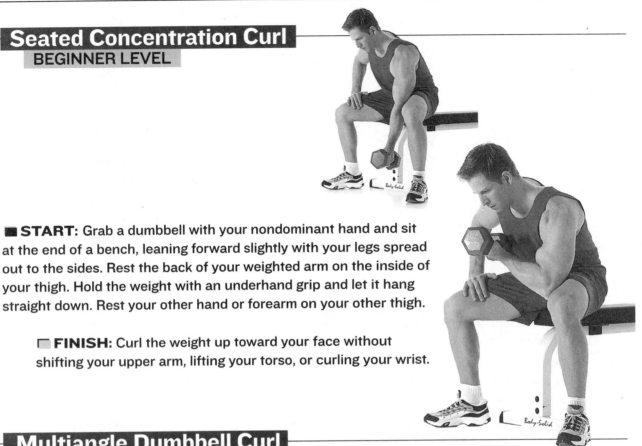

Seated Concentration Curl
BEGINNER LEVEL

■ **START:** Grab a dumbbell with your nondominant hand and sit at the end of a bench, leaning forward slightly with your legs spread out to the sides. Rest the back of your weighted arm on the inside of your thigh. Hold the weight with an underhand grip and let it hang straight down. Rest your other hand or forearm on your other thigh.

☐ **FINISH:** Curl the weight up toward your face without shifting your upper arm, lifting your torso, or curling your wrist.

Multiangle Dumbbell Curl
INTERMEDIATE LEVEL

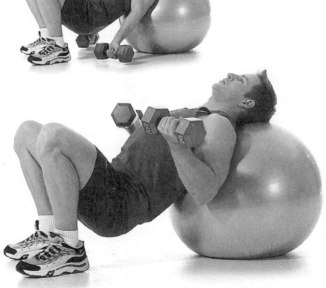

■ **START:** Lie with your head, neck, and upper back completely in contact with a Swiss ball. Keep your feet flat on the floor, and bend your knees as you lower your hips until you're mimicking the in-cline-curl position. With an underhand grip, hold two dumbbells straight down, at arm's length.

☐ **FINISH:** Do an incline curl with your el-bows braced against the ball, at your sides. At the top of the curl, raise your hips up until they're just slightly lower than parallel to the floor—almost the flat-press position. Then slowly lower the weights until your arms hang nearly straight down. Lower your hips to the starting position.

Swiss-Ball Preacher Curl
INTERMEDIATE LEVEL

■ **START:** Place a pair of dumbbells on the floor in front of a ball. Kneel directly behind the ball, and drape your arms over it to grab the dumbbells in an underhand grip.(You can also use a neutral or overhand grip.) Let your weight move back toward your heels as you brace your triceps on the ball, forearms down.

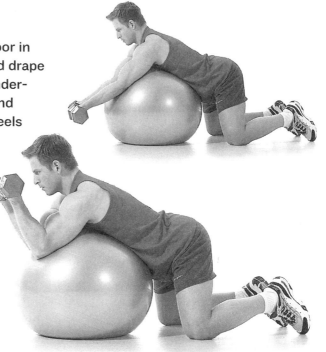

▢ **FINISH:** Keep your back straight as you curl the weights up until your forearms are just short of perpendicular to the floor. (Lifting them higher is too easy to be of any benefit—all that does is move the weights horizontally.)

Standing Concentration Curl
INTERMEDIATE-TO-ADVANCED LEVEL

■ **START:** Take a wide stance (about twice shoulder-width) over a dumbbell on the floor. Bend forward at the hips to a flat-back position and grab the dumbbell with your nondominant hand, placing your other hand on the middle of your opposite thigh to support your back. Keep your back flat, and let your weighted arm hang directly underneath your shoulder.

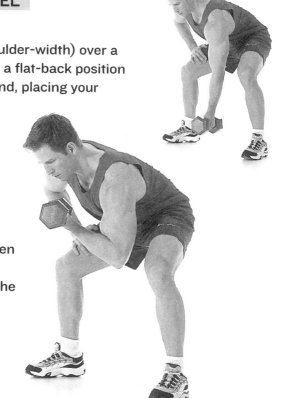

▢ **FINISH:** Curl the weight toward your face, moving only your forearm and making sure your elbow doesn't move back. Stop when the weight is about chin-high, pause, and slowly return to the starting position. Finish the set with that arm and then repeat with the other.

Hammer Curl
INTERMEDIATE-TO-ADVANCED LEVEL

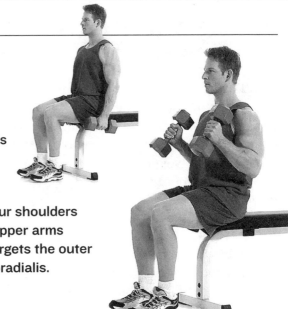

■ **START:** Sitting or standing, hold a pair of dumbbells with a neutral grip and let them hang at arm's length.

▢ **FINISH:** Slowly curl the weights up toward your shoulders without changing your wrist position. Keep your upper arms tucked against your sides throughout. This grip targets the outer head of the biceps, the brachialis, and the brachioradialis.

VARIATIONS

We won't do the entire list, but just about any variation that you can do with an underhand (supinated) grip you can also do with the hammer grip. Try alternating, piston-style, and inclined variations (especially inclined, since that position already stresses the outer head of the biceps).

45-Degree Prone Curl
ADVANCED LEVEL

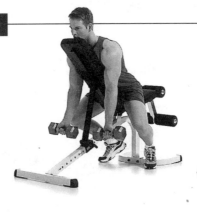

■ **START:** Grab two dumbbells with an underhand grip and lean against a 45-degree incline bench with your arms hanging straight down.

▢ **FINISH:** Curl the weights straight up, keeping your upper arms perpendicular to the floor and your wrists in a fixed position.

VARIATIONS

Same as before: You can do these with a hammer grip, with supination, alternating, piston-style, or Zottman-style. Mix 'em, match 'em, trade 'em with your friends.

Zottman Curl
ADVANCED LEVEL

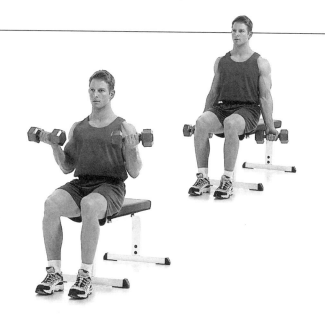

■ **START:** Position yourself as you would for a seated or standing curl: Hold two dumbbells straight down with an underhand grip.

▢ **FINISH:** Perform a standard curl. After squeezing your biceps at the top, turn the weights around so your palms face forward. Then lower the weights, taking care to resist gravity on the way down. At the bottom position, switch back to the original supinated grip.

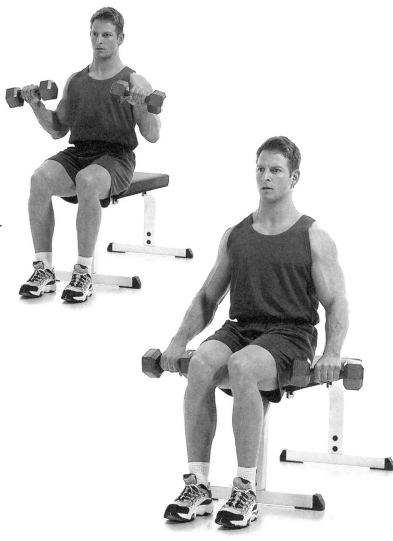

EXERCISES FOR THE FOREARMS

Wrist Curl
BEGINNER LEVEL

■ START: Hold two dumbbells with an underhand (supinated) grip and kneel on the floor, facing the long side of a bench. Position your forearms on the bench so the dumbbells hang off the other side. Open your palms to let the weights roll down to your fingertips.

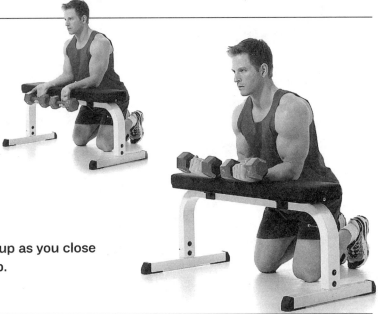

◻ FINISH: Roll the weights back up as you close your fingers and curl your wrists up.

VARIATION
Unilateral Wrist Curl

It's just as effective to do a set with one hand and then with the other. This is also useful for evening out muscle size and strength imbalances.

Wrist Extension
BEGINNER LEVEL

■ START: Get in the same position as for the wrist curl, but use an overhand (pronated) grip to target your wrist extensors instead of your wrist flexors.

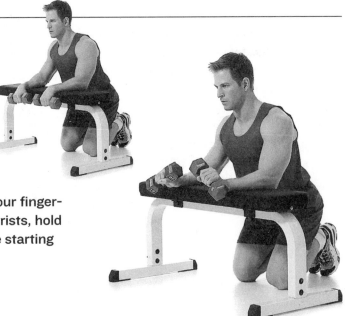

◻ FINISH: No rolling the weights to your fingertips for this one. Just bend back your wrists, hold the extended position, and return to the starting position.

VARIATION
Unilateral Wrist Extension

Again, you can work with one dumbbell, switching sides after completing your set with one hand.

LOWER BODY

To work their quadriceps, hamstrings, calves, and gluteals, beginners should select one knee-dominant, two hip-dominant, and one calf exercise. Do 1 or 2 sets of 12 to 15 repetitions of each.

Intermediate and advanced lifters should perform two knee-dominant, two hip-dominant, and both calf exercises. Do 2 or 3 sets of 8 to 12 reps of each exercise.

BEGINNER

KNEE-DOMINANT
- Squat ----------------(page 152)
- Sumo squat -----------(page 152)

HIP-DOMINANT
- Reverse lunge ---------(page 158)
- Leg curl --------------(page 158)

CALVES
- Seated calf raise -------(page 161)

INTERMEDIATE

KNEE-DOMINANT
- Split squat -------------(page 153)
- Front squat -----------(page 153)
- Lunge ----------------(page 155)

HIP-DOMINANT
- Decline leg curl --------(page 159)
- Romanian deadlift ------(page 159)

CALVES
- Unilateral standing calf raise -----------------(page 162)

ADVANCED

KNEE-DOMINANT
- Unilateral squat -------(page 154)
- Bulgarian split squat ---(page 154)
- Swiss-ball Bulgarian split squat ---------------(page 155)
- Side lunge ------------(page 156)
- 45-degree traveling lunge -------------------(page 157)

HIP-DOMINANT
- Unilateral Romanian deadlift --------------(page 159)
- Power clean ----------(page 160)

KNEE-DOMINANT EXERCISES

Squat
BEGINNER LEVEL

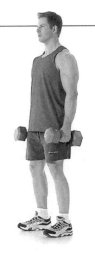

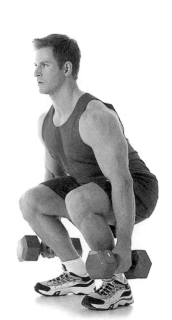

■ **START:** Stand holding two dumbbells at your sides at arm's length, your feet shoulder-width apart. Pull your shoulder blades back.

☐ **FINISH:** Bend your knees and lower your body as if you were sitting back into a chair. Stop when the tops of your thighs are parallel to the floor. The object is to keep your lower back in its naturally arched alignment and your knees from moving forward past your toes. Return to the starting position.

Sumo Squat
BEGINNER LEVEL

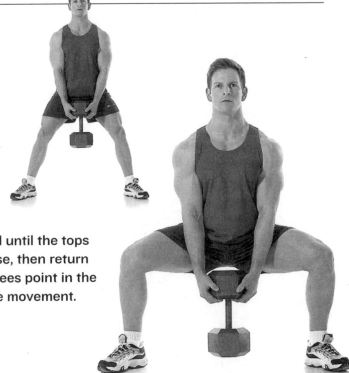

■ **START:** Take a wide stance (about twice shoulder-width) and point your toes outward at 10 and 2 o'clock. Pick up a heavy dumbbell, and hold one end at arm's length with both hands on the inner part of the upper weight plate so it points to the floor between your legs. Pull your shoulder blades back and lift your torso up.

☐ **FINISH:** Bend your knees and descend until the tops of your thighs are parallel to the floor. Pause, then return to the starting position. Make sure your knees point in the same direction as your toes throughout the movement.

Split Squat
INTERMEDIATE LEVEL

■ **START:** Grab two dumbbells and let them hang at your sides as you place one foot about 3 feet in front of the other, toes facing forward. Your front foot should be flat on the floor, but only the ball of your back foot should touch the ground. To help your balance, align your feet with their corresponding buttocks, not with each other.

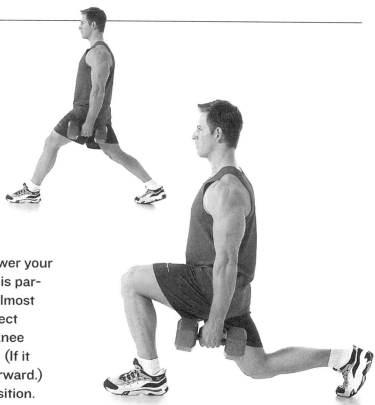

☐ **FINISH:** Bend both knees and lower your body until the top of your front thigh is parallel to the floor and your rear knee almost touches the floor. Keep your torso erect throughout, and don't let your front knee move past your toes as you descend. (If it does, move your front foot farther forward.) Pause, then return to the starting position.

Front Squat
INTERMEDIATE-TO-ADVANCED LEVEL

■ **START:** Grab a pair of dumbbells with a neutral grip and rest the ends on the meatiest parts of your shoulders (not the collarbones, in other words). Your upper arms should be parallel to the floor.

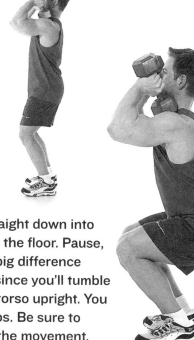

☐ **FINISH:** Bend your knees and lower your body straight down into a sitting position until your upper thighs are parallel to the floor. Pause, then return to the starting position. You should feel a big difference here: You have to pay more attention to your posture since you'll tumble forward if you don't keep your back straight and your torso upright. You should also feel more of the exercise in your quadriceps. Be sure to keep your upper arms parallel to the floor throughout the movement.

Unilateral Squat
ADVANCED LEVEL

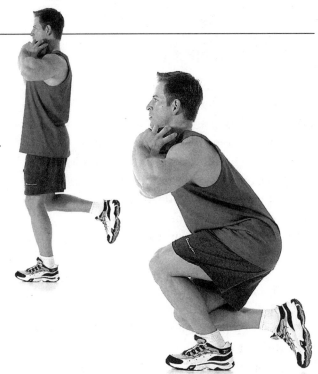

■ **START:** Stand with your legs shoulder-width apart. With two hands, hold a dumbbell against your upper chest, just under your chin. Bend your dominant knee about 90 degrees so your foot is halfway between the floor and your butt.

▢ **FINISH:** Bend your other knee and squat down until that thigh is parallel to the floor. Pause, then return to the starting position. Keep your torso as upright as possible throughout. Finish the set, then repeat with your other leg. (And, yes, you are basically standing on one leg at a time, and this is as tough as it sounds.)

Bulgarian Split Squat
ADVANCED LEVEL

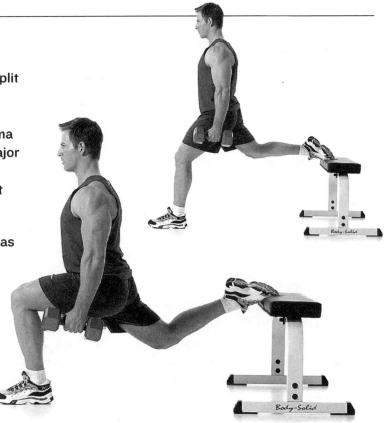

■ **START:** Same as for the standard split squat on page I53, except you rest your back toes on a bench or step, and start with fairly light weights—the microtrauma induced by this exercise can feel like major surgical rearrangement of your muscle fibers the day after you try it for the first time.

▢ **FINISH:** Lower yourself as far as you can without discomfort. Your range of motion will be limited by your hip-flexor and quadriceps flexibility. Pause, then return to the starting position.

VARIATION
Swiss-Ball Bulgarian Split Squat

Assume the Bulgarian split-squat position with the lower shin and instep of your back leg resting on a ball instead of on a bench. The ball will make balance a bigger factor as you do the exercise. If necessary, put the ball in a corner or anchor it with a few dumbbells.

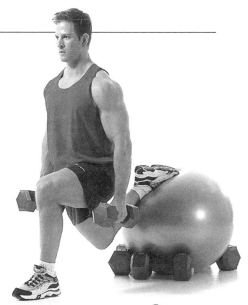

Lunge
INTERMEDIATE LEVEL

■ **START:** Stand with your feet hip-width apart, and hold two dumbbells at your sides.

▢ **FINISH:** Take a bold stride forward, far enough so that your front thigh ends up parallel to the floor with your knee over (not past) your toes. Quickly push back up to the starting position. Alternate legs, or finish your reps with one leg before switching.

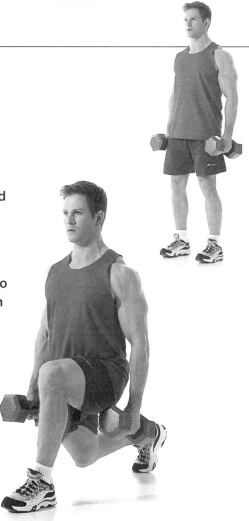

RESIDENTIAL RESISTANCE PROGRAMS

Side Lunge
ADVANCED LEVEL

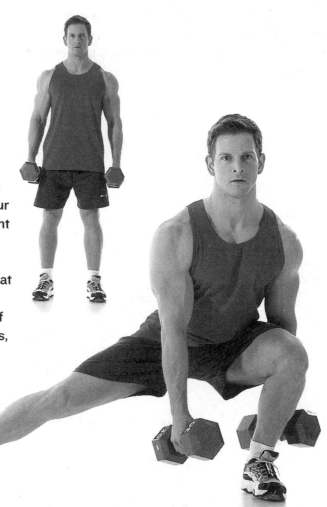

■ **START:** Same as for the standard lunge.

☐ **FINISH:** Step 2 feet or so to the side, keeping your toes pointed forward as your knee bends to get you into what you might call a side-squat position. Your thigh should end up parallel to the floor (although it may take some time to reach that flexibility level), with the dumbbells hanging on either side of it. Push yourself back up quickly, then either alternate legs, or finish your reps with one leg before switching.

45-Degree Traveling Lunge
ADVANCED LEVEL

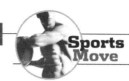

Sports Move

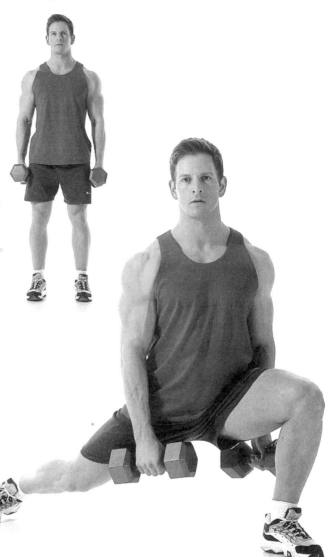

■ **START:** Same as for the standard lunge.

☐ **FINISH:** Lunge-step out at a 45-degree angle—forward and to the side—with your front thigh ending up parallel to the floor and your front knee over your toes. Then, instead of pushing back with your front foot, step forward with your back foot so you end up in the starting position a few feet northeast or northwest of where you started. Do the next rep with the other foot, angling toward the other side, like you're doing a drunken wedding march. Keep alternating until you finish your reps—or until you hit a wall.

HIP-DOMINANT EXERCISES

Reverse Lunge
BEGINNER LEVEL

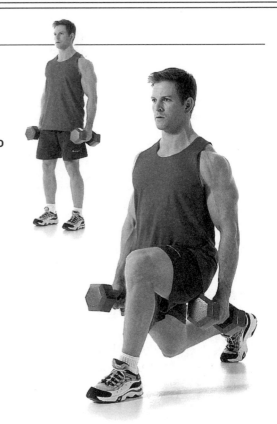

■ **START:** Stand with two dumbbells hanging at arm's length. Pull your shoulder blades back and your belly in so your torso stays erect throughout the movement.

◻ **FINISH:** Step back 2 to 3 feet (depending on your leg length) with one foot, allowing only the ball of that foot to touch the floor behind you. As (not after) you step, lower the knee of your receding leg to 2 or 3 inches above the floor. Your front leg should end up bent about 90 degrees, with that knee over the toes. Quickly switch direction and push yourself back up.

Leg Curl
BEGINNER LEVEL

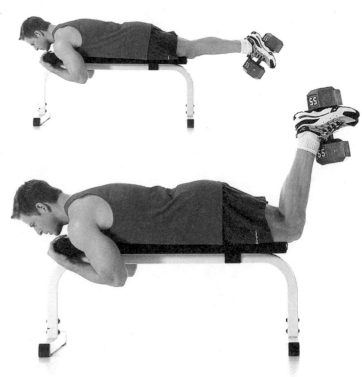

■ **START:** Set a dumbbell between the insteps of your feet and lie facedown on a flat bench. (This is tricky at first. If you can get someone to help you with it, you'll save yourself a few minutes of cursing.) Grab the front or sides of the bench for support.

◻ **FINISH:** Keeping your hips down on the bench, curl the weight up toward your buttocks. Stop when your lower legs point straight up, and without pausing, immediately lower the weight slowly. *Note:* This is technically a knee-dominant exercise, since your hips aren't involved. It does work the hamstrings, which also act to extend the hip; so that's why we put it in this section. Same with the decline leg curl on the next page.

Decline Leg Curl
INTERMEDIATE LEVEL

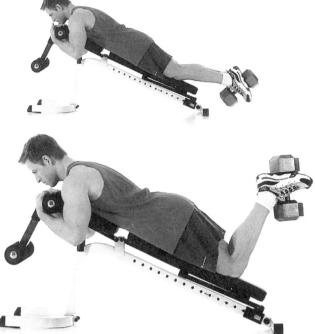

■ **START:** You need a bench that declines—or a flat bench you can tilt with phone books or a sturdy crate under the front end to simulate a decline bench. Same setup as for the leg curl, except you won't be able to straighten your knees completely—your feet would rest on the floor.

▢ **FINISH:** Curl the weight up toward your buttocks. Stop when your lower legs point straight up. Immediately lower the weight slowly, without letting it touch the floor.

Romanian Deadlift
INTERMEDIATE-TO-ADVANCED LEVEL

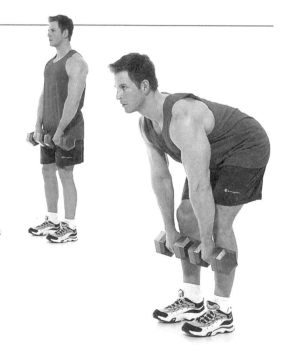

■ **START:** Stand with your feet shoulder-width apart, your knees slightly bent, and two dumbbells hanging down at arm's length in front of your thighs. Retract your shoulder blades and pull in your stomach.

▢ **FINISH:** Bend forward at the hips until the weights are at about midshin level and your torso is as close to parallel to the floor as possible. Pause, then press your heels against the floor as you lift your torso back to the starting position. Keep your back slightly arched throughout the exercise.

ADVANCED VARIATION
Unilateral Romanian Deadlift

Make it tougher by lifting one foot a few inches off the floor and keeping it there throughout the movement.

Power Clean
ADVANCED LEVEL

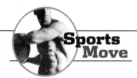

Sports Move

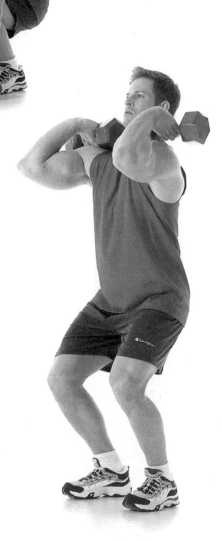

■ **START:** Assume the bottom position of a squat, thighs parallel to the floor. Grip a pair of dumbbells with an overhand grip as they rest on the floor in front of your feet. Keep your torso erect and a slight arch in your lower back.

▢ **FINISH:** Driving with your legs, straighten yourself in an explosive movement as you drag the weights up along the front of your body to chest height. As you go up on the balls of your feet, quickly drop underneath the weights and "catch" them on your shoulders with your elbows high. Immediately lower them in front of you and descend to the starting position.

EXERCISES FOR THE CALVES

Seated Calf Raise
BEGINNER LEVEL

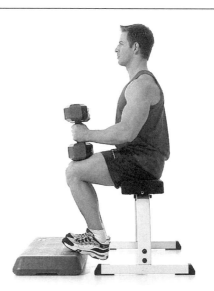

■ **START:** Grab a pair of dumbbells and sit at the end of a bench with the balls of your feet on an aerobics step or wooden block and your heels hanging off. (A couple of phone books will also work.) Hold the end of a dumbbell on top of each thigh, down near the knee. The dumbbells should be vertical, held in a neutral grip. Let your heels drop as low as possible.

▢ **FINISH:** Push your heels up as high as you can. Pause, then repeat.

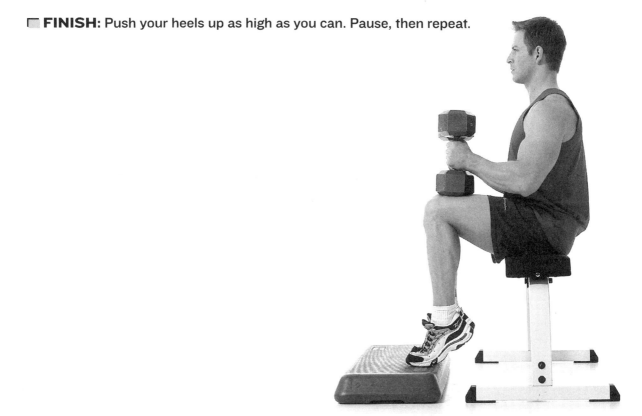

Unilateral Standing Calf Raise
INTERMEDIATE LEVEL

■ **START:** Grab a dumbbell in your nondominant hand and stand on the ball of that foot on a step or wooden block. Rest the instep of your other foot across the Achilles tendon of your working ankle. Hold on to something sturdy with your free hand if you need to. Lower your working heel off the edge of the step as far as your calf will stretch.

☐ **FINISH:** Push your working heel straight up as high as you can. Pause, then return to the starting position. Finish the set with that leg, then repeat with the other.

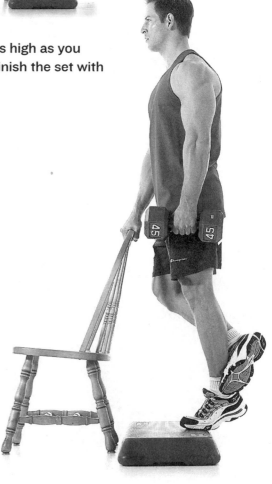

CHAPTER 8

ONE BARBELL, ONE BENCH, ONE BODY

Now for the big cannon in your home-workout arsenal: the barbell, in all its glory. We're talking here about the very symbol of manly strength, the icon of testosterone-building power. According to some guys, you're not really working out unless you're pumping a barbell up and down.

We're not saying we agree with that. As we've stated approximately 117 times already, you can build muscle by lifting any random heavy object. We will say this: If you want a measure of strength that you can compare against universal standards, you need an Olympic barbell. That's the 7-foot, 44-pound bar used in every gym, every high school and college weight room, every weight-lifting and powerlifting competition.

With a universal barbell come universal rites of passage. Though we've never done a survey, we suspect that every serious musclehead can tell you where he was the first time he did bench presses with a 45-pound plate on each side of the bar (a poundage that's rounded up to 135 pounds). The day he can put two 45-pound plates on each side and crank out a true repetition with 225 pounds is his entry into a power fraternity. And if he ever graduates to three plates on each side—315—he knows he's earned a special place within the union of ironworkers.

Strength and muscle are linked, of course, so handling poundages that would shame an anvil salesman also builds the type of muscles that captivate female eyeballs from 50 paces.

In fact, the only drawback to working exclusively with a barbell is the lack of versatility on upper-body exercises. Your range of motion is limited since the bar stops when it hits your chest or shoulders. And sometimes even that limited range of motion isn't particularly friendly to your joints. Your shoulders are by nature fragile and unstable, and forcing them to move a heavy, inflexible object overhead is sometimes asking for trouble in the form of chronic, painful overuse injuries.

Versatility is less of an issue when you do lower-body exercises with a barbell. Once you get the hang of them, you'll find that barbell squats and deadlifts use your knee, hip, and lower-back joints in the ways nature meant for them to be used. We'll go even further here and say that the barbell is the best tool for working your lower body, even if it comes in second, behind dumbbells, for working upper-body muscles.

That isn't to say that the barbell can't provide variety for your upper body. Here are a few variables you can play with to build more muscle and give your joints a break.

Grip. Switching from a pronated (overhand) to a supinated (underhand) grip invariably changes the angle of pull. And though the neutral (palms-facing) grip doesn't usually make sense with a barbell, we'll occasionally recommend a "false" grip, with your thumb on the same side of the bar as the rest of your fingers rather than hooked around the bar in a "full" grip.

Hand position. A wide (twice shoulder width) grip has a different effect on your muscles than a close (narrower than shoulder width) grip, as does anything in between.

Body position. Do the same movement from another position and you hit a different part of the targeted muscle. A well-known example is the bench press for your chest, which you can do flat, declined, or inclined. (The same options are available with any type of strength-training equipment, of course.)

Bar position. Some exercises differ from each other only in where you position the bar. For example, both versions of the shoulder press—the military press and the behind-the-neck press—involve pushing the bar overhead with your shoulder and triceps muscles. The behind-the-neck version tends to put your shoulder joint in a very biomechanically disadvantageous position. In English, that means it can be uncomfortable and even painful for some. Many fitness organizations go so far as to list it as a contraindicated exercise. We suggest that you go ahead and try it—you'll know early on whether it's a good idea to include it in your regular routine. If it hurts, steer clear of it. The same goes for any other bar position.

Angle of movement. As with bar position, you can sometimes change the pattern of movement to get a different effect from a barbell exercise. On a bench press, you can bring the bar down to your collarbones instead of to the middle of your chest. Again, not every angle works for every body, so you have to try them all to figure out which movement patterns work wonders and which wreak havoc. If it's painful, don't do it. No matter what your limitations, we offer two guarantees: A barbell offers benefits for everybody. And a barbell-built body will get noticed—from any angle.

A word on hardware: Though we ran down all the options in chapter 4, in this chapter we assume that you've opted for a 7-foot Olympic barbell and that you have enough weights for maximum lifts. Further, we presume that you have either a bench with adjustable uprights or a power rack.

We're also going to show some exercises using an EZ-curl bar. To save you a trip back to chapter 4, an EZ-curl bar is a W-shaped barbell that shifts the angle of pull for a lot of arm exercises. It's an optional but useful tool.

MIDSECTION

As you've probably guessed, barbells don't exactly lend themselves to abdominal exercises. Beginners should refer back to the body-weight ab programs in chapter 6. Intermediate and advanced guys can supplement the body-weight movements with 1 or 2 sets of 8 to 12 repetitions of the following exercises.

INTERMEDIATE	ADVANCED
Barbell rollout ----------(page 166) Full-contact twist -------(page 166)	On-your-feet barbell rollout ---------------(page 166)

EXERCISES FOR THE MIDSECTION

Barbell Rollout
INTERMEDIATE LEVEL

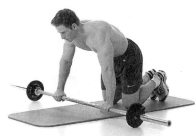

■ **START:** Load a pair of small (2½- or 5-pound) plates onto a barbell. Kneel on an exercise mat or towel with your shoulders directly over the bar. Grab the bar with an overhand, shoulder-width grip. Put your butt in the air. Start with your back in a somewhat-rounded position, allowing it to extend into a more neutral position as you execute the movement.

□ **FINISH:** Roll the bar out in front of you, holding your knees in place as your hips, torso, and arms go forward. Keeping your arms taut, advance as far as you can without arching your back or touching the floor with anything above your knees. Pause for a split second, then pull back to the starting position, feeling your abs contracting forcefully as you do.

ADVANCED VARIATION
On-Your-Feet Barbell Rollout

If you're strong enough, do this on the balls of your feet instead of on your knees.

Full-Contact Twist
INTERMEDIATE LEVEL

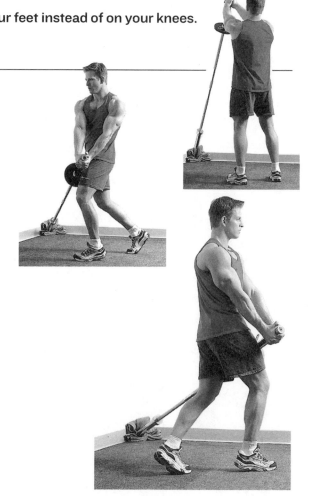

■ **START:** Load a barbell lightly on one end. Wrap the other end in a towel and stick it into a corner of your workout room. Stand facing the loaded end, lock your fingers around the end of the bar (in front of the plate), and hold it in front of your face.

□ **FINISH:** Pivot your feet and torso simultaneously to move the top of the bar down and to your nondominant side so it ends up just above your nondominant knee. Feel your torso muscles work as you lift the bar up and then down toward your other knee. That's 1 repetition. *Caution:* Make sure your shoes and the floor allow smooth pivots on the balls of your feet. On carpet, for example, you may want to be in your stocking feet.

CHEST AND UPPER BACK

The presses and rows in this section are great for upper-torso development. Beginners should do 1 or 2 sets of 8 to 10 reps of two kinds of bench presses. The back exercises—rows and the pullover—aren't particularly beginner-friendly, and the rows are tough on anyone who has back problems. We strongly recommend that you get a chinup bar (or a power rack with a chinning bar, if you have the headroom) and use it as described in chapter 6. Chinups and pullups are superior to pullovers, and reverse pushups are a back-friendly, beginner-friendly variation on the barbell rows described in this chapter. If you can manage rows, do 2 or 3 sets of 8 to 10 reps each of two different types.

Intermediates can do 2 to 4 sets of 6 to 10 reps each of two presses, two rows, and the pullover. Advanced lifters can pick the same combination of exercises but do 3 to 5 sets of 4 to 8 reps.

BEGINNER

CHEST
- Bench press ----------(page 168)
- Feet-up bench press ---(page 168)

INTERMEDIATE

CHEST
- Close-grip bench press -----------------(page 168)
- Incline bench press -----(page 169)
- Decline bench press ----(page 169)

UPPER BACK
- Pronated bent-over row -----------------(page 170)
- Supinated bent-over row -----------------(page 170)
- EZ-curl pullover --------(page 172)
- Swiss-ball EZ-curl pullover --------------(page 172)

ADVANCED

CHEST
- Wide-grip bench press ---------------(page 168)
- Reverse-grip bench press --------------------(page 168)
- Altered-angle bench press --------------------(page 168)

UPPER BACK
- T-bar row -------------(page 171)
- Pullover ---------------(page 171)

EXERCISES FOR THE CHEST

Bench Press
BEGINNER LEVEL

■ **START:** Lie on a bench with your head, torso, and hips pressed against it and your feet spread wide and flat on the floor. Grab the barbell with a full (thumbs wrapped around the bar) overhand grip. Place your hands slightly wider than shoulder-width apart, remove the bar from the uprights, and hold it with straight arms over your collarbone. Pull your shoulder blades together in back.

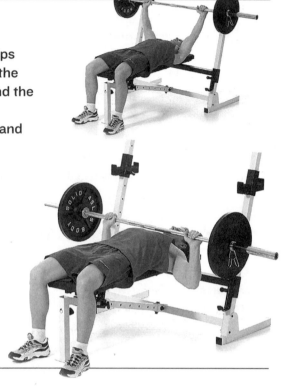

□ **FINISH:** Lower the bar, slowly and in control, to just above your nipples. Then press it up and just slightly back so it finishes above your collarbone again. Stop just short of locking your elbows, and keep your shoulder blades pulled back.

BEGINNER-TO-INTERMEDIATE VARIATION
Feet-Up Bench Press

If lower-back discomfort is a problem for you, put your feet up on the bench, or lift them up in the air. Even if you have no back problems, this is a fun variation to try; it requires more balance and forces you to maintain an abdominal contraction throughout the exercise.

INTERMEDIATE-TO-ADVANCED VARIATION
Close-Grip Bench Press

Place your hands less than shoulder-width apart—down to about 8 inches—to shift emphasis to your triceps. (You'll find variations later in this chapter.) The narrower your grip, the harder the exercise is on your wrists. Advanced lifters can try this on a decline bench to hit the pecs.

ADVANCED VARIATIONS
Wide-Grip Bench Press

A wide grip—twice shoulder-width—helps you isolate your pectoral muscles. Your range of motion is shorter, so you use your shoulders and triceps less. This is also very effective on an incline.

Reverse-Grip Bench Press

Grab the bar with a shoulder-width, underhand grip. This targets your front delts and triceps.

Altered-Angle Bench Press

Lower the bar toward your throat rather than your nipples, forcing your elbows out to the sides. This changes the angle of pull on your pecs and increases demand on your shoulders.

Incline Bench Press
INTERMEDIATE-TO-ADVANCED LEVEL

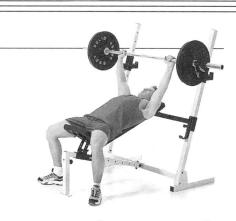

■ **START:** If your incline bench adjusts, set it at between 10 and 30 degrees to target your upper chest. (A steeper angle shifts emphasis to your delts.) With your head, torso, and hips pressed to the bench and your feet flat on the floor, use a full overhand grip that's slightly wider than shoulder-width to hold the barbell at arm's length above your chin.

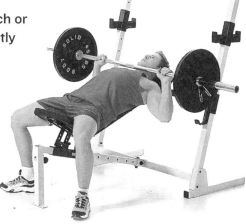

▢ **FINISH:** Lower the bar, in control, to within an inch or two of your collarbone. Then press it up and very subtly back so that it finishes above your chin.

Decline Bench Press
INTERMEDIATE-TO-ADVANCED LEVEL

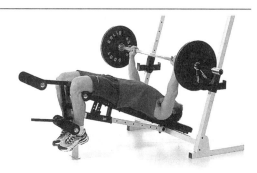

■ **START:** Lie on a decline bench with your lower shins hooked beneath the leg supports at the end. Hold the barbell with a full, overhand grip that's slightly wider than shoulder-width. Set it up directly over your lower chest.

▢ **FINISH:** Lower the bar slowly and in control to just an inch or two above your chest before pausing momentarily and then pressing it back up.

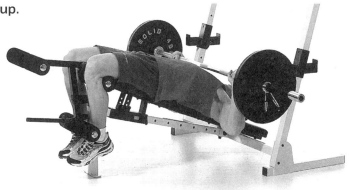

EXERCISES FOR THE UPPER BACK

Pronated Bent-Over Row
INTERMEDIATE-TO-ADVANCED LEVEL

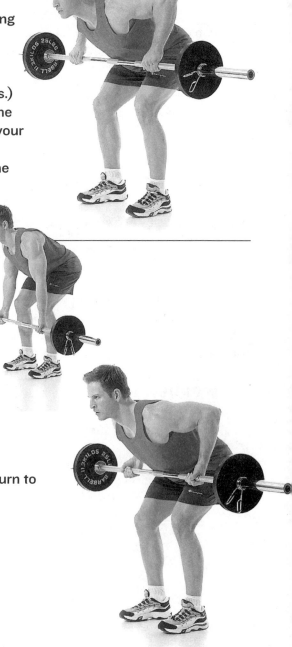

■ **START:** Stand with your feet shoulder-width apart and your knees bent 15 to 30 degrees. Keep your torso straight with a slight arch in your back as you lean forward at the hips. Try to get your torso close to parallel to the floor. Grab the barbell off the floor with a false (thumbs in line with the rest of your fingers) overhand grip that's slightly wider than shoulder width. Let the bar hang at arm's length in front of you.

◻ **FINISH:** Retract your shoulder blades to start pulling the bar up to the lower part of your sternum (breast-bone). (Imagine that your arms are just along for the ride; otherwise, you'll use them as the prime movers and get less of a workout for your middle-back muscles.) Pause at the top, with your chest sticking out toward the bar. Slowly return to the starting position. Try to keep your torso in the same position throughout the movement. (That's the purpose of the bent knees—they provide the suspension your torso needs to remain steady.)

Supinated Bent-Over Row
INTERMEDIATE-TO-ADVANCED LEVEL

■ **START:** This row puts your biceps in a stronger position, allowing them to help out with the exercise. That means you can start with a little more weight on the barbell than you'd use for the pronated bent-over row. Assume the same stance, but hold the bar directly under your shoulders with an underhand, full (thumbs opposing your fingers) grip.

◻ **FINISH:** Pull the bar to your navel, pause, then return to the starting position.

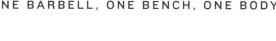

T-Bar Row
ADVANCED LEVEL

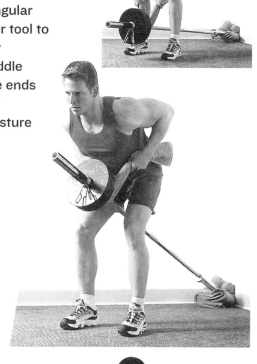

■ **START:** Wrap one end of the bar in an old towel and stuff it into a corner. If you have something heavy—a dumbbell or sandbag—to put over the bar to steady it, use it. Before you load the other end of the bar, wrap a workout towel around it. (If you have a triangular handle for cable rows or lat pulldowns, that's an even better tool to put on the bar.) Then load the end with 25-pound or lighter plates—bigger ones will restrict your range of motion. Straddle the bar so that you face away from the corner, and grab the ends of the towel or the handle with a neutral grip. Get into the starting position described for the other rows, with your posture a bit more upright and your elbows in closer to your torso.

◻ **FINISH:** Pull the bar up until your hands touch your abdomen. Pause, then slowly return to the starting position. Keep your knees bent, your back slightly arched, and your elbows close to your torso throughout.

Pullover
ADVANCED LEVEL

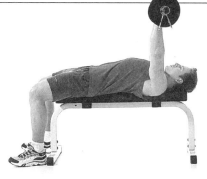

■ **START:** Set the barbell on the floor, perpendicular to one end of a bench. Lie on the bench with your head at the end by the bar. Reach back and grab the bar with a full, overhand grip that's just a bit narrower than shoulder width. Lift the bar over your upper chest, with your elbows slightly bent. Set your feet on the floor or bench, whichever you prefer.

◻ **FINISH:** Lower the bar back behind your head until your arms are in line with your neck. Pause, then pull the bar back up over your chest. Keep your elbows bent at the same angle throughout the movement.

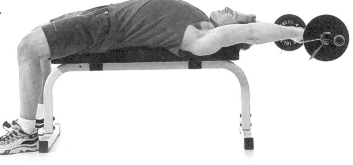

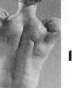
Pullover

EZ-Curl Pullover

You can do this one with an EZ-curl bar, which should reduce the strain on your wrists.

Swiss-Ball EZ-Curl Pullover

Holding the EZ-curl bar, lie with your head, neck, and upper back in contact with a Swiss ball. Bridge your hips up so they're parallel to the floor and your knees are bent 90 degrees. Then extend your arms directly over your chest. From this position, do standard pullovers without letting your hips dip below the level of the ball.

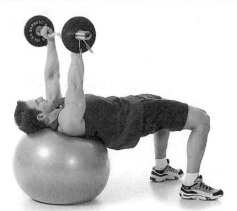

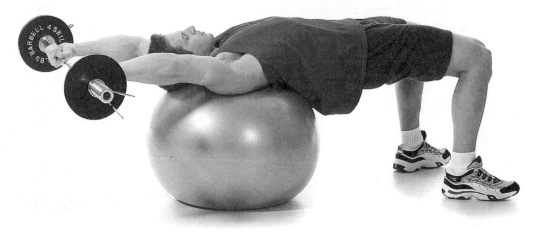

SHOULDERS AND ARMS

For a solid all-barbell arms-and-shoulders workout, beginners should do 1 or 2 sets of 8 to 10 reps of a shoulder press, an upright row or shrug, a triceps movement, and a biceps exercise.

Intermediate and advanced lifters should select one explosive lift (either the hang clean or Neider press), one press, one shrug or upright row,

two triceps movements, and two biceps movement. The front raise and the forearm exercises are optional; if you choose to do the latter, pick only one. If you're at the intermediate level, do 2 or 3 sets of 6 to 10 reps per exercise. If you're more advanced, do 3 or 4 sets of 4 to 8 reps for each. If time is an issue, do fewer sets of the arm exercises.

BEGINNER

SHOULDERS
- Upright row ---------(page 174)
- Military press -------(page 174)
- Front shrug ---------(page 179)

TRICEPS
- Lying triceps extension -------------------(page 180)
- Lying triceps extension with EZ-curl bar ---(page 180)

BICEPS
- Standing curl -------(page 183)
- EZ standing curl -------------------(page 183)

FOREARMS
- Wrist curl ----------(page 187)
- Reverse wrist curl ---(page 187)

INTERMEDIATE

SHOULDERS
- Seated military press ------(page 174)
- Behind-the-neck press ----(page 175)
- Seated behind-the-neck press --------------------(page 175)
- Hang clean --------------(page 176)
- Front raise --------------(page 177)
- Neider press -------------(page 177)
- Reverse shrug ------------(page 179)

TRICEPS
- Decline lying triceps extension -------------(page 180)
- Swiss-ball lying triceps extension with EZ-curl bar ---------(page 180)
- Close-grip bench press ----(page 181)
- French press -------------(page 182)
- Swiss-ball EZ French press -------------------(page 182)

BICEPS
- Narrow-grip standing curl --(page 183)
- Extended-wrists standing curl -----------(page 183)
- Reverse curl -------------(page 184)
- Preacher curl ------------(page 184)
- Swiss-ball preacher curl --(page 185)
- Wide- or narrow-grip preacher curl ----------(page 185)

FOREARMS
- Standing wrist curl -------(page 188)

ADVANCED

SHOULDERS
- Swiss-ball seated military press ----------------(page 175)
- Incline front raise ------(page 177)
- Cuban press -----------(page 178)
- Push press ------------(page 178)
- Push jerk -------------(page 178)
- Overhead shrug -------(page 179)

TRICEPS
- Incline lying triceps extension -------------(page 181)
- Decline close-grip bench press ----------------(page 181)

BICEPS
- Reverse-grip preacher curl with EZ bar ------(page 185)
- Prone 45-degree curl --(page 185)
- Prone 45-degree curl with extended wrists ------(page 185)
- Drag curl -------------(page 186)

EXERCISES FOR THE SHOULDERS

Upright Row
BEGINNER LEVEL

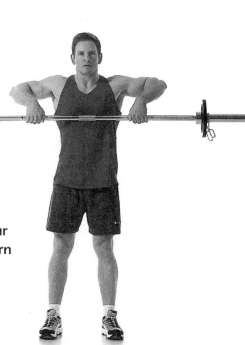

■ **START:** Grab the barbell with a false, overhand grip that's shoulder width or a little wider. Stand and let the bar hang at arm's length in front of your thighs.

▢ **FINISH:** Pull the bar up to your lower chest, or until your upper arms are parallel to the floor. Pause, then slowly return to the starting position.

Military Press
BEGINNER LEVEL

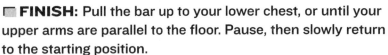

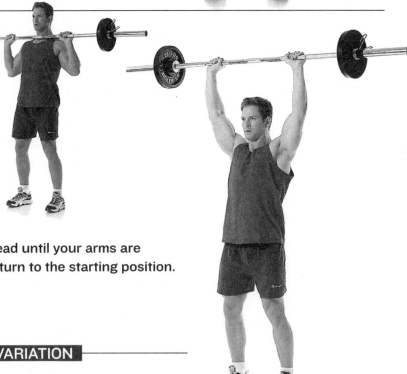

■ **START:** Grab the barbell with a full, overhand grip that's shoulder width or a little wider. Stand and hold the bar at collarbone level, with your back in its natural alignment and your knees slightly bent.

▢ **FINISH:** Press the bar overhead until your arms are straight but not locked. Slowly return to the starting position.

INTERMEDIATE-TO-ADVANCED VARIATION
Seated Military Press

Do the same movement while seated at the end of a bench, without a back support.

ADVANCED VARIATION
Swiss-Ball Seated Military Press

Simply perform the military-press movement while sitting on a ball, taking extra care not to let your back arch too much.

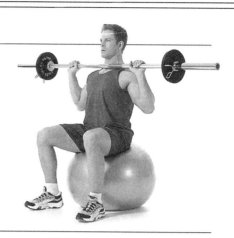

Behind-the-Neck Press
INTERMEDIATE-TO-ADVANCED LEVEL

■ **START:** Grip the bar as you would for a military press, but hold it behind your head, just above (not touching) the base of your neck.

▢ **FINISH:** Press the bar up, pause, then slowly lower it to the starting position without letting it drift backward. *Note:* This is one of those exercises that many experts nowadays tell you not to do, because of the stress on your shoulders. As previously noted, any overhead press—in front of the neck or behind—can be stressful for some guys. Other guys are able to do all the pressing variations pain-free. Our advice is to start with light weights until your body finds its groove. And stay within your comfort zone. If a shoulder press feels like it's pulling apart your shoulder joints, it's not right for you.

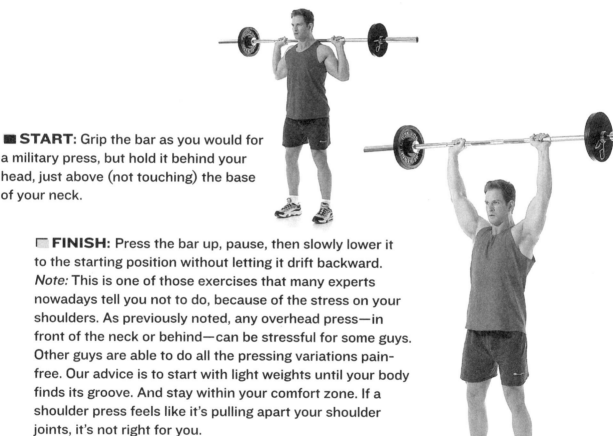

VARIATION
Seated Behind-the-Neck Press

Do the same movement while sitting, without a back support.

Hang Clean
INTERMEDIATE-TO-ADVANCED LEVEL

Sports Move

■ **START:** Grab the barbell with a full, overhand, shoulder-width grip. Set your feet shoulder-width apart, with your knees bent about 30 degrees, and bend forward at the hips as you hold the bar at arm's length, just below your knees.

☐ **FINISH:** This is a multipart sequence that you execute quickly and powerfully. First, dip your knees, as if you were about to jump. Quickly reverse the motion, as if you were jumping *and* trying to throw the bar over your shoulders. As you rise on the balls of your feet, shrug your shoulders. With all this upward momentum generated by your traps and lower body, pull the bar up to shoulder level as fast as you can. Finally, dip down with your knees and hips as you "catch" the bar on your shoulders. The bar will roll to the ends of your fingers, your wrists will bend back, and your upper arms should end up parallel to the floor, in front of your torso. Quickly return to the starting position—this is one exercise in which there's no benefit to pausing and slowly lowering the weight. Work on your form with light weights for several weeks before attempting this with heavier loads. You'll know you've got it right when the bar snaps into place on your shoulders on each repetition.

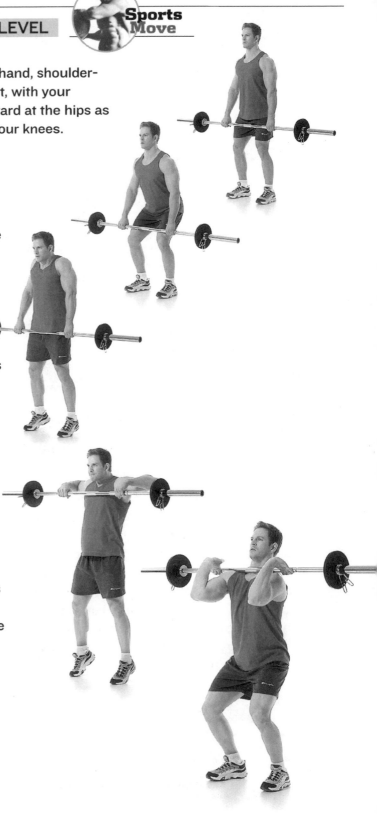

Front Raise
INTERMEDIATE-TO-ADVANCED LEVEL

■ **START:** Grab an EZ-curl bar with a full, overhand, shoulder-width grip, and stand with the barbell hanging in front of your thighs. Set your feet shoulder-width apart with your knees slightly bent, and lean forward very slightly at the hips (to help you avoid leaning back as you lift). Pull in your abs and tighten all your upper-body muscles, and slightly bend your elbows.

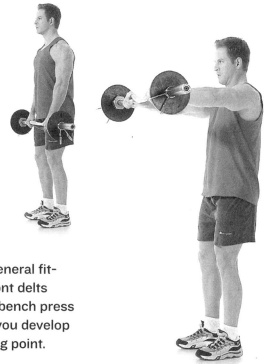

▢ **FINISH:** Raise the bar in front of you until your arms are parallel to the floor. Pause, then return to the starting position. *Note:* Don't attempt this exercise without a specific purpose. If you're lifting for general fitness, it's not very useful or necessary, since your front delts tend to get a lot of work. If you're trying for a bigger bench press and you tend to get stuck halfway up, this can help you develop the shoulder strength to get you through that sticking point.

ADVANCED VARIATION
Incline Front Raise

Do the same movement while lying on a steeply inclined (around 75 degrees) bench. You'll sacrifice range of motion but make the exercise much tougher.

Neider Press
INTERMEDIATE-TO-ADVANCED LEVEL

Sports Move

■ **START:** Grab a relatively light bar with a full overhand grip that's a bit wider than shoulder width. Stand and hold it at your chest with your elbows out to the sides and your knuckles pointing straight ahead—from the waist up, you should look like you're about to do a bench press, except you're vertical instead of horizontal.

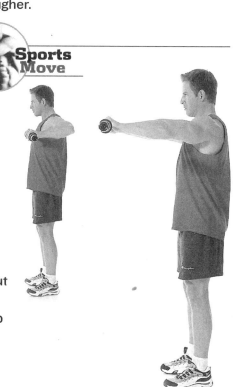

▢ **FINISH:** Explosively press the bar forward (not up) until your arms are straight in front of you. Do this without letting the bar dip down (that's why you're using a lighter load). Quickly pull it back and repeat. Work hard but keep the bar under control—don't slam it off your chest.

Cuban Press
ADVANCED LEVEL

■ **START:** Use a very lightly loaded (or unloaded) barbell for this shoulder warmup exercise. Stand in the finishing position of an upright row: bar at chest level in an overhand grip, forearms pointing down, and upper arms parallel to the floor.

▭ **FINISH:** Without moving your upper arms or your elbows, rotate your forearms until they point straight up (or almost straight up) instead of straight down. Then press the bar overhead, without locking your elbows. Pause, lower the press, then reverse the forearm rotation to return to the starting position.

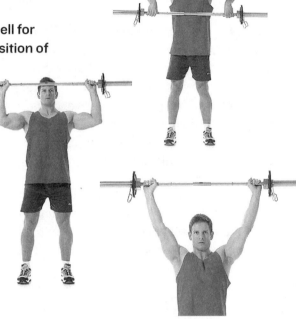

Push Press
ADVANCED LEVEL

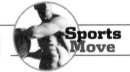
Sports Move

■ **START:** Load the barbell with more weight than you would for the more traditional shoulder presses, and rest it on the fronts of your shoulders—though it will be the backs of your hands, not the bar itself, that actually touch your anterior deltoids. Keep your arms close to your body.

▭ **FINISH:** Bend your knees and lower yourself to the half-squat position, then immediately drive yourself up with your legs as you thrust the weight toward the ceiling until you are up on your toes and your arms are straightened above you. Slowly return to the starting position.

VARIATION
Push Jerk

Same as above, but step forward with one foot as you push the weight overhead. Step back, then lower the weight. Alternate feet either with each rep or with each set.

Front Shrug
BEGINNER LEVEL

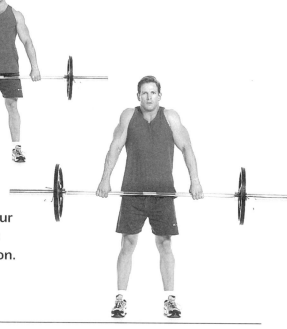

■ **START:** Grab the barbell with a full, over-hand, shoulder-width grip, and stand with the bar at arm's length against your front thighs.

▢ **FINISH:** Shrug your shoulders straight up toward your ears, keeping your arms straight and your head still. Pause when your shoulders are as high as they can go, then slowly return to the starting position.

INTERMEDIATE VARIATION
Reverse Shrug

Same grip and same motion, but hold the barbell down behind you.

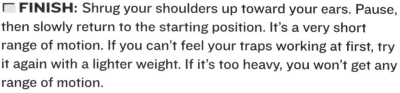

Overhead Shrug
ADVANCED LEVEL

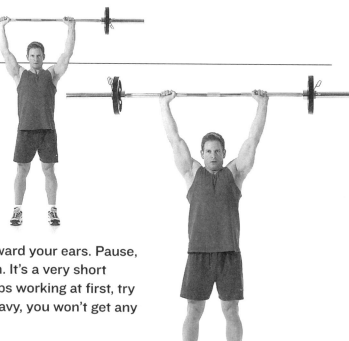

■ **START:** Load the bar with relatively light plates, and grab it with a full, overhand, shoulder-width grip. Stand, press it over your head, and hold it there with straight arms.

▢ **FINISH:** Shrug your shoulders up toward your ears. Pause, then slowly return to the starting position. It's a very short range of motion. If you can't feel your traps working at first, try it again with a lighter weight. If it's too heavy, you won't get any range of motion.

EXERCISES FOR THE TRICEPS

Lying Triceps Extension
BEGINNER LEVEL

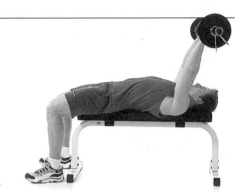

■ **START:** Grab the barbell with a full, overhand grip that's just narrower than shoulder width. Lie on a bench holding the bar over your eyes with straight arms. Your upper arms aren't perpendicular to your torso in this position, but this angle makes the exercise harder for your triceps (since they're starting in a prestretched position) and easier on your elbows.

▢ **FINISH:** Bend at your elbows as you lower the bar until it almost touches your head. Pause, then lift it back to the starting position. Keep your upper arms in the same position throughout the exercise.

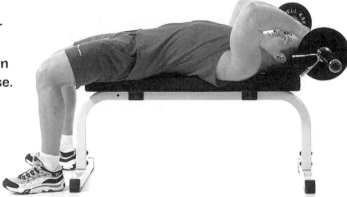

BEGINNER VARIATION
Lying Triceps Extension with EZ-Curl Bar

We highly recommend using an EZ-curl bar to ease the strain on your wrists.

INTERMEDIATE VARIATIONS
Decline Lying Triceps Extension

Use a decline bench instead of a flat bench, to increase the demand on your triceps.

Swiss-Ball Lying Triceps Extension with EZ-Curl Bar

Use an EZ-curl bar to do triceps extensions while lying with your head, neck, and shoulder blades in contact with a ball, your lower back off the ball, your feet shoulder-width apart, your hips parallel to the floor, and your knees bent 90 degrees.

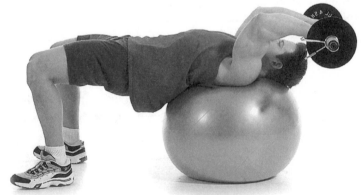

ADVANCED VARIATION
Incline Lying Triceps Extension

If you're trying to build triceps strength to improve your bench press, this is an interesting alternative. It feels odd at first and can be tough on your elbows, but you should feel (and see) a difference in your triceps' size and strength after a couple of workouts.

Close-Grip Bench Press
INTERMEDIATE LEVEL

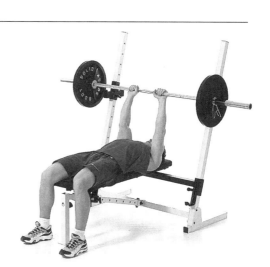

■ **START:** Lie on a bench and grab the barbell with a full, overhand grip that's narrow enough (just less than shoulder-width) to shift the emphasis from your pecs to your triceps but not so narrow as to strain your wrists and elbows. With straight arms, hold the bar over your chest.

▢ **FINISH:** Slowly lower the bar until it almost touches your lower chest. Pause, then press back up to the starting position.

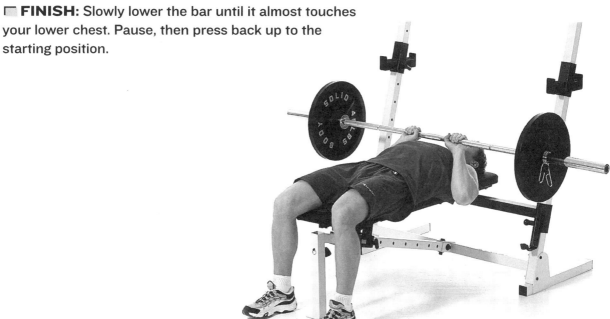

ADVANCED VARIATION
Decline Close-Grip Bench Press

This move simulates a dip (page 278), for lower-chest action.

French Press
INTERMEDIATE-TO-ADVANCED LEVEL

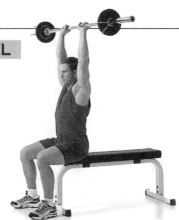

■ **START:** Grab the barbell with a full, overhand grip that's just narrower than shoulder width. Stand, or sit on the end of a bench. Hold the bar over your head with your arms straight but your elbows unlocked. Your upper arms should be just outside your ears.

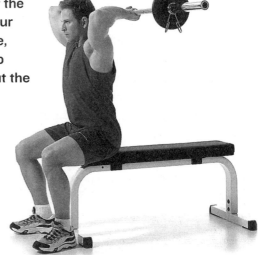

□ **FINISH:** Bend your elbows and slowly lower the bar toward the back of your neck. Stop when your forearms are just past parallel to the floor. Pause, then press back up to the starting position. Keep your upper arms in the same position throughout the exercise.

INTERMEDIATE VARIATION
Swiss-Ball EZ French Press

Use an EZ-curl bar rather than a straight bar as you sit on a ball to do standard French presses.

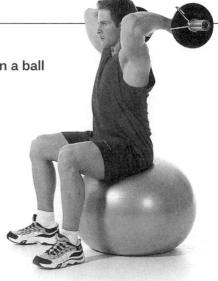

EXERCISES FOR THE BICEPS

Standing Curl
BEGINNER LEVEL

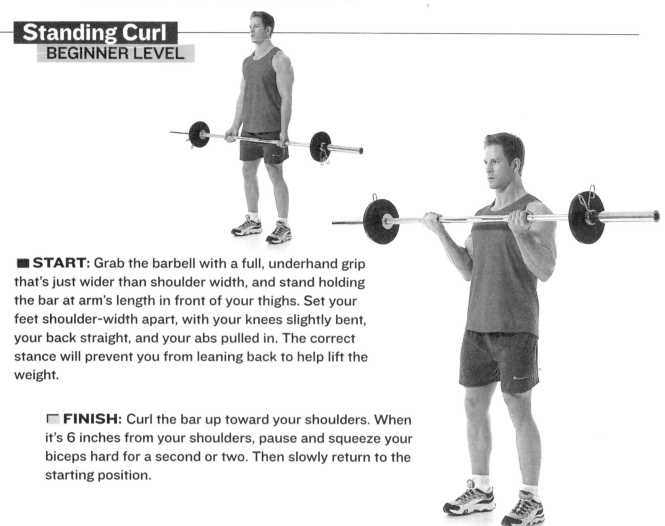

■ **START:** Grab the barbell with a full, underhand grip that's just wider than shoulder width, and stand holding the bar at arm's length in front of your thighs. Set your feet shoulder-width apart, with your knees slightly bent, your back straight, and your abs pulled in. The correct stance will prevent you from leaning back to help lift the weight.

□ **FINISH:** Curl the bar up toward your shoulders. When it's 6 inches from your shoulders, pause and squeeze your biceps hard for a second or two. Then slowly return to the starting position.

BEGINNER VARIATION
EZ Standing Curl

Using an EZ-curl bar eases the strain on your wrists and also increases the demand on your brachioradialis, which is another arm-flexor muscle.

INTERMEDIATE VARIATIONS
Narrow-Grip Standing Curl

Move your hands in to shoulder width or slightly closer to shift demand from the inner portion to the outer portion of the biceps.

Extended-Wrists Standing Curl

Bending your wrists back slightly, with the heel of your hand leading the movement, can increase the demand on the biceps by taking the wrist flexors (forearm muscles) out of the movement.

Reverse Curl
INTERMEDIATE-TO-ADVANCED LEVEL

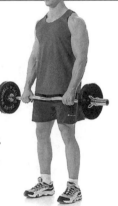
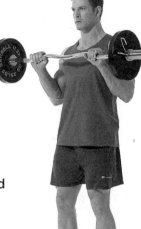

■ **START:** Use the same starting position and slight forward lean as in the regular standing curl, but switch to a pronated (overhand) grip on an EZ-curl bar. (We think it's too tough on your wrists to do this with a straight bar.)

☐ **FINISH:** Curl the weight up to bring the backs of your hands toward your shoulders. Stop 6 inches away and pause. Then return to the starting position. The reverse grip shifts the emphasis of the exercise from your biceps to your brachialis and forearms.

Preacher Curl
INTERMEDIATE-TO-ADVANCED LEVEL

■ **START:** A preacher bench shifts the angle so the first part of the curl is harder and the last part is easier. Some believe this helps the biceps grow longer, but we disagree. However, this exercise does help your biceps get bigger and stronger. Gravity works hard against your biceps in the first few inches of this movement, a very different effect from a standard curl. Here's how to do the exercise: Grab a barbell or EZ-curl bar with a shoulder-width, underhand grip, and position yourself on the preacher bench so the top of the pad almost touches your armpits. Start with your upper arms against the pads and your elbows slightly bent.

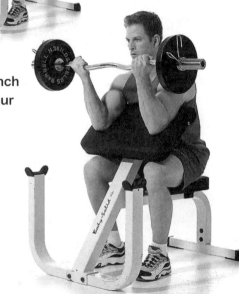

☐ **FINISH:** Keep your back straight as you curl the weight up until your forearms are just short of perpendicular to the floor (anything higher is too easy to bother with—it's just moving the bar horizontally). Return to the starting position.

INTERMEDIATE VARIATION
Swiss-Ball Preacher Curl

Position a loaded EZ-curl bar on the floor in front of a ball. Kneel behind the ball and let your torso rest on it as you drape your arms over to grab the bar with an underhand grip. Let your weight move back toward your heels as you brace your triceps on the ball, forearms down. Then curl the bar as in the standard preacher curl.

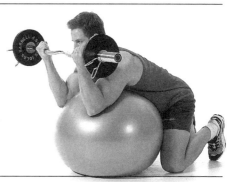

INTERMEDIATE-TO-ADVANCED VARIATION
Wide- or Narrow-Grip Preacher Curl

You can widen or narrow your grip to shift the emphasis from the inner (short) head to the outer (long) head. Remember, the narrower the grip, the more the long head works.

ADVANCED VARIATION
Reverse-Grip Preacher Curl with EZ Bar

Shift the emphasis to your brachialis and forearms with an overhand grip. Don't try this with a straight barbell; it's too tough on your wrists.

Prone 45-Degree Curl
ADVANCED LEVEL

■ **START:** Grab a barbell or EZ-curl bar with an underhand, shoulder-width grip, and lie on your chest on an incline bench set at 45 degrees. Hold the bar at arm's length below your shoulders.

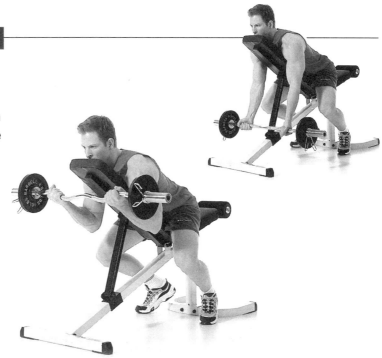

□ **FINISH:** Curl the bar up as high as you can without allowing your upper arms to move forward. Pause at the top and contract your biceps. Slowly return to the starting position.

VARIATION
Prone 45-Degree Curl with Extended Wrists

Bend back your wrists so the heels of your hands lead the movement. This makes the exercise tougher on your biceps.

Drag Curl
ADVANCED LEVEL

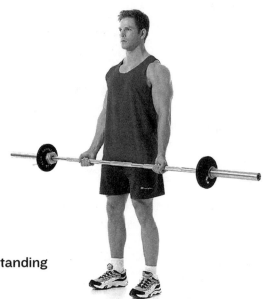

■ **START:** Set up as you would for the standing curl on page 183.

□ **FINISH:** Instead of curling the bar up, move your elbows up and back (but not out), letting the bar "drag" up the front of your body without ever quite touching your torso. Stop when your elbows are as high as they'll go. Pause, then return to the starting position.

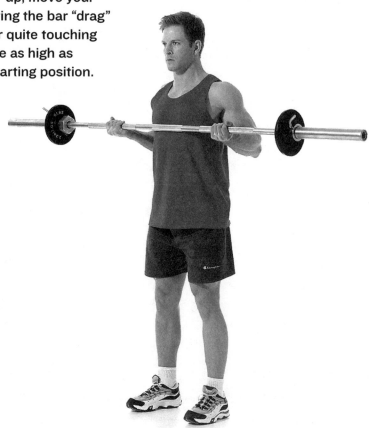

EXERCISES FOR THE FOREARMS

Wrist Curl
BEGINNER LEVEL

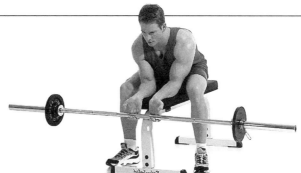

■ **START:** Grab the barbell with an underhand grip, your hands a few inches apart. Straddle a bench and, with your back flat, rest your forearms on it, letting your hands and the bar hang off the end. Allow your wrists to bend back and the barbell to roll to the ends of your fingers.

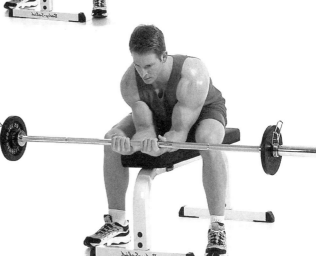

☐ **FINISH:** Close your fingertips as you curl your palms toward your biceps. Pause, reverse the motion, and let the bar roll back to your fingertips.

Reverse Wrist Curl
BEGINNER LEVEL

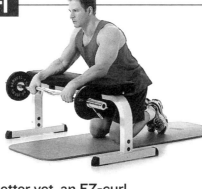

■ **START:** Grab a barbell or, better yet, an EZ-curl bar with an overhand grip and kneel facing the long side of a bench. Rest your forearms on the bench with your wrists hanging off the other side. Lower the bar as far as possible.

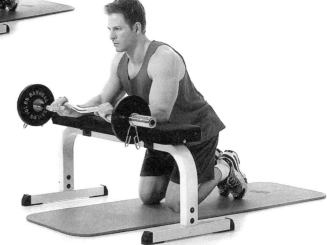

☐ **FINISH:** Raise the bar by bringing the backs of your hands toward your elbows.

Standing Wrist Curl
INTERMEDIATE-TO-ADVANCED LEVEL

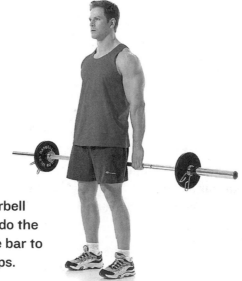

■ **START:** Using an overhand grip, let the barbell hang behind your back as if you were going to do the reverse shrug described on page 179. Allow the bar to roll down so you're holding it with your fingertips.

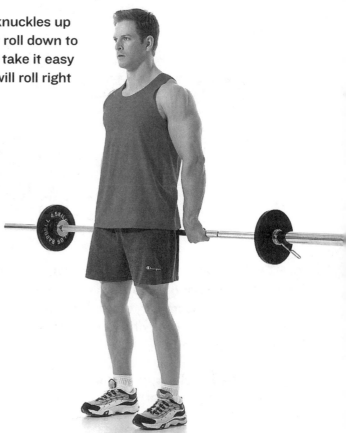

▢ **FINISH:** Close your hands and curl your knuckles up toward your forearms. Pause, then let the bar roll down to your fingertips again. (Obviously, you want to take it easy on the weight load here. Otherwise, that bar will roll right past your fingertips to the floor.)

LOWER BODY

We all dream of bulging biceps and a 32-inch waist bristling with abdominal segments that look like those on Batman's suit. We all start weight training with the idea that we'll get these things with curls and crunches. The reality is that the biggest muscles on your body are below the waist. (No, that doesn't include your man muscle.) The squats and deadlifts in this section will produce shifts in your metabolism and hormones that will make the mirror muscles possible.

Beginners should do 1 or 2 sets of 10 to 12 reps each of one knee-dominant and two hip-dominant movements, as well as one calf exercise. None of the knee-dominant exercises with a barbell is suitable for beginners, who have to start with the body-weight lunge and squat in chapter 6.

Intermediate-level lifters should do 2 to 4 sets of 8 to 10 reps each of two knee-dominant and two hip-dominant movements, as well as one calf exercise. Advanced lifters should use the same exercise-selection guidelines as intermediates, but do 3 to 5 sets of 4 to 8 reps of each.

BEGINNER	INTERMEDIATE	ADVANCED
KNEE-DOMINANT	**KNEE-DOMINANT**	**KNEE-DOMINANT**
Back squat with heel support (page 191)	Lunge (page 190)	45-degree lunge (page 190)
	Traveling lunge (page 190)	Front squat (page 192)
HIP-DOMINANT	Back squat (page 191)	Overhead squat (page 193)
Reverse lunge (page 196)	Front squat with lifting straps (page 192)	Hack squat (page 193)
Stepup (page 196)	Split squat (page 194)	Bulgarian split squat (page 194)
Side stepup (page 197)		Jump squat (page 195)
	HIP-DOMINANT	Side lunge (page 195)
CALVES	Alternating stepup (page 197)	
Seated calf raise (page 202)	Crossover stepup (page 197)	**HIP-DOMINANT**
	Cardio stepup (page 197)	Unilateral deadlift (page 198)
	Deadlift (page 198)	Suitcase deadlift (page 198)
	Sumo deadlift (page 198)	Unilateral Romanian deadlift (page 199)
	Romanian deadlift (page 199)	Snatch-grip Romanian deadlift (page 199)
		Good morning (page 199)
		Power clean (page 200)
		Muscle snatch (page 201)
		CALVES
		Standing calf raise (page 202)

KNEE-DOMINANT EXERCISES

Lunge
INTERMEDIATE LEVEL

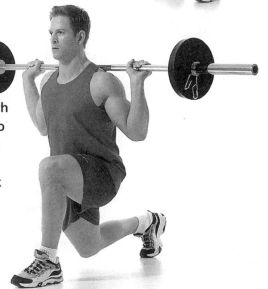

■ **START:** Take a shoulder-width stance and rest the barbell across your traps.

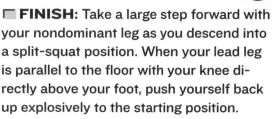

□ **FINISH:** Take a large step forward with your nondominant leg as you descend into a split-squat position. When your lead leg is parallel to the floor with your knee directly above your foot, push yourself back up explosively to the starting position.

INTERMEDIATE VARIATION
Traveling Lunge

Instead of pushing back up from the down position, bring your back leg forward to get to the starting position a few feet ahead of where you started. Execute the next lunge with your other leg. Continue alternating legs as you lunge across the room.

ADVANCED VARIATION
45-Degree Lunge

Work your inner thighs more by stepping out at a 45-degree angle from your body as you execute your lunge. Be sure to point your toes in the direction you're stepping, and make sure your knee stays over your toes.

Back Squat
INTERMEDIATE-TO-ADVANCED LEVEL

■ **START:** Set your barbell on the squat supports so you have to bend your knees slightly to step under it and set it on your shoulders. (You don't want to have to lift it up to the supports at the end of a set—you may not be able to reach them.) Position yourself under the bar so it rests on the backs of your shoulders and your trapezius, not your neck. (When you pull your shoulder blades back, your traps should form a nice shelf for the bar. It shouldn't hurt at all— if it does, it's a sure sign you're doing something wrong.) Hold the bar with a wide, overhand grip, straighten your legs to lift it off the rack, step back, and set your feet shoulder-width apart with your knees slightly bent and your lower back in its naturally arched position.

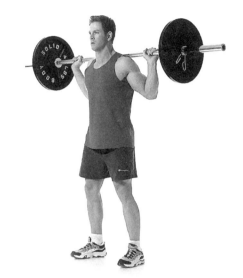

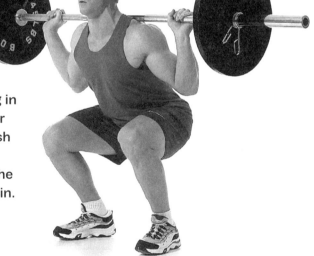

☐ **FINISH:** Initiating the descent at the hips, not the knees, lower yourself as though sitting in a chair behind you. Stop when the tops of your thighs are parallel to the floor, pause, then push back up to the starting position. Your knees should stay in line with your feet throughout the movement—they shouldn't splay out or pinch in.

BEGINNER VARIATION
Back Squat with Heel Support

If you're new to squatting, you'll have a hard time keeping your heels on the floor where they belong. Better flexibility is the ultimate answer. Until you develop that, you can place a wooden plank or a small weight plate or two under your heels to compensate.

Front Squat
ADVANCED LEVEL

■ **START:** This more upright version will stress your quads more than the back squat, so use a lighter weight. Grab the barbell in an overhand, shoulder-width grip. Bring your elbows forward so your palms face up. (If you've done the hang clean and power clean described elsewhere in this book, you'll recognize this as the "catch" position of those lifts.) Rest the bar on your front delts.

☐ **FINISH:** Start the descent with your hips, as described for the back squat on the previous page, and keep your elbows high as you lower yourself until your upper thighs are parallel to the floor. Pause, then push yourself back up to the starting position. You'll need some practice to develop a comfort level with this exercise, but it's worth the trouble. Besides strengthening your quads, it de-emphasizes your lower back—if you lean forward at all, the weight falls on the floor. It also helps you develop your form in either version of the clean. You get more comfortable "racking" the weight on your shoulders.

INTERMEDIATE VARIATION
Front Squat with Lifting Straps

Wrist discomfort is common with this movement. Avoid it by investing in a pair of lifting straps that you loop around the bar where you'd grip it. Hold the straps in a pulled-up position as you rest the bar on the fronts of your shoulders. Yes, we realize that back in chapter 4 we said we didn't like straps. They're okay in this case, however, because you use them just to make it easier to balance the weight, not to help lift it.

Overhead Squat
ADVANCED LEVEL

■ **START:** This exercise has a long learning curve: It requires a lot of balance as well as tremendous strength and flexibility in your back and shoulders. Before you try it with challenging weights, you may first want to try it with a broomstick, then a standard barbell (if you have one) or EZ-curl bar, then an unloaded Olympic bar. Press the bar overhead with a full, overhand grip that's slightly wider than shoulder width. Lock out your elbows, and pull your upper arms back so they're next to your ears. Set your feet shoulder-width apart with your knees slightly bent and your lower back in its naturally arched position.

◻ **FINISH:** Slowly descend until your thighs are parallel to the floor. Pause, then push back up to the starting position.

Hack Squat
ADVANCED LEVEL

■ **START:** This one is rough on your knees, so do it only occasionally or for short training cycles; avoid it entirely if you have a history of knee problems. Set the barbell on the floor behind a pair of large weight plates. Stand with your feet about shoulder-width apart and your heels up on the weight plates. Squat down, grab the bar with a shoulder-width, underhand grip, then stand up so the bar rests behind your hamstrings.

◻ **FINISH:** Descend toward the floor with your arms straight and your torso erect. Stop when the tops of your thighs are parallel to the floor and the bar is grazing your Achilles tendons. Pause, then return to the starting position.

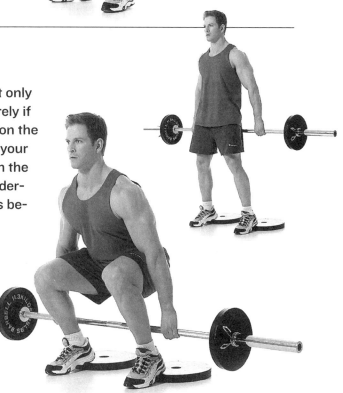

Split Squat
INTERMEDIATE-TO-ADVANCED LEVEL

■ **START:** Rest the barbell on your traps and stand with one foot 2½ to 3 feet in front of the other, each in line with its corresponding buttock.

□ **FINISH:** Keep your upper body erect as you descend until the top of your front thigh is parallel to the ground. Pause, then press back up to the starting position.

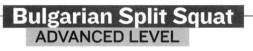

Bulgarian Split Squat
ADVANCED LEVEL

■ **START:** Rest a barbell on your traps and stand with the instep of one foot on a bench or sturdy stool 2½ to 3 feet behind you.

□ **FINISH:** Do a split squat, descending until the top of your front thigh is parallel to the floor. Pause, then push back up to the starting position.

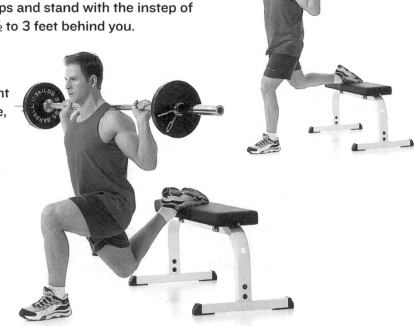

Jump Squat
ADVANCED LEVEL

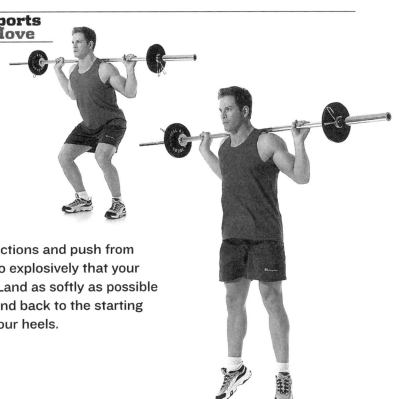

■ **START:** Use a light weight—perhaps one-third of what you'd work with on back squats—and go for speed and power. Stay away from this one if you've had back problems. Set up for a back squat with the barbell resting on your traps. Then squat down quickly until your thighs are at a 45-degree angle with the floor.

▢ **FINISH:** Immediately change directions and push from your calves to straighten your body so explosively that your feet come off the floor a few inches. Land as softly as possible on your toes, then immediately descend back to the starting position as you shift your weight to your heels.

Side Lunge
ADVANCED LEVEL

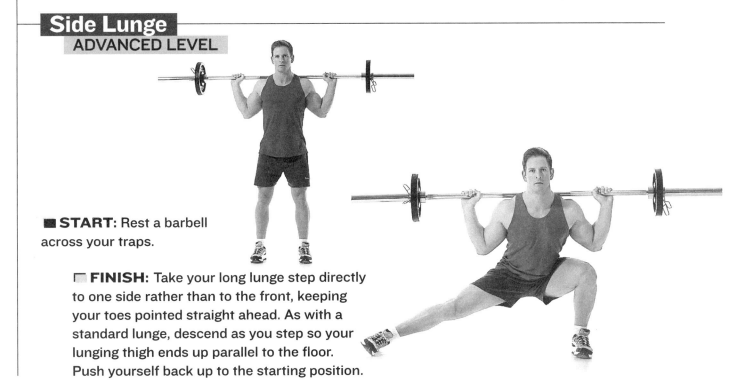

■ **START:** Rest a barbell across your traps.

▢ **FINISH:** Take your long lunge step directly to one side rather than to the front, keeping your toes pointed straight ahead. As with a standard lunge, descend as you step so your lunging thigh ends up parallel to the floor. Push yourself back up to the starting position.

HIP-DOMINANT EXERCISES

Reverse Lunge
BEGINNER LEVEL

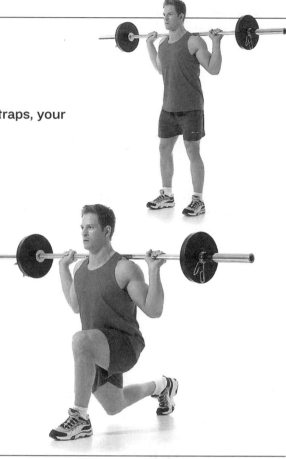

■ **START:** Stand with a barbell resting across your traps, your feet about hip-width apart.

☐ **FINISH:** With your nondominant leg, take a large lunging stride backward so that only the ball of that foot touches the floor. Simultaneously sit back into the lunge until your back knee is just an inch or two off the floor while your front leg is bent 90 degrees, thigh parallel to the floor and shin perpendicular. Push off from your front leg to return to the starting position.

Stepup
BEGINNER LEVEL

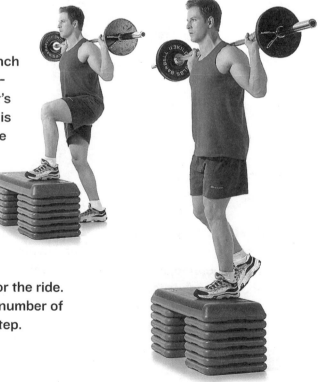

■ **START:** Stand in front of a sturdy step or bench with a barbell resting on your traps. Put your nondominant foot flat on the step—that's the leg that's going to do the work. Make sure your lower back is in its naturally arched position, your shoulders are pulled back, and your eyes face forward.

☐ **FINISH:** Push down through your working heel to lift your other leg and brush the step with that foot. Then return to the starting position. It's important to keep all your weight on your working foot—your other foot is just along for the ride. Finish the set, then switch and do the same number of repetitions with your dominant foot on the step.

BEGINNER VARIATION
Side Stepup

Stand to the side of the step and lift a foot onto it. Do your stepup laterally. This puts the emphasis on your outer-thigh and outer-gluteal muscles.

INTERMEDIATE VARIATIONS
Alternating Stepup

Start with both feet on the floor in front of the step. Step up with one foot, lower it, then step up with the other and lower it. That's one repetition. Don't underestimate the challenge to your balance and stamina with this variation—choose a light weight to start.

Crossover Stepup

Stand sideways to one side of a step with the barbell on your back. Step up with the foot that's farthest from the step, crossing that foot in front of your other leg. Push up with the crossing leg and just drag the other along for the ride. Then return to the starting position. When you finish all the reps with one leg, move to the other side of the step and step up and across with your other leg. Don't try this with a lot of weight until you're comfortable with the movement.

Cardio Stepup

Do the standard stepup, but step all the way on and all the way off the bench each time without pausing between reps. You'll use momentum and sacrifice strength gains, but you'll get that heart rate up.

Deadlift

INTERMEDIATE-TO-ADVANCED LEVEL

■ **START:** Load a barbell and set it on the floor. Squat in front of it with your feet shoulder-width apart. Grab it overhand with your hands just outside your legs, your shoulders over or just behind the bar, your arms straight, and your back flat or slightly arched. (Your exact position depends on your unique biomechanics.)

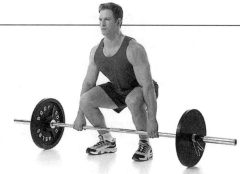

□ **FINISH:** Simple as it sounds, all you really do is stand up. The key is to push with your heels and pull the weight to your body as you stand. As you get better at the lift and use heavier weights, you'll develop tremendous strength and muscle mass on the back of your body—middle traps, lower back, gluteals, hamstrings. Pause with the weight (don't lean back), then slowly return to the starting position. Pause with the weight on the floor and reset your body over the bar. You defeat the purpose of the *dead*lift if you use momentum to knock out reps.

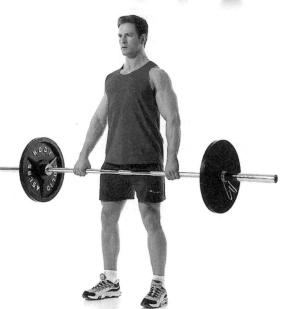

INTERMEDIATE-TO-ADVANCED VARIATION
Sumo Deadlift

Squat over the barbell with a stance that's wider than shoulder width, and turn your toes out at about a 45-degree angle. Use a shoulder-width grip as you perform a deadlift. The upright stance afforded by the foot position of this variation means you get less hip and more inner-thigh work.

ADVANCED VARIATIONS
Unilateral Deadlift

From the standard deadlift starting position, grab the bar with your nondominant hand and perform a deadlift, taking extra care to keep your shoulders and hips from leaning in one direction or the other. Return to the starting position. Finish the set with that side, then repeat with the other.

Suitcase Deadlift

Set the barbell lengthwise outside your nondominant foot, with the middle of the bar next to your leg. Grab it with your nondominant hand and perform a unilateral deadlift as described above. Keep your posture as upright as possible. Return to the starting position. Finish the set with that side, then repeat with the other.

Romanian Deadlift
INTERMEDIATE-TO-ADVANCED LEVEL

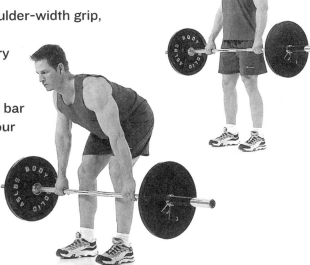

■ **START:** Grab the barbell with an overhand, shoulder-width grip, and stand holding it at arm's length in front of your thighs. Set your feet shoulder-width apart with a very slight bend in your knees. Pull your shoulders back.

▢ **FINISH:** Bend over at the hips to lower the bar down your legs, toward the floor. Stop when your torso is parallel to the floor or when you can't go lower without rounding your back. Pause, then push down with your heels to return to the starting position. Keep your knees bent at the same angle and your shoulder blades pulled back throughout.

ADVANCED VARIATIONS
Unilateral Romanian Deadlift

If your balance is good, increase the challenge by lifting your dominant foot a few inches off the floor and keeping it there as you do the movement with your nondominant leg. Finish the set with that side, then repeat with the other.

Snatch-Grip Romanian Deadlift

Widen your grip to twice shoulder width.

Good Morning
ADVANCED LEVEL

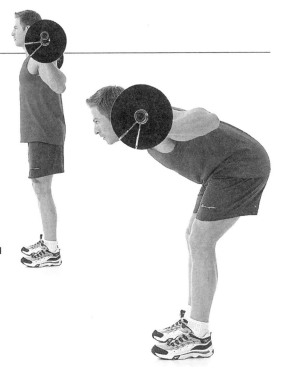

■ **START:** Stand holding a light barbell across your traps, and set up as you would for the back squat on page 191.

▢ **FINISH:** Lean forward from the hips until your torso is just about parallel to the floor—or until you can go no farther without losing the arch in your lower back. Push with your heels to straighten back up to the starting position.

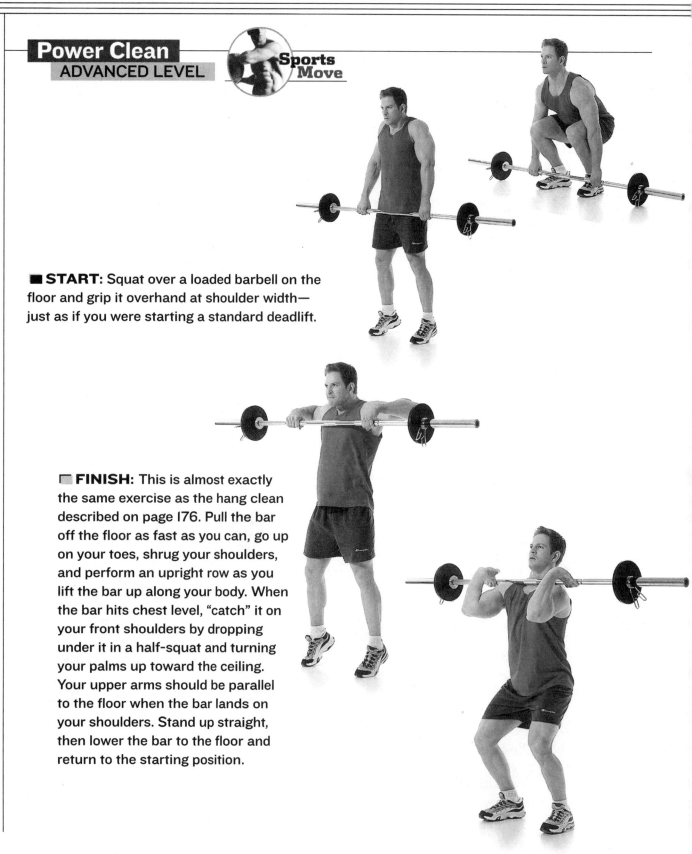

Power Clean
ADVANCED LEVEL

Sports Move

■ **START:** Squat over a loaded barbell on the floor and grip it overhand at shoulder width— just as if you were starting a standard deadlift.

▢ **FINISH:** This is almost exactly the same exercise as the hang clean described on page 176. Pull the bar off the floor as fast as you can, go up on your toes, shrug your shoulders, and perform an upright row as you lift the bar up along your body. When the bar hits chest level, "catch" it on your front shoulders by dropping under it in a half-squat and turning your palms up toward the ceiling. Your upper arms should be parallel to the floor when the bar lands on your shoulders. Stand up straight, then lower the bar to the floor and return to the starting position.

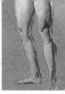

Muscle Snatch
ADVANCED LEVEL

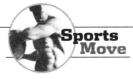

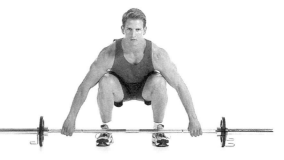

■ **START:** Use light weight for this one—it's a speed-and-technique move. Get in the same starting position as for the deadlift and power clean, but use a wide (twice shoulder-width) grip.

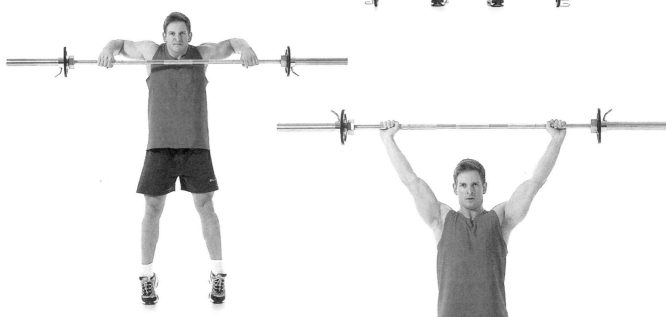

☐ **FINISH:** The first part of the lift is exactly like the power clean, using almost every muscle, from your calves to your traps, to move the bar up as fast as possible. Instead of "racking" the bar on your shoulders, as in a power clean, snap it overhead once it reaches chest level. Quickly return to the starting position.

Note: There are two differences between this exercise and the snatch used in Olympic weight lifting: First, you don't drop under the bar in a full squat to catch it. You can try it that way if you want, but it's very tough on your knees. It's also very hard to support a weight overhead in that position, as you learned if you tried the overhead squat described on page 193. The second difference is that in the muscle snatch you don't have to get the weight overhead with straight arms. It's okay to finish with a press, though that isn't allowed in Olympic lifting.

EXERCISES FOR THE CALVES

Seated Calf Raise
BEGINNER LEVEL

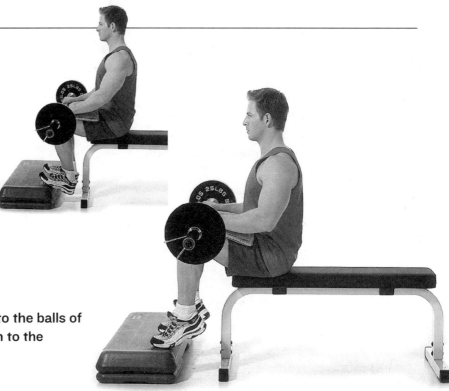

■ **START:** Sit at the end of a bench with the balls of your feet on a step, a wooden block, or a couple of phone books about a foot in front of you. Put a towel or sweatshirt over the tops of your knees and rest a barbell across them. Hold it there with your hands. With your torso erect, allow your heels to drop as low as they'll go.

◻ **FINISH:** Press back up to the balls of your feet. Pause, then return to the starting position.

Standing Calf Raise
ADVANCED LEVEL

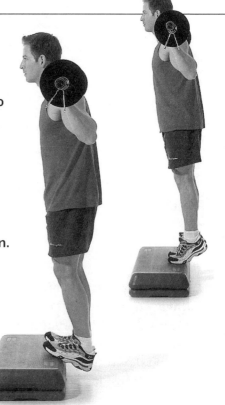

■ **START:** This one demands some balance since you have no free hand with which to steady yourself. Resting a light barbell across your traps, stand on a low step with your heels off the edge. Keep your knees straight (but not locked) and your torso erect as you rise on the balls of your feet as high as you can.

◻ **FINISH:** Lower your heels as far past the level of the step as possible. Pause, then return to the starting position.

CHAPTER 9

PULLEY FOR YOU: THE MOST VERSATILE UPGRADE

We won't yank you on this one: Serious muscle is built with barbells and dumbbells. We have yet to meet a successful athlete, strongman, or really well-built guy who did the majority of his construction work with cables or machines. That said, we should add that we know of few accomplished muscleheads who reached their goals using nothing but free weights. Anyone who has access to a cable system tends to use it.

Here are a few reasons why: First, cables offer a versatility that you usually sacrifice when opting for a machine over free weights. With cables, you can do more exercises, at more angles, with more variations than with any other form of resistance. We'll show you more than 50 exercises (not to mention variations on those exercises, which we didn't bother counting) that you can do on any home cable-machine setup. And we could've shown you at least 50 more.

A second benefit of a cable system is constant tension. You may think you get enough of that from your job, wife, and kids, but that's not the kind of tension we're talking about. Say you're doing a dumbbell fly: You have lots of tension on your muscles in the first two-thirds of the movement, when you're moving the weights against gravity. In the last part of the exercise, you're moving the weights horizontally, so gravity couldn't care less. At the top of the movement, with the weights over your chest, you're resting. Not so with a cable system: At the top of a movement, the tension remains high, so your muscles work hard through the entire range of motion.

The third plus is safety and function. Injuries are a real concern with barbells, a bit less of a problem with dumbbells, and no problem at all with cables. If you do get hurt while using free weights, cable exercises are sensible and highly recommended rehabilitation tools. They allow for multi-dimensional ranges of motion that are easy on your joints and as tough as you want them to be on your muscles.

Not a bad set of benefits for a simple system based on moving a cable around a pulley to elevate a stack of metal plates. And not bad at all for a relatively modest piece of home gym equipment that usually takes up fewer cubic feet than Dennis Rodman's stereo speakers.

Now for the inconveniences: Cable exercises work better for some body parts than others. They're great for your upper back, for example, which is why the strongest lifters in the world add cable exercises to their workouts. Cables provide an unending smorgasbord of exercises for your shoulders and arms, along with some of our favorite abdominal moves. Unfortunately, it's nearly impossible to get a challenging chest or quadriceps workout with cables. And though you can do some

interesting exercises for your gluteals, hamstrings, and lower back, they fall into the category of supplemental, rather than main-event, movements.

What the heck, you can't have it all. (Actually, you can—but that's the subject of chapter 11.)

While most of the exercises in this chapter involve a simple cable system that allows you to use a high or low pulley, we couldn't resist the temptation to throw in some exercises using a cable-crossover apparatus. We love crossover machines with a passion that sometimes disturbs us. (Our therapist is helping us work through it.) We do realize that few of you will be able to outfit your home gyms with two towers standing about $9\frac{1}{2}$ feet apart, so we included the unilateral versions of those crossover movements, just to keep it fair.

Finally, we assume you have a variety of handles for your cable system: a long straight bar (for lat pulldowns and wide-grip rows), a shorter straight bar, a straight bar with vertical handles (for wide neutral grips), a triangle handle (for narrow neutral grips), a rope handle, an EZ-curl bar, and one or more stirrup handles (the ones shaped like the letter *D*). Some of the exercises require a flat bench. And a pair of ankle straps is a worthwhile extra. One big tip applies to all cable exercises: Make sure there's tension on your muscles before you start a set or repetition. That means you may have to adjust your stance a foot or two one way or another at the start to make sure there's no slack in the cable (or cables, if you're lucky enough to have a crossover. Did we mention how much we love those things?).

MIDSECTION

What these exercises lack in number they make up for in quality. They're fun, they're challenging, and they hit your abs in ways they've never been hit. Again, we suggest that beginners start with the body-weight exercises in chapter 6. Intermediate and advanced lifters should choose one move for the rectus abdominis and one for the obliques, doing 2 or 3 sets of 10 to 12 reps per exercise.

EXERCISES FOR THE RECTUS ABDOMINIS

Lying Cable Crunch
INTERMEDIATE LEVEL

■ **START:** Attach a rope handle to the low pulley. Lie on the floor with your head near the low pulley, your knees bent, and your feet flat on the floor. Hold the handle over your chest so the crotch (where it splits off from one rope into two) is at the base of your neck.

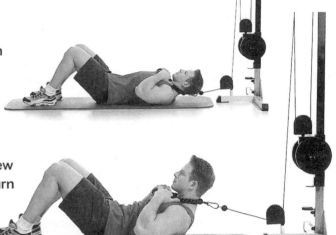

▢ **FINISH:** Crunch your rib cage toward your pelvis, lifting your shoulder blades a few inches off the floor. Pause, then slowly return to the starting position.

Standing Cable Crunch
INTERMEDIATE LEVEL

■ **START:** Attach a rope handle to the high pulley. Stand with your back to the pulley, and hold one leg of the handle on top of each shoulder. Set your feet shoulder-width apart, with your knees bent slightly.

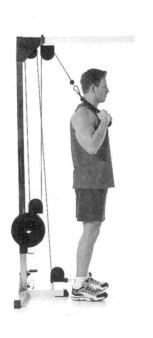

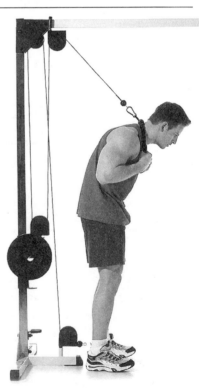

▢ **FINISH:** Bend forward at the waist, rounding your back and aiming your chest toward your pelvis. Keep the ropes in a fixed position relative to your shoulders throughout. There's no benefit to pulling the rope down farther with your arms. Pause in the lowest position possible, then slowly return to the starting position.

VARIATION
Twisting Cable Crunch

Same movement, but twist at the waist and move your nondominant shoulder toward your opposite knee. Pause, return to the starting position, then lower your other shoulder toward its opposite knee. That's I repetition. You can also combine the straight-down and twisting movements in I set.

Kneeling Cable Crunch
INTERMEDIATE LEVEL

■ **START:** Attach the rope handle to the high pulley. Face the machine, grab the ropes, and kneel in front of the weight stack with your buttocks near your heels but not resting on them. Hold the ropes at the sides of your face with your elbows pointing straight down to the floor.

□ **FINISH:** Crunch your rib cage toward your pelvis without moving any other part of your lower body from its original position. Pause when your elbows approach your knees, then slowly return to the starting position.

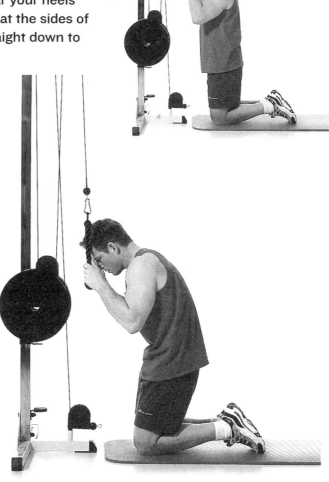

VARIATION
Twisting Kneeling Cable Crunch

Same movement, but twist at the waist and bring your nondominant shoulder toward the opposite knee. Pause, straighten, then lower your other shoulder toward its opposite knee. That's I repetition. You can also combine the straight-down and twisting movements in the same set.

Reverse Cable Crunch
INTERMEDIATE LEVEL

■ **START:** Loop the ankle straps around your ankles, face the weight stack, and attach the straps to the low pulley. Lie on the floor with your feet closer to the weight stack. Lift your feet off the floor so your legs form 90-degree angles at the hips and knees. Lay your arms on the floor at your sides, palms down.

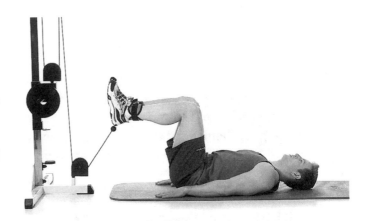

☐ **FINISH:** Slowly roll your hips up until your knees come within a few inches of your chest. Pause, then slowly return to the starting position. A good way to develop a feel for this exercise is to imagine a bucket of water glued to your pelvis. Try to empty the bucket onto your chest. When you have it right, your tailbone will rise just a few inches off the floor. That's how you'll know your abs are doing all the work.

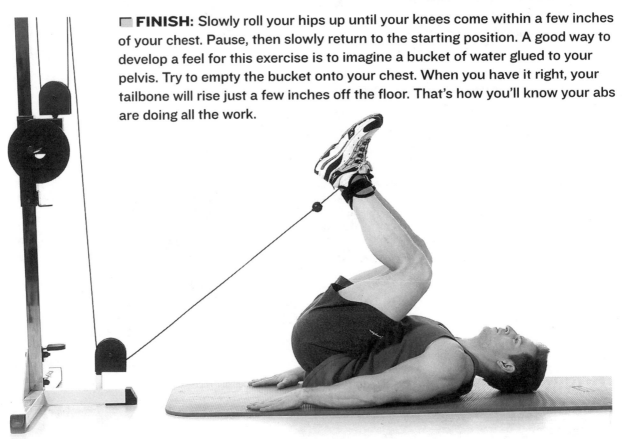

Kneeling Three-Way Cable Crunch
ADVANCED LEVEL

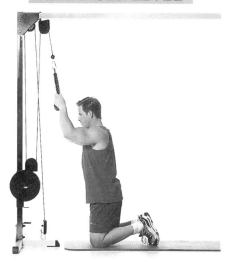
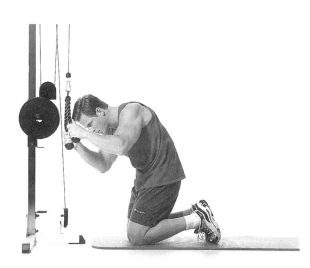

■ **START:** Attach a rope handle to the high pulley. Kneel facing the pulley, and grab the ends of the rope with your palms facing each other. Hold the pulley in front of your face with your elbows slightly bent.

☐ **FINISH:** Bend forward at the waist, rounding your back and aiming your chest at your pelvis. Stop when you feel a full contraction in your abdominal muscles. Return to the starting position, then repeat the movement, this time aiming your chest toward your left knee. Stop when you feel a full contraction in your left obliques. Return, then repeat the movement to your right. That's I repetition.

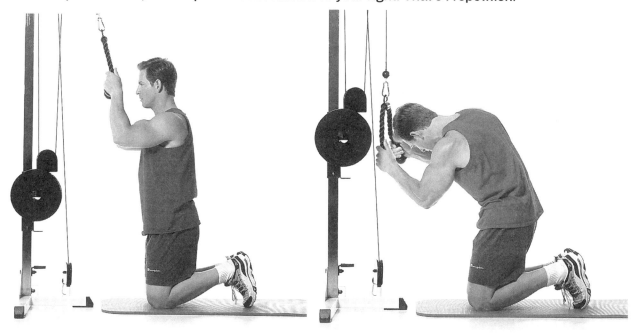

Barbell Cable Rollout
ADVANCED LEVEL

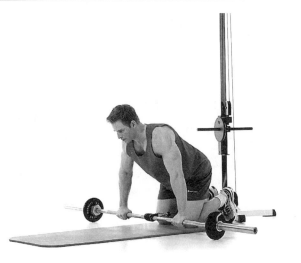

■ **START:** Put an ankle strap around the middle of a barbell and attach it to the low pulley. Select a light cable weight. Kneel on an exercise mat with your back to the weight stack and the cable between your legs. Grab the bar with an overhand, shoulder-width grip.

▢ **FINISH:** Roll the bar away from you and follow it with straight arms as far forward as you can go, then roll it back. The cable helps you pull the weight back but adds resistance to the negative portion of the exercise, providing a new challenge for your muscles. For variety, try it to the other way: Kneel on the opposite side of the bar, facing the weight stack, so you have resistance pulling it toward you but none rolling it out.

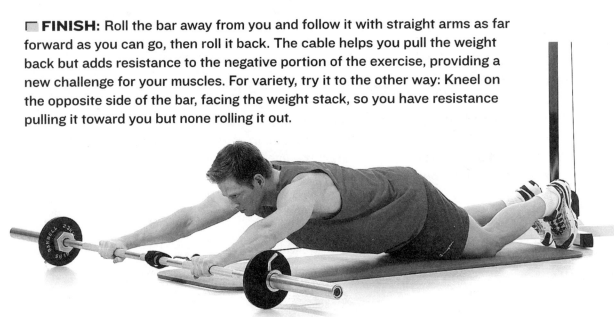

EXERCISES FOR THE OBLIQUES

Standing Oblique Crunch
INTERMEDIATE LEVEL

■ START: Attach a stirrup handle to the high cable and stand sideways to the weight stack. Grab the handle with your inside hand and pull it down so your palm is in line with your head and your elbow points straight down.

▢ FINISH: Crunch your rib cage sideways toward your hip bone on the same side as the arm holding the pulley, keeping your hand in the same position relative to your head. Pause, then slowly straighten your back. Finish the repetitions on that side, then repeat with your opposite side toward the weight stack.

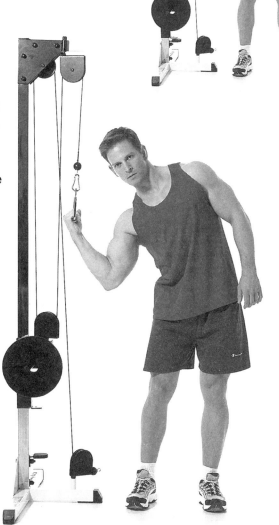

High Woodchopper
ADVANCED LEVEL

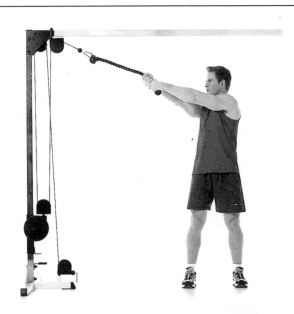

■ **START:** Attach a rope handle to the high cable. Grab the rope with a hand-over-hand grip, and stand sideways, about 3 feet from the weight stack. Hold the rope over your inside shoulder, as if it were an ax you were about to swing.

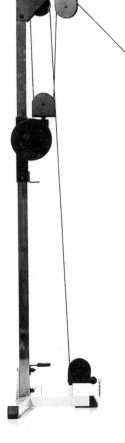

▢ **FINISH:** Bend and twist at the waist, bringing your hands down and across your torso so they end up on the far side of your outside calf. Let your feet pivot slightly with the movement, to protect your knees. Pause at the bottom, then slowly straighten back to the starting position. Finish the reps on that side, then repeat with your opposite side toward the weight stack.

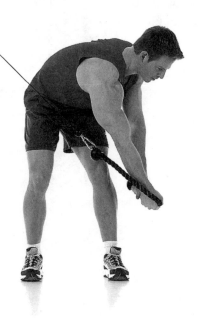

Low Woodchopper
ADVANCED LEVEL

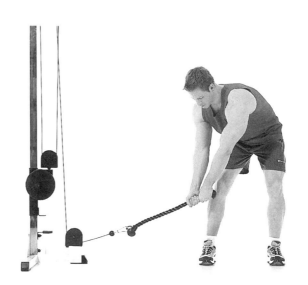

■ START: Attach the rope handle to the low cable. Grab the rope with a hand-over-hand grip, and stand sideways, about 3 feet from the weight stack. Hold the rope just outside the thigh nearest the weight stack. Bend your knees and keep your chest up.

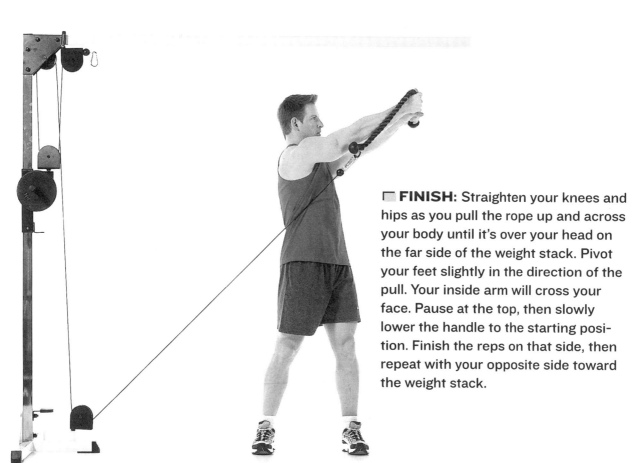

□ FINISH: Straighten your knees and hips as you pull the rope up and across your body until it's over your head on the far side of the weight stack. Pivot your feet slightly in the direction of the pull. Your inside arm will cross your face. Pause at the top, then slowly lower the handle to the starting position. Finish the reps on that side, then repeat with your opposite side toward the weight stack.

CHEST AND UPPER BACK

Beginners should do 1 or 2 sets of 10 to 12 reps of one fly or crossover, one pulldown, and one row. It wouldn't hurt to add a set or two of pushups, since cable chest exercises aren't the best for building muscle and strength.

Intermediate and advanced lifters can do 2 or 3 sets of 8 to 10 reps of a press, fly, or crossover movement, one pulldown, one row, and one rear lateral exercise. Add a dip or advanced pushup variation from chapter 6 to help hit your chest.

BEGINNER

CHEST
- Unilateral high cable fly ------------------(page 215)
- Staggered unilateral high cable fly ---------(page 215)
- Standing high cable crossover -------(page 216)

UPPER BACK
- Lat pulldown ------(page 223)
- Supinated lat pulldown ------------------(page 224)
- Neutral-grip lat pulldown ------------------(page 224)
- Supinated cable row -------------(page 226)
- Neutral-grip pronated cable row --------(page 227)
- Close-grip pronated cable row -------(page 227)

INTERMEDIATE

CHEST
- Chest-level standing high cable crossover --------------------(page 216)
- Unilateral low cable fly ---------(page 217)
- Standing low cable crossover -----(page 218)
- Cable fly ----------------------(page 219)
- Incline cable fly -----------------(page 219)
- Decline cable fly ----------------(page 219)
- Swiss-ball cable fly ------------(page 220)
- Swiss-ball incline cable fly -------(page 220)
- Swiss-ball decline cable fly ------(page 221)

UPPER BACK
- Wide-grip lat pulldown ----------(page 224)
- Mixed-grip lat pulldown ---------(page 224)
- Unilateral lat pulldown ----------(page 224)
- Behind-the-neck lat pulldown ----(page 224)
- Double pulldown ----------------(page 225)
- Pronated cable row ------------(page 227)
- Wide-grip pronated cable row ----(page 227)
- Rope-handle pronated cable row -(page 227)
- Unilateral cable row -----------(page 228)
- Neutral-grip unilateral cable row -(page 228)
- Supinated-grip unilateral cable row --------------------(page 228)
- Standing unilateral high row -----(page 229)
- Bent-over row -----------------(page 230)
- Standing pullover ---------------(page 231)
- Bent-over rear lateral raise ------(page 232)
- Unilateral bent-over rear lateral raise ------------------(page 232)
- Standing rear lateral raise ------(page 233)
- Unilateral standing rear lateral raise -----------------(page 233)
- Lying pullover ------------------(page 234)

ADVANCED

CHEST
- Swiss-ball unilateral cable fly ----------(page 221)
- Dumbbell cable press -------------(page 222)

UPPER BACK
- Incline lying pullover ----------(page 234)

EXERCISES FOR THE CHEST

Unilateral High Cable Fly
BEGINNER LEVEL

■ **START:** Attach a stirrup handle to the high pulley and stand sideways to the weight stack. Grab the handle with your inside hand. Take a couple steps away from the stack and perhaps a step back; you want to start with tension in the cable so there's resistance throughout the movement. Pull your shoulders back, and place your free hand on your hip. Keep a slight bend in your working elbow.

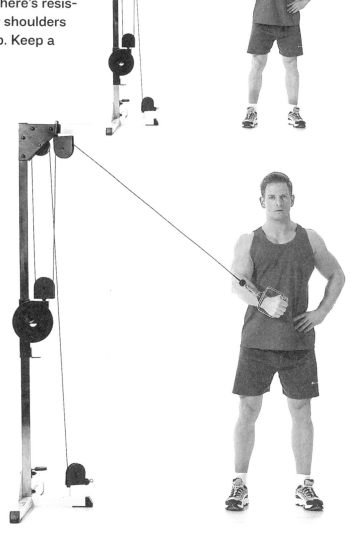

□ **FINISH:** Bring the cable handle down and across your body in a wide, arcing motion, without changing the angle in your elbow. Stop before your working shoulder pulls forward (at about the midpoint of your body)—you want your shoulders and hips to stay in the same position throughout. Pause, then slowly return to the starting position. Finish the reps with that arm, then turn around and repeat with the other.

VARIATION
Staggered Unilateral High Cable Fly

For better balance, stand with the foot that's farthest from the weight stack slightly in front of the foot that's closer. Then bend your forward leg. It also helps to use your free hand to hold the opposite thigh.

Standing High Cable Crossover
BEGINNER LEVEL

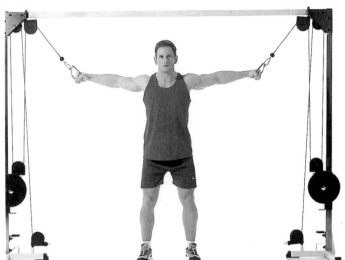

■ **START:** This is the bilateral version of the unilateral high cable fly. Attach stirrup handles to both high pulleys, and follow the same setup as for the unilateral version. Take special care to pull back your shoulder blades and keep your elbows slightly bent.

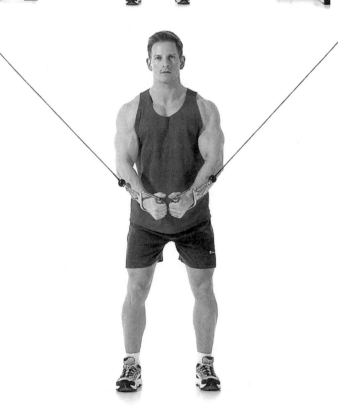

□ **FINISH:** Pull the handles down in a wide arc in front of your body until your hands meet about a foot or so in front of your midsection. Pause, squeeze your pecs together, then slowly return to the starting position.

INTERMEDIATE VARIATION
Chest-Level Standing High Cable Crossover

As you pull, keep your hands higher so they finish in front of your chest instead of your midsection. This takes the emphasis off your lower chest and spreads it over the entire pectoralis major.

Unilateral Low Cable Fly
INTERMEDIATE LEVEL

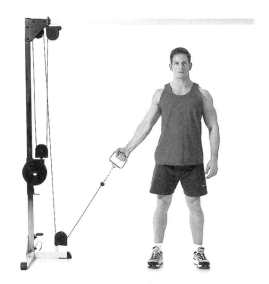

■ **START:** Attach a stirrup handle to the low pulley, then set up as you would for the unilateral high cable fly.

◻ **FINISH:** Without increasing the bend in your elbow, bring the handle up and across your body in a wide arc until your working hand is in front of the opposite cheek. Then lower to the starting position.

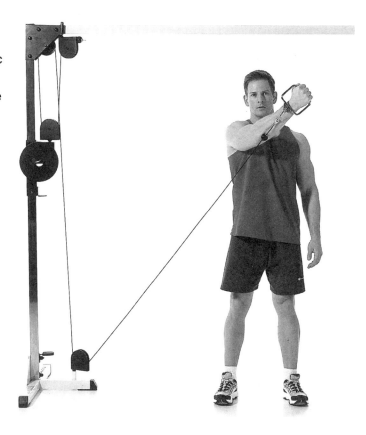

Standing Low Cable Crossover
INTERMEDIATE LEVEL

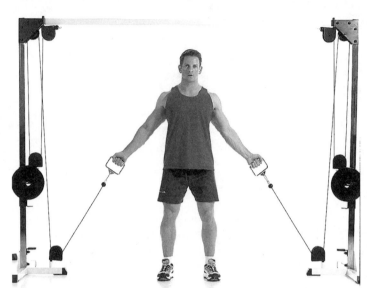

■ **START:** Here's the bilateral version of the low cable fly. Attach the stirrup handles to the low pulleys, and setup as for the low fly.

▢ **FINISH:** Bring your hands up in a wide arc until they're in front of your face. Squeeze your pecs together, then slowly return to the starting position.

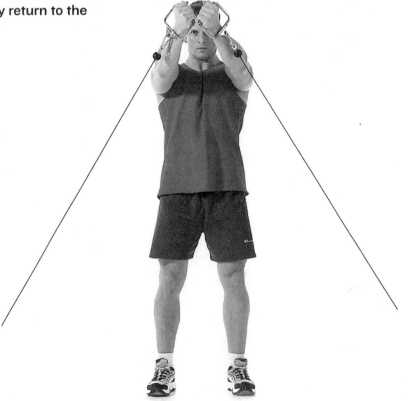

Cable Fly
INTERMEDIATE LEVEL

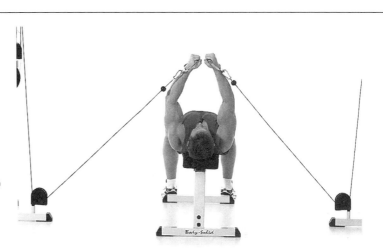

■ **START:** Attach stirrup handles to the low pulleys of a cable-crossover machine. Put a bench between the columns and lie on it. Grab the handles and hold them directly over the middle of your chest, with just a slight bend in your elbows.

▢ **FINISH:** Lower your arms down and back toward your ears until your elbows are about even with the bench. Pause before bringing the handles up in a wide, arcing motion.

VARIATIONS
Incline Cable Fly

To move emphasis to your upper pecs, use an incline bench, starting and finishing with the handles over your upper chest or collarbone.

Decline Cable Fly

To move emphasis to your lower pecs, use a decline bench, starting and finishing with the handles over your lower chest.

Cable Fly

VARIATIONS

Swiss-Ball Cable Fly

Place a Swiss ball between the columns of the crossover station, grab the low-cable stirrup handles, then lie on the ball with only your shoulder blades touching it. Your knees should be bent 90 degrees, and your torso and thighs should be parallel to the floor. Then do a standard cable fly.

Swiss-Ball Incline Cable Fly

Start with your head and neck raised off the ball and your back completely in contact with it so that your back is slightly arched. Keep your feet flat on the floor, and bend your knees as you lower your hips until you're simulating the incline-bench position. You're ready to fly.

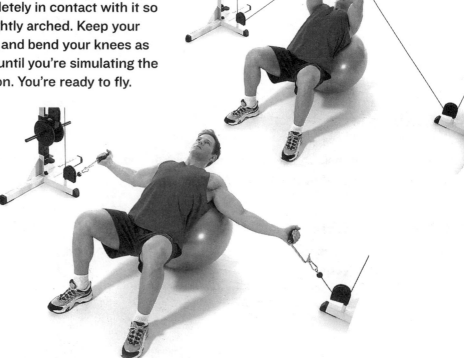

Swiss-Ball Decline Cable Fly

Hook your insteps beneath some heavy dumbbells on the floor as you lie far enough back on the ball that your chest is slightly lower than your hips. Keep your back flat and your neck in line with your spine. Then do the decline-fly variation.

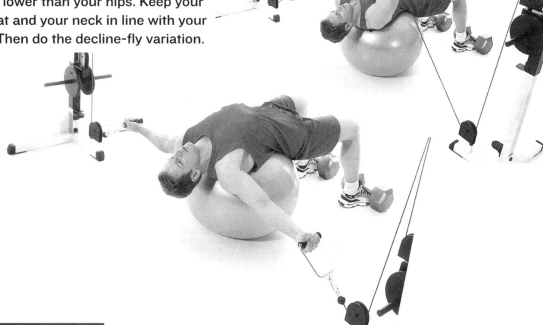

ADVANCED VARIATION
Swiss-Ball Unilateral Cable Fly

Place the ball in front of a stirrup handle attached to the low pulley. Position yourself sideways to the weight stack and lie on the ball, getting into either the flat position pictured on the opposite page, or the incline or decline variations just described. Grab the handle with your inside hand, and hold your outside thigh with your outside hand for stability. Then do a standard cable fly with your working arm, taking care not to turn on the ball to help get the weight moving.

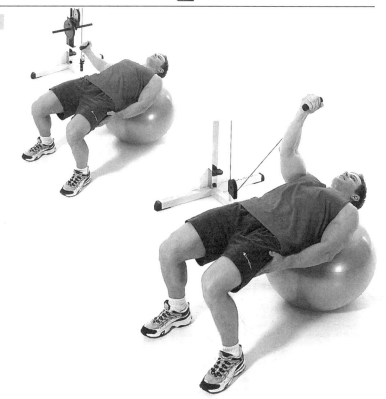

Dumbbell Cable Press
ADVANCED LEVEL

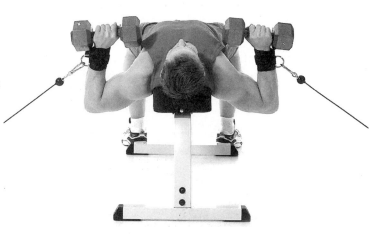

■ **START:** You need ankle straps, dumbbells, a cable-crossover machine, a bench, and a little bit of patience as you get yourself into position. (Besides that, it's a snap.) Put the bench between the pulleys. Select fairly light weights on the stacks. Fasten the straps to your wrists, hook the straps to the low pulleys, pick up two light to moderate dumbbells, lie on the bench, and hold the dumbbells at the sides of your chest.

□ **FINISH:** Execute a standard dumbbell press, as described on page 122. The extra challenge, of course, is the simultaneous vertical resistance from the dumbbells and horizontal resistance from the cables. Pause, then slowly lower the weights to the starting position.

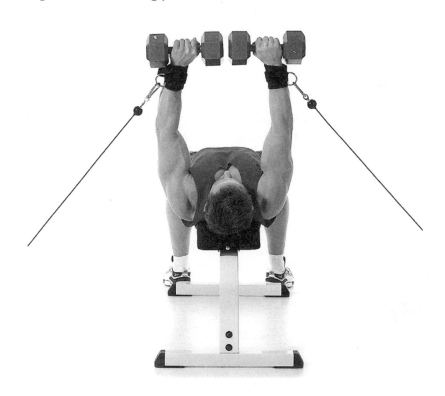

EXERCISES FOR THE UPPER BACK

Lat Pulldown
BEGINNER LEVEL

■ **START:** Attach the long straight bar to the high cable and slide a bench underneath it. Sit on the bench, and grab the bar with a false (thumb on the same side as your fingers), overhand, shoulder-width grip. Keep your arms straight and your torso upright or leaning back slightly.

▢ **FINISH:** Pull your shoulder blades together and down, stick your chest out, and pull the bar to your chest. Pause with the bar an inch or two off your chest, then slowly let it rise to the starting position. Keep your chest out.

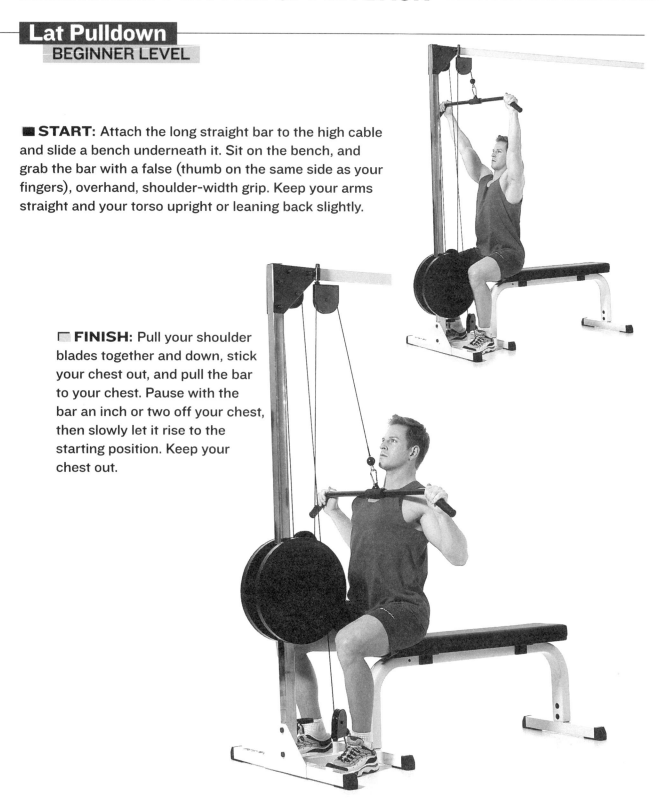

Lat Pulldown

BEGINNER VARIATION
Supinated Lat Pulldown

A false underhand grip results in the easiest pulldown because the best angle of pull for your biceps. The closer your hands are to each other, the more the biceps are involved.

BEGINNER-TO-INTERMEDIATE VARIATION
Neutral-Grip Lat Pulldown

Use either of the neutral-grip handles (the straight bar with vertical handles, or the triangle handle) to put your arms in a stronger position. While you'll be able to use more weight, remember that your arms bear some of that extra weight. When you use the narrow grip, your chest also does some of the work. Keep in mind the extra muscle involvement, and don't make these neutral-grip movements the only back exercises you do.

INTERMEDIATE VARIATIONS
Wide-Grip Lat Pulldown

A wider-than-shoulder-width false grip cuts your range of motion slightly but helps you feel the exercise more in your lats and less in your arms.

Mixed-Grip Lat Pulldown

Just like it sounds: one hand over the bar, one under. The only advantage is the spice of variety.

Unilateral Lat Pulldown

Use a stirrup handle to do your pulldowns one hand at a time. The movement will be more of an arc.

INTERMEDIATE-TO-ADVANCED VARIATION
Behind-the-Neck Lat Pulldown

This has been a "thou shalt not" exercise for so many years that, in many gyms, the pulldown stations are set up for pulldowns to the front only, so you can't do a behind-the-neck pulldown unless you contort your neck. At home, however, it's easier to position your bench so you get a straight angle of pull from the bar to the back of your neck without flexing your neck forward. Even at home, you still have to take precautions, particularly if you have limited shoulder-joint flexibility. Our advice: If you can do this exercise with good posture and no discomfort in your shoulder joints, it's a good one to work into the mix.

Double Pulldown
INTERMEDIATE LEVEL

■**START:** Attach the stirrup handles to the high pulleys of the crossover machine. Grab a handle with each hand (palms facing forward) and kneel between the two stations so that your arms and body form the letter Y. (We apologize for any disco flashbacks this may induce.) Pull your shoulders back and push your chest forward.

▢**FINISH:** Pull the handles down until your upper arms meet your torso. Pause, then slowly return to the starting position.

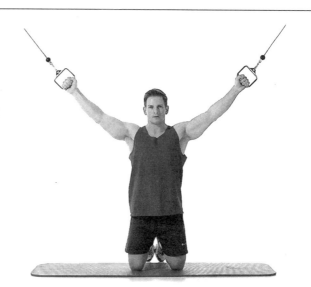

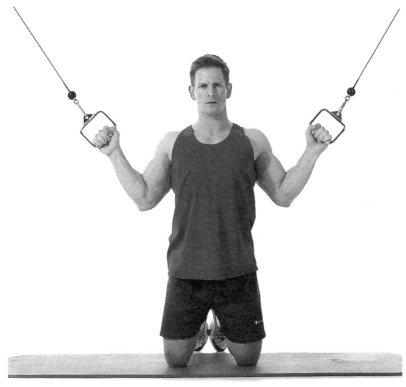

Supinated Cable Row
BEGINNER LEVEL

■ **START:** Attach a short straight bar to the low pulley and grab it with a false, underhand (supinated) grip that's shoulder-width or narrower. Sit on the floor about 2½ feet in front of the pulley, with your arms straight, knees bent, feet flat on the floor, and torso erect.

▢ **FINISH:** Pull the bar to your waist, keeping your elbows close to your torso. The movement is easier than the pronated (overhand) version because your biceps are in a stronger position and pull more of the load.

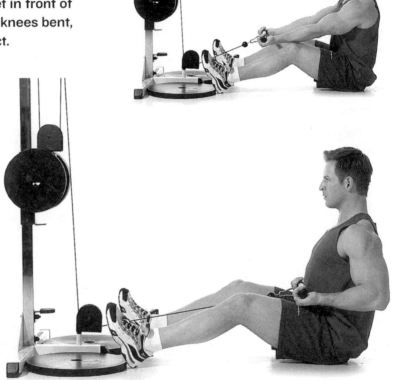

Pronated Cable Row
INTERMEDIATE LEVEL

■ **START:** Attach a short straight bar to the low pulley, and set a pair of 45-pound weight plates on the floor to either side of the pulley. Grab the bar with a false, overhand, shoulder-width grip. Sit on the floor about 2½ feet in front of the low pulley, with your arms straight, your feet braced against the weight plates, and your torso erect.

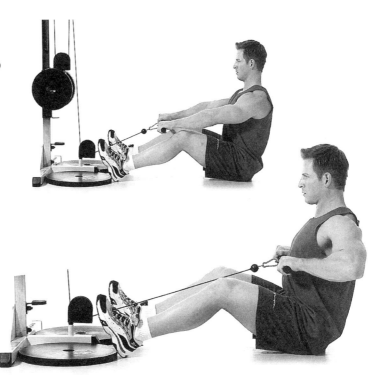

▢ **FINISH:** Start the movement by pinching your shoulder blades together in back, then pull the bar to the lower part of your sternum. Keep your elbows up. Pause, then slowly return to the starting position.

BEGINNER VARIATIONS
Neutral-Grip Pronated Cable Row

Use the straight bar with vertical handles at each end.

Close-Grip Pronated Cable Row

Let your elbows brush past your rib cage as you pull the bar to your abdomen. The more belly you have, the shorter your range of motion on this one.

INTERMEDIATE VARIATIONS
Wide-Grip Pronated Cable Row

Use a wider grip (you may need a longer bar to do it) to shorten your range of motion, shifting more work to your lats and taking some from your arms.

Rope-Handle Pronated Cable Row

Use the rope handle instead of a straight bar, and pull the handle to your neck instead of your sternum. This shifts work to your rear delts and upper traps.

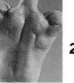

Unilateral Cable Row
INTERMEDIATE LEVEL

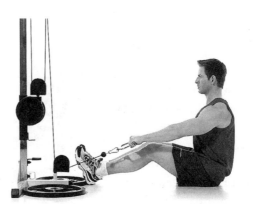

■ **START:** Attach a stirrup handle to the low pulley. Grab it overhand with your non-dominant hand and sit in the same position as for the supinated and pronated cable rows. Place your free hand on your thigh or on the floor next to you for balance.

☐ **FINISH:** Pull the handle to the lower side of your rib cage, keeping your elbow out away from your body and your torso stationary. Pause, then slowly return to the starting position. Finish the set with that arm before repeating with the other arm.

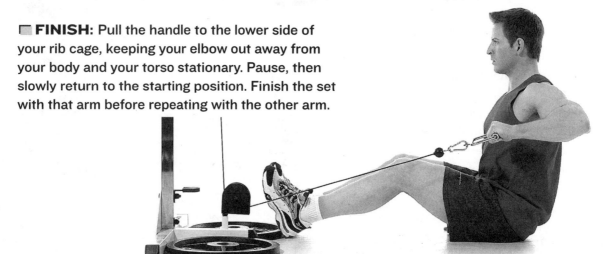

VARIATIONS

Neutral-Grip Unilateral Cable Row

Hold the handle so your palm faces sideways. Your elbow will be between your shoulder and waist as you pull back the handle.

Supinated-Grip Unilateral Cable Row

Hold the handle underhand, and keep your elbow close to your rib cage as you pull back the handle.

Standing Unilateral High Row
INTERMEDIATE LEVEL

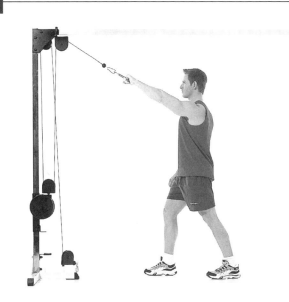

■ **START:** Attach a stirrup handle to the high pulley. With your nondominant hand, grab the handle with an overhand grip. Face the weight stack with your opposite leg slightly bent and a foot or two in front of your nondominant leg. Position yourself so your working arm and the cable form a straight line.

□ **FINISH:** Pull the handle straight down and back until the it reaches your chest and your elbow is behind your torso. Pause, then slowly re-turn to the starting position. Finish the set with that arm, then repeat with the other.

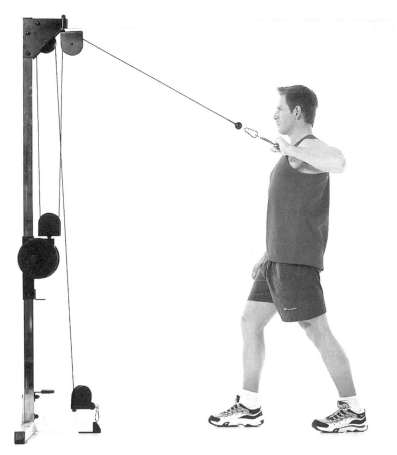

Bent-Over Row
INTERMEDIATE LEVEL

■ **START:** Attach the short straight bar to the low pulley. Face the weight stack and grab the bar with an underhand grip. Stand about 2 feet from the weight stack and bend over about 45 degrees at the hips, keeping your lower back slightly arched and your knees bent.

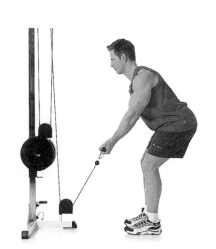

□ **FINISH:** Pinch your shoulder blades together behind you, then pull the bar up toward your abdomen until the base of your hands make contact with your torso. Keep your elbows close to your sides. Pause, then return to the starting position.

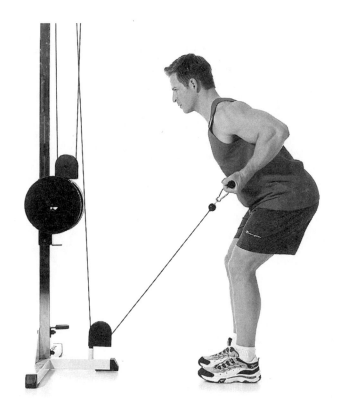

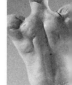

Standing Pullover
INTERMEDIATE LEVEL

■ **START:** Attach the rope handle to the high pulley. Grab the ends of the rope and stand facing the weight stack, 3 to 3½ feet in front of it. Bend forward at the hips about 45 degrees, with your lower back slightly arched and your knees bent. Your upper arms should be along-side your ears and straight.

◻ **FINISH:** Pull the handles down in a smooth, arcing motion until they touch your thighs. Keep your arms straight and the rest of your body in the same posi-tion. Pause, then slowly return to the starting position.

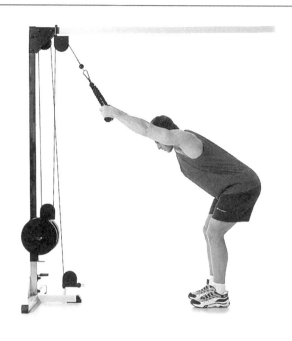

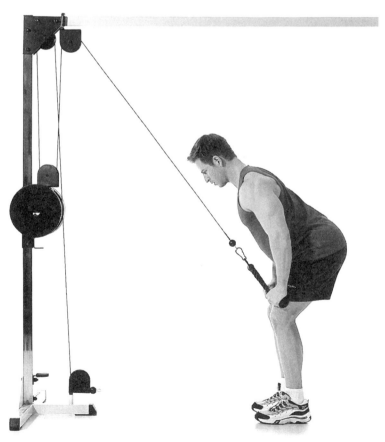

Bent-Over Rear Lateral Raise
INTERMEDIATE LEVEL

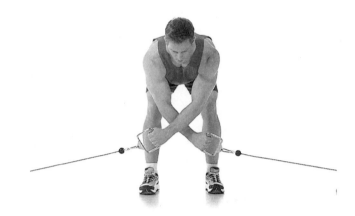

■ **START:** Attach the stirrup handles to the low pulleys of the cable-crossover machine. Grab the handles with a crossover grip—left hand holding the handle from the right-side column, right hand holding the left-side cable. Stand in the middle with your torso bent forward almost parallel to the floor. Hold the handles down directly beneath your shoulders. Keep your back slightly arched and your elbows slightly bent.

▢ **FINISH:** Pull the handles up in a wide arc until your upper arms are parallel to the floor. Keep the same bend in your elbows as you work—no increase, no decrease. Pause, then slowly lower the handles to the starting position.

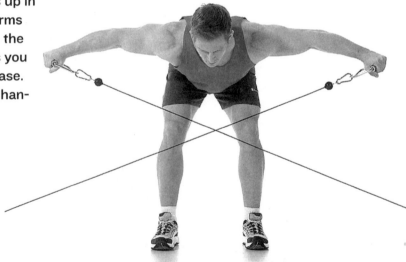

VARIATION
Unilateral Bent-Over Rear Lateral Raise

If you don't have a crossover machine, you can do this one side at a time by assuming the bent-over position sideways to the single-pulley station.

Standing Rear Lateral Raise
INTERMEDIATE LEVEL

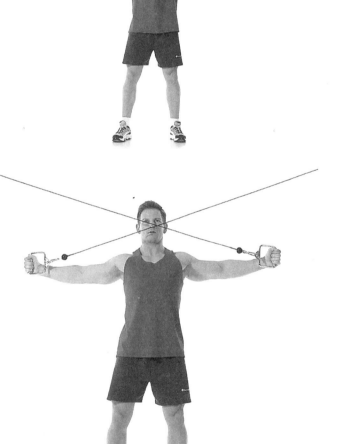

■ **START:** Attach the stirrup handles to the high pulleys of the crossover machine. Stand between the stacks and hold the handles with a crossover grip. Stretch out your arms in front of your face and slightly bend your elbows.

▢ **FINISH:** Pinch your shoulder blades back together, then pull the handles back until your palms face forward at shoulder level and your arms are even with your torso. Pause, then slowly return to the starting position.

VARIATION
Unilateral Standing Rear Lateral Raise

Do this one side at a time by standing sideways at the weight stack and pulling the handle across your body.

Lying Pullover
INTERMEDIATE-TO-ADVANCED LEVEL

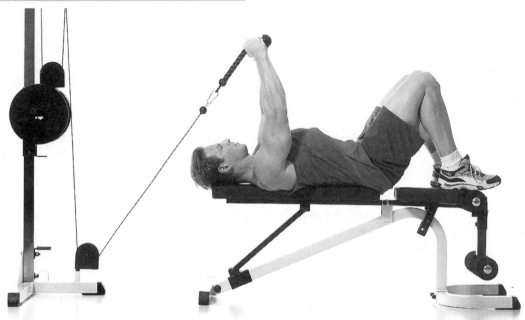

■**START:** Attach the rope handle to the low pulley. Set one end of your bench about 2 feet from the pulley—the cable, when extended, should bisect the bench lengthwise. Lie on the bench with your head at the end near the pulley. Reach behind you, grab the ends of the rope with your palms facing each other, and hold the rope over your chest at arm's length or with a slight bend in your elbows. (You may need to pull the bench out farther to keep the cable from parting your hair, if you have any; scraping your skull, if you don't.) Put your feet up on the bench to keep your lower back from arching.

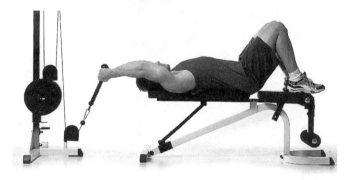

▢ **FINISH:** Without bending your elbows beyond their starting angle, slowly lower the handles behind your head until your arms are parallel to the floor. Pause, then return to the starting position.

ADVANCED VARIATION
Incline Lying Pullover

Set the bench at a slight incline—15 to 30 degrees. When you lower your arms behind your head, stop when they're at a 45-degree angle to the floor.

SHOULDERS AND ARMS

For a complete shoulders-and-arms workout, beginners should do 1 or 2 sets of 10 to 15 reps of one trapezius exercise (such as the upright row or cable shrug), one shoulder-isolation movement (lateral raise), one external rotation, one triceps pushdown, and a biceps curl.

Intermediate and advanced guys should do the same exercises, adding a triceps extension and reverse-grip or neutral-grip curl (such as the rope curl). Do 2 or 3 sets of 8 to 10 reps per exercise. Advanced lifters using heavier weights can cut down the reps to 6 to 10.

As in the barbell workout, whatever your skill level, you may do one forearm exercise if you like.

EXERCISES FOR THE SHOULDERS

Upright Row
BEGINNER LEVEL

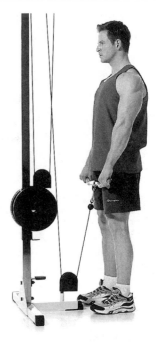

■ **START:** Attach an EZ-curl bar to the low cable. (A straight bar is okay, although it's not as easy on your wrists). Stand facing the weight stack, about a foot in front of it. Grab the bar with an overhand, shoulder-width grip, and hold it at arm's length, in front of your thighs.

▢ **FINISH:** Pull the bar up until your upper arms are parallel to the floor (no higher). Pause, then slowly lower the bar back to the starting position.

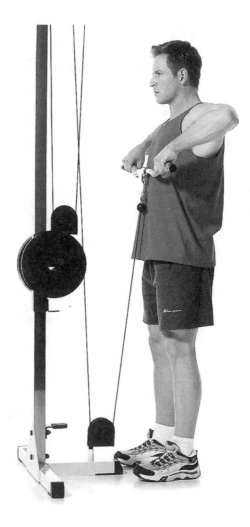

VARIATION
Stand-Back Upright Row

For more shoulder comfort, stand 2 to 3 feet away from the stack. This shifts some of the work to your rear delts and traps. Your elbows come back as well as up, and your forearms are almost parallel to the floor at the top position.

Cable Shrug
BEGINNER LEVEL

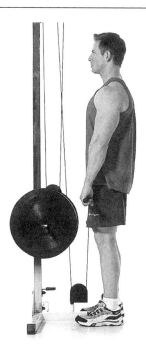

■ **START:** Attach a straight bar to the low pulley. Grab the bar with an overhand, shoulder-width grip, stand facing the weight stack, and hold the bar at arm's length in front of your thighs.

◻ **FINISH:** Shrug your shoulders up toward your ears, keeping your arms and neck straight. (Don't bend your elbows, in other words, or flex your neck forward.) Pause, then return to the starting position.

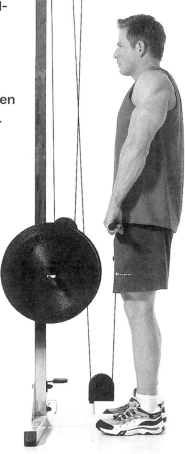

Lateral Raise
BEGINNER LEVEL

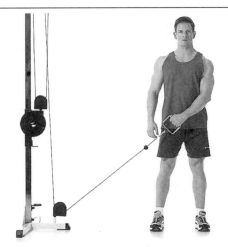

■ **START:** Attach a stirrup handle to the low pulley. Grab the handle with your nondominant hand and stand sideways to the cable column so your dominant side is toward the weight stack. Hold the handle near your stack-side hip, with your elbow slightly bent, as if you were about to pull a sword from a scabbard.

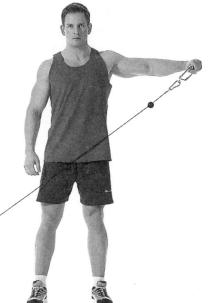

□ **FINISH:** Raise the handle up and across your body until your arm is parallel to the floor and the cable is right against your body. (You'll figure out the best position by trial and error—you may get a better feel for the exercise by standing closer to or farther from the weight stack, or by raising your arm at a higher angle.) Pause, then return to the starting position. Finish the set with that arm, then switch and repeat with your other arm.

BEGINNER VARIATION
Bilateral Lateral Raise

Attach the stirrup handles to both low cables of the crossover machine. Grab the handles with a crossover grip and stand between the towers. Lean forward slightly and execute the move the same way you would with one arm.

INTERMEDIATE VARIATION
Lean-Away Lateral Raise

Position your feet very close to the low cable attachment, hold on to the station rack with your free hand, and lean away from the apparatus until your nonworking arm is completely straight. (If you let go, you'd fall sideways.) The angle increases the load on your delts as you execute the raise.

Front Raise
BEGINNER LEVEL

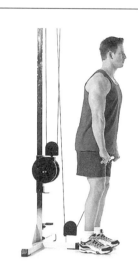

■ **START:** Attach the straight bar to the low pulley and grab it with an overhand, shoulder-width grip. Stand facing away from the cable station so that you're straddling the cable and holding the bar at arm's length in front of your thighs. Lean forward a bit (chest over toes), and bend your knees slightly.

□ **FINISH:** Raise the bar out in front of you until it's level with your shoulders. Pause, then return to the starting position. The cable travels between your legs, so be careful.

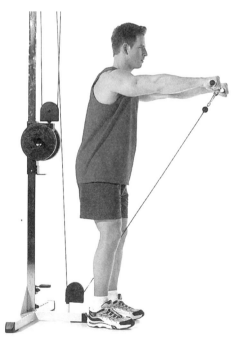

VARIATION
Unilateral Front Raise

Attach a stirrup handle to the low pulley and stand with your back to it and slightly to the side of it so your working arm lines up directly in front of the cable. Start with the handle at arm's length at your side, and keep your arm straight as you lift the handle out in front of you until it's at shoulder level.

Kneeling External Rotation
BEGINNER LEVEL

■ **START:** You'll need a rolled-up workout towel for this one. Attach a stirrup handle to the low pulley, grab the handle with your nondominant hand, and kneel sideways to the cable column so your dominant side is toward the weight stack. Bend your nondominant arm 90 degrees so the elbow braces the towel against your hip. Your forearm should be parallel to the floor, in front of your abdomen.

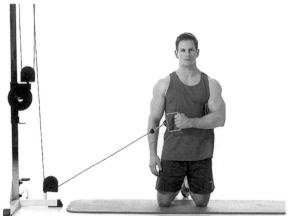

☐ **FINISH:** Pull the handle out and away from your torso, keeping the towel pinned against your hip with your elbow, as if you were opening a door. Pause when your forearm is as far to the side as it will go, then return to the starting position. Finish the set with that arm, then switch and repeat with your other arm.

Kneeling Internal Rotation
BEGINNER LEVEL

■ **START:** You'll need a rolled-up workout towel for this one. Attach a stirrup handle to the low pulley. Grab the handle and kneel sideways to the weight stack with your working side closest to it, 2½ to 3 feet away. Bend your arm 90 degrees so your elbow braces the towel against your rib cage. The knuckles of your working hand should point toward the weight stack, and your forearm should be perpendicular to your torso.

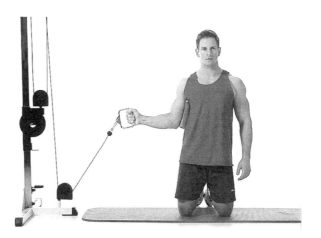

▢ **FINISH:** Pull the handle across your torso until your forearm touches your abs. Pause, then return to the starting position. Finish your set with that arm, then repeat with your other arm.

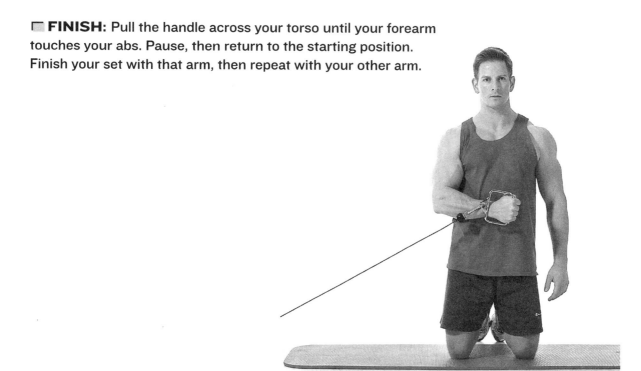

Standing External Rotation
INTERMEDIATE LEVEL

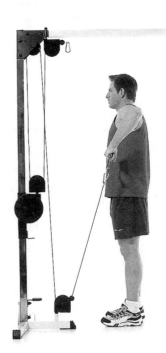

■ **START:** Attach a stirrup handle to the low pulley. Grab the handle with your nondominant hand and stand facing the weight stack, about a foot away. Lift your working arm into the finishing position of an upright row: upper arm parallel to the floor and forearm pointing straight down.

▢ **FINISH:** Without allowing your upper arm to move up or down, rotate it so your forearm points toward the ceiling. Pause, then return to the starting position. Finish your set with that arm, then repeat with your other arm.

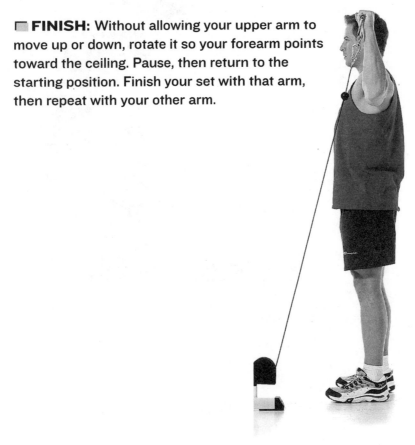

Standing Sideways External Rotation
ADVANCED LEVEL

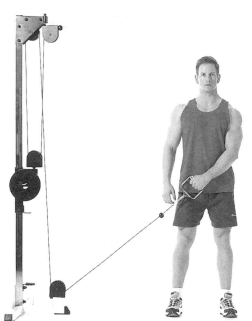

■ **START:** Attach a stirrup handle to the low pulley. Grab the handle with your nondominant hand and stand sideways to the weight stack so your dominant side is closest to it. Bend your working elbow not quite 90 degrees, with the inside of that forearm facing the side of your torso.

☐ **FINISH:** Pull the handle out and up so your hand is just above your head. You should look like you're about to throw a pitch, or like you've just hit a tennis backhand. Pause, then return to the starting position. Finish your set with that arm, then repeat with your other arm.

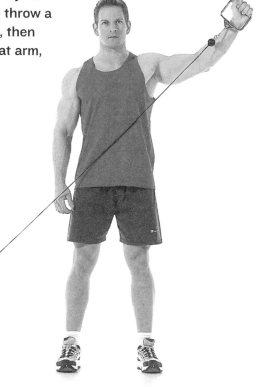

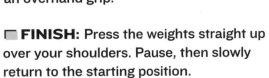

Seated Shoulder Press
ADVANCED LEVEL

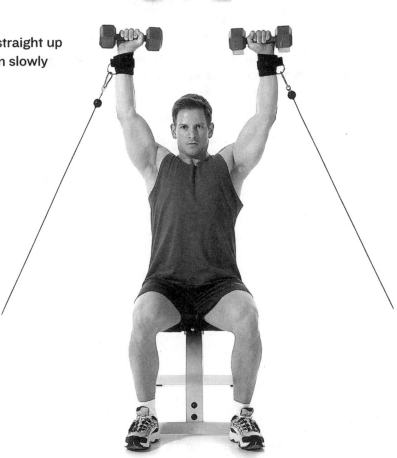

■ **START:** Set a bench between the columns of a crossover machine and put a pair of dumbbells on the floor next to it. Put ankle straps on your wrists and attach them to the low pulleys. Straddle the bench and pick up the dumbbells. Hold them at jaw level with an overhand grip.

▢ **FINISH:** Press the weights straight up over your shoulders. Pause, then slowly return to the starting position.

VARIATION
Unilateral Seated Shoulder Press

Same setup, but lift with the arm closest to the weight stack, and grab the side of the bench with your opposite hand for balance.

EXERCISES FOR THE TRICEPS

Kickback
BEGINNER LEVEL

■ **START:** This is a simple exercise, despite a deceptively complex setup: Attach an ankle strap to the low pulley. Stand facing the weight stack, a few feet away from it and slightly off-center so your nondominant shoulder is in line with the cable. Move your opposite foot forward a step and bend that knee. Step back with your other foot and keep that leg straight. Bend forward at the hips until your torso is parallel to the floor, and grab the strap with your nondominant hand, using a neutral grip. Rest your free forearm on its corresponding knee. Pull back your working arm so your upper arm is parallel to the floor and against your torso. Your elbow should point backward; your forearm should point down.

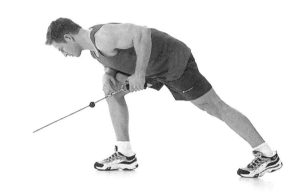

☐ **FINISH:** Straighten your working arm, keeping the rest of your body—especially your working upper arm—in the original position. Pause, then return to the starting position. Finish the set with that arm, then repeat with your other arm.

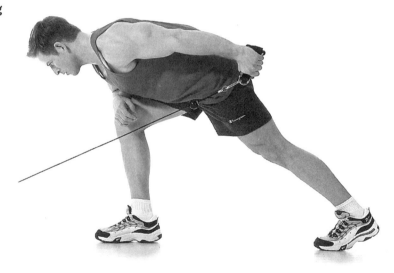

Pushdown
BEGINNER LEVEL

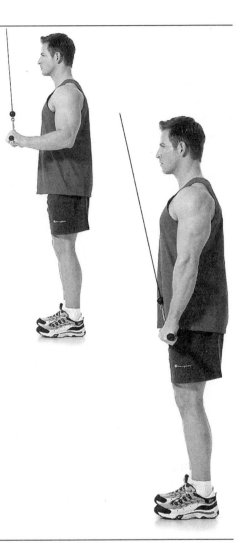

■ **START:** Attach an EZ-curl bar to the high pulley. Grab the bar with an overhand grip, your hands 6 to 12 inches apart. Stand facing the weight stack with your feet about a foot or so away from it. Tuck your elbows close to your sides, and pull down the bar so your forearms are just above parallel to the floor.

▢ **FINISH:** Push down the bar until your arms are straight. Keep everything else—shoulders, back, upper arms—in their original positions. Pause, then slowly return to the starting position.

BEGINNER VARIATION
Straight-Bar Pushdown

This will switch you from a close, semineutral grip to a pronated, shoulder-width grip that emphasizes the medial triceps head. The movement is the same.

INTERMEDIATE VARIATIONS
Supinated-Grip Straight-Bar Pulldown

An underhand grip on the straight bar is easier on your wrists but requires more muscular control. You'll have to use less weight.

Rope Pushdown

If you want to use the rope attachment, use less weight and move your hands apart as you pull down. Ideally, your palms should face each other at the beginning of the movement but face the floor at the end.

Crossover Pushdown
INTERMEDIATE LEVEL

■ **START:** Attach stirrup handles to the high pulleys of the crossover machine, grab them with a crossover grip, and stand in the middle of the station with your forearms crossed in front of your chest.

▢ **FINISH:** Straighten your arms so they end up about a foot outside your hips, as if you were carrying two shopping bags. Keep your upper body in the same posture throughout the movement. Pause, then return to the starting position.

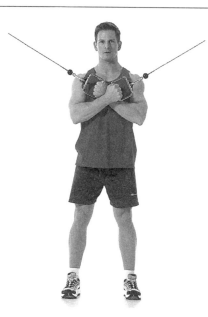

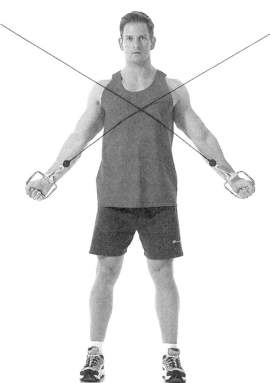

ADVANCED VARIATION
Unilateral Crossover Pushdown

When you have one weight stack instead of two, stand as shown above, but hold the handle with the arm farthest from the weight stack. Do all your reps with that arm, then switch.

Lying Triceps Extension
INTERMEDIATE LEVEL

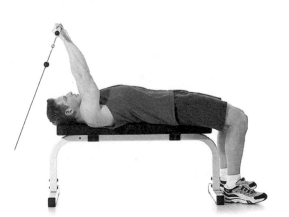

■ **START:** Place your bench perpendicular to the low cable station. Attach either the rope handle or EZ-curl bar to the low pulley. Grab the attachment, and lie on the bench with your head close to the weight stack. Hold the attachment at arm's length above your forehead.

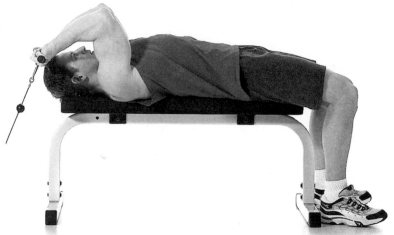

▢ **FINISH:** Lower your forearms behind you until the backs of your hands nearly touch the crown of your head. Pause, then return to the starting position. Try to keep your upper arms in the same position throughout the exercise.

Overhead Triceps Extension
INTERMEDIATE LEVEL

■ **START:** Attach the rope handle or EZ-curl bar to the low pulley. Grab the attachment, and sit on your bench (or stand) with your back to the weight stack. Lift the attachment overhead so your upper arms are perpendicular to the floor, with your biceps facing your ears.

□ **FINISH:** Lower your forearms behind your head until they're just below parallel to the floor—no farther. Pause, then return to the starting position.

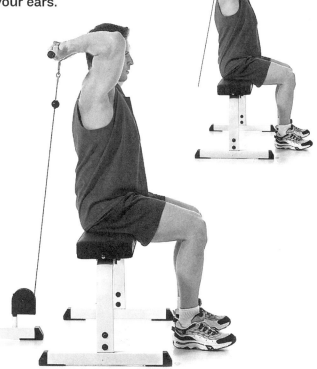

VARIATION
Swiss-Ball Overhead Triceps Extension

Simply do the seated version while perched on the ball rather than on a bench. Just make sure you place the ball close enough to the low cable that you can maintain a near vertical line when you extend your arms, without the ball touching the cable station.

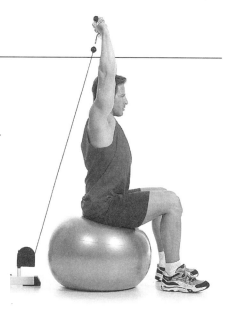

Bent-Over Triceps Extension
INTERMEDIATE LEVEL

■ **START:** Attach the rope handle or EZ-curl bar to the high pulley. Stand with your back to the weight stack, about a foot or two in front of it, and reach back to grab the attachment. Bend over at the hips until your torso and upper arms are parallel to the floor. (Stagger your stance, putting one foot in front of the other, for balance.) Your upper arms should be next to your ears, with your elbows bent 90 degrees and the attachment just above the back of your head.

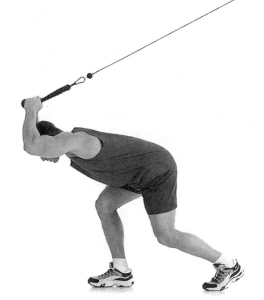

☐ **FINISH:** Straighten your arms. Pause, then return to the starting position.

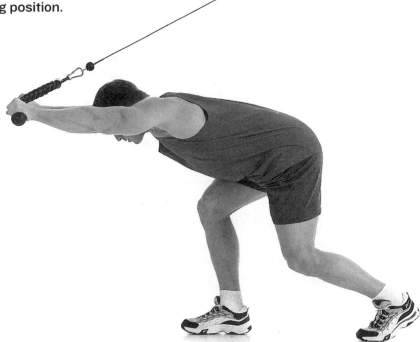

EXERCISES FOR THE BICEPS

Standing Curl
BEGINNER LEVEL

■ **START:** Attach a straight bar to the low pulley. Stand facing the weight stack, and grab the bar with a wide, underhand grip. Hold it at arm's length in front of your thighs, with your knees slightly bent, your back straight, and your shoulders back.

▢ **FINISH:** Curl the bar until your forearms are almost perpendicular to the floor. Pause, then return to the starting position.

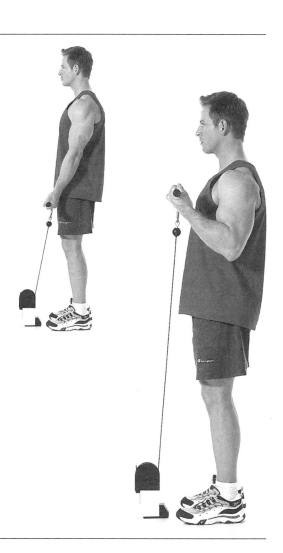

BEGINNER VARIATIONS
Narrow-Grip Standing Curl

Move your hands closer together to shift demand from the inner to the outer portion of the biceps.

Semisupinated-Grip Standing Curl

To move more work to the brachialis and make the curl easier on your wrists, use an EZ-curl bar to position your hands at 45-degree angles, between a supinated and neutral grip.

INTERMEDIATE VARIATIONS
Rope-Handle Standing Curl

Use the rope attachment and a neutral grip to move even more work to the brachialis.

Reverse-Grip Standing Curl

Use an EZ-curl bar and an overhand (pronated) grip for maximum brachialis involvement.

Lying Curl
INTERMEDIATE LEVEL

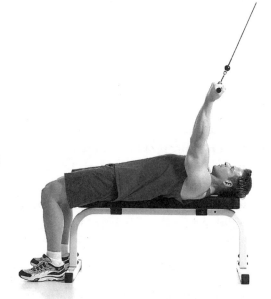

■ **START:** To put more emphasis on the short (inside) head of your biceps, attach a straight bar to the high pulley, and set a bench beneath it. Grab the bar with an underhand grip, and lie on the bench with your head close to the weight stack. Hold the bar with straight arms over your chest.

▫ **FINISH:** Curl the bar toward your forehead, trying to keep your upper arms in their original position. Stop before the bar touches your head, pause, and allow it to rise until your arms are almost straight but not fully locked out.

INTERMEDIATE VARIATION
Lying Curl with Grip Adjustments

The narrow, semisupinated, neutral, and reverse grips described as variations of the standing curl will work here as well.

Preacher Curl
INTERMEDIATE LEVEL

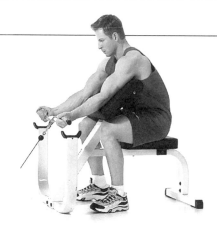

■ **START:** Attach the EZ-curl bar to the low pulley. Set up a preacher bench so you'll face the weight stack while lifting. Grab the bar with an underhand grip as you sit at the bench, your upper arms resting on the pad. Start with your arms almost straight.

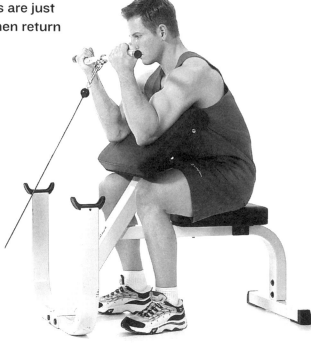

▢ **FINISH:** Curl the bar until your forearms are just short of perpendicular to the floor. Pause, then return to the starting position.

VARIATION
Swiss-Ball Preacher Curl

Attach the EZ-curl bar to the low pulley, put the ball in front of the weight stack, kneel behind the ball and rest your triceps on the front of it. Then do a standard preacher curl.

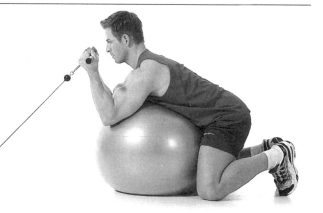

Crucifix Curl
ADVANCED LEVEL

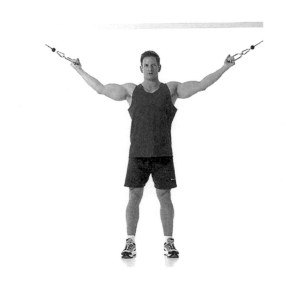

■ **START:** Attach the stirrup handles to the high pulleys of the crossover machine. Grab the handles underhanded, and stand between the towers. Hold your arms out so your upper arms are parallel to the floor and your elbows are bent slightly.

▢ **FINISH:** Curl both handles up toward your head, keeping your upper arms parallel to the floor. Pause, then slowly return to the starting position.

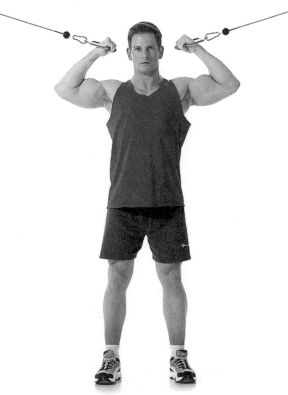

VARIATION
Unilateral Crucifix Curl

Work one arm at a time by standing sideways to the weight stack, grabbing one high handle, and taking a step or two away from the station. Put your nonworking hand on your hip for balance.

EXERCISES FOR THE FOREARMS

Standing Wrist Curl
BEGINNER LEVEL

■ **START:** Attach a straight bar to the low pulley and stand with your back to the weight stack. Grab the bar with a pronated grip (your palms facing the weight stack), and hold it behind you so it almost touches your hamstrings. Roll the bar down to your fingertips.

◻ **FINISH:** Roll the bar back up with your fingers, and flex your wrists so your hands curl up toward your butt. Pause, then return to the starting position.

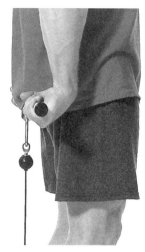

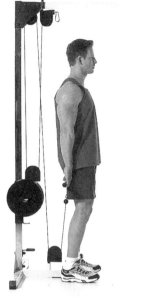

Kneeling Wrist Curl
BEGINNER LEVEL

■ **START:** Attach a straight bar to the low pulley, and place a bench crossways in front of the cable column. Grab the bar with an underhand grip, kneel next to the far side of the bench (so it's between you and the weight stack), and rest your forearms on the bench with your wrists hanging off the other side. Roll the bar down to your fingertips.

◻ **FINISH:** Roll the bar back up, and flex your wrists so your palms curl up toward your elbows. Pause, then return to the starting position.

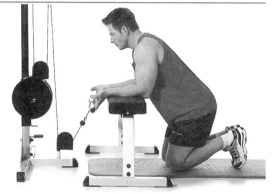

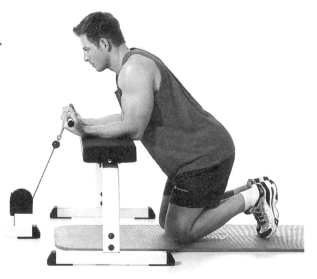

Reverse Wrist Curl
BEGINNER LEVEL

■ **START:** Attach an EZ-curl bar to the low pulley. Set up as for the kneeling wrist curl, but hold the bar with an overhand grip.

□ **FINISH:** Raise the bar by bringing the backs of your hands toward your elbows. Pause, then return to the starting position.

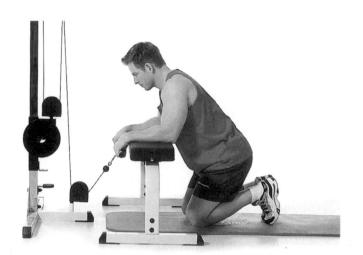

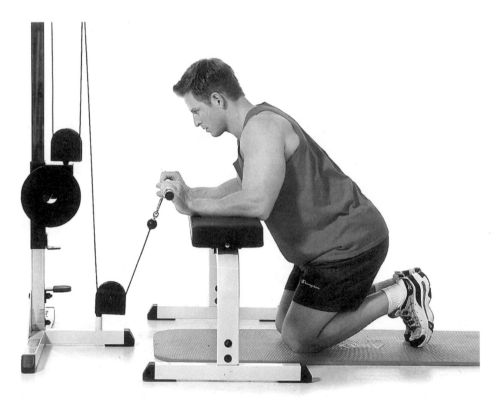

LOWER BODY

We recommend that you use the lower-body cable exercises in this section to complement or add variety to a routine based on free weights or the body-weight exercises in chapter 6. If you insist on doing your lower-body work exclusively with cables, here's your program.

Beginners should do 1 or 2 sets of 12 to 15 repetitions of one knee-dominant and two hip-dominant movements, plus a calf exercise.

Intermediate and advanced lifters should do 2 or 3 sets of 10 to 12 reps of two knee-dominant and two hip-dominant movements, plus two calf exercises. If you're using heavy weights at the advanced level, you can take the reps down to 8 to 10.

BEGINNER

KNEE-DOMINANT
— Split squat ------------(page 258)

HIP-DOMINANT
— Lying leg curl ----------(page 262)
— Unilateral lying
  leg curl --------------(page 262)
— Towel-assisted lying
  leg curl --------------(page 262)
— Standing hip extension --(page 263)

CALVES
— Seated calf raise -------(page 268)

INTERMEDIATE

KNEE-DOMINANT
— Lunge -----------------(page 259)
— Diagonal rotation
  squat ----------------(page 260)

HIP-DOMINANT
— Standing adduction -----(page 264)
— Standing abduction -----(page 265)
— Reverse lunge ----------(page 266)

CALVES
— Standing unilateral
  calf raise -------------(page 269)

ADVANCED

KNEE-DOMINANT
— Bulgarian split squat ---(page 261)

HIP-DOMINANT
— Pull-through ----------(page 267)

KNEE-DOMINANT EXERCISES

Split Squat
BEGINNER LEVEL

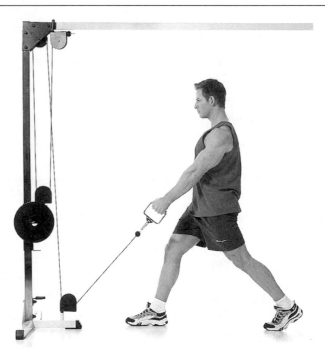

■ **START:** Attach a stirrup handle to the low pulley. Grab the handle with your nondominant hand using a neutral grip, and stand facing the weight stack with your dominant foot about 2½ feet away from it and your nondominant foot about 2 feet behind it. (Line up your feet with their corresponding buttocks, not with each other.) Extend your arm straight out and pull your shoulders back. Face your shoulders and hips squarely toward the cable station.

□ **FINISH:** Lower your body until the top of your forward thigh is parallel to the floor and your rear knee almost touches the floor. Return to the starting position. Finish the set, then switch legs and repeat.

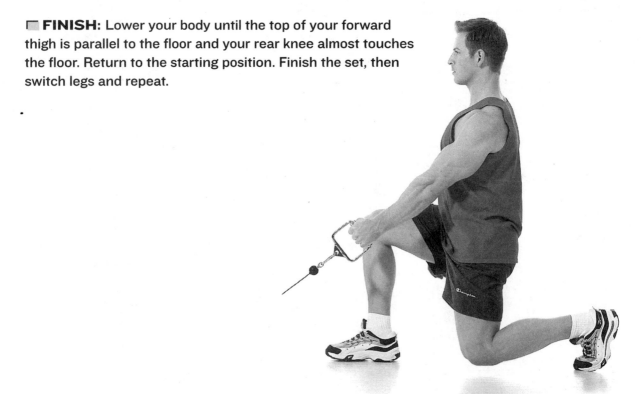

Lunge
INTERMEDIATE LEVEL

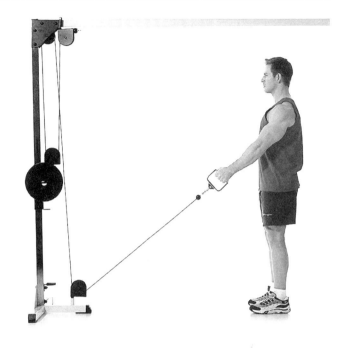

■ **START:** Same setup as for the split squat, except you stand with your feet parallel and hip-width apart, 3 to 3½ feet in front of the weight stack.

▢ **FINISH:** Stride toward the weight stack with one leg, finishing with your back straight, your forward knee over that ankle, and the top of your forward thigh parallel to the floor. Push back up to the starting position, finish the set, then repeat with your other leg. Start with light weights, no matter how strong you are. Cable lunges challenge your balance, since you work against two forms of resistance: the cable that pulls you forward, and gravity, which pulls you down.

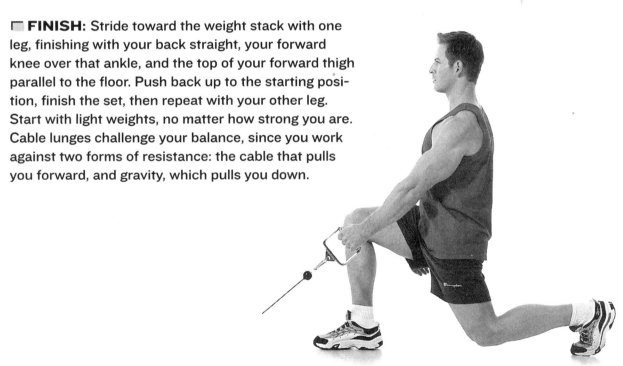

Diagonal Rotation Squat
INTERMEDIATE-TO-ADVANCED LEVEL

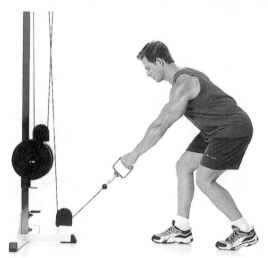

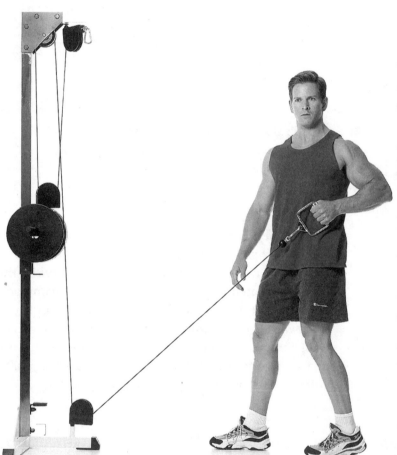

■ **START:** Attach a stirrup handle to the low pulley. Grab the handle with your nondominant hand and stand facing the weight stack with your dominant foot about 12 inches in front of your nondominant one. Plant your forward foot flat on the floor, supporting your weight on that leg. Only the toes of your rear foot should touch the floor—use them just for balance. Your working arm and the cable should form a straight line from shoulder to pulley. Squat down and bend forward at the hips so your rear knee is bent about 45 degrees and your torso forms a 45-degree angle with the floor.

☐ **FINISH:** Stand, pull the handle to the side of your rib cage, and twist to the left. Pause, then slowly return to the starting position. Finish the set on that side before repeating on the other.

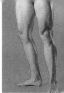

Bulgarian Split Squat
ADVANCED LEVEL

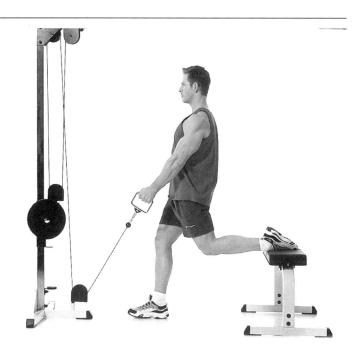

■ **START:** Same setup as for the split squat and lunge, except you place a bench 2 to 3 feet behind you. Stand with one foot forward and the instep of your other foot up on the bench.

□ **FINISH:** Lower your body until the top of your forward thigh is parallel to the floor. Pause, and push back up to the starting position. Finish the set, then switch legs and repeat.

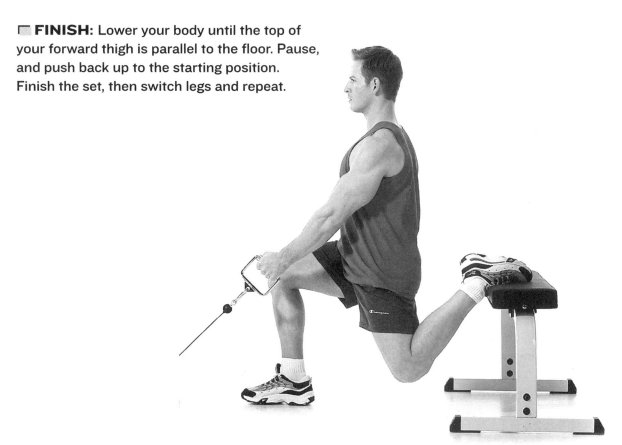

HIP-DOMINANT EXERCISES

Lying Leg Curl
BEGINNER LEVEL

■ **START:** Position the end of a bench 2½ to 3 feet from the low pulley. Use an aerobics step, a wooden box, weight plates, sandbags, phone books, or any other sturdy platform to raise the far end of the bench so it slants down toward the pulley. Attach the ankle straps to your ankles, then hook both straps to the pulley. Lie facedown on the bench with your head at the high end and your knees hanging off the low end.

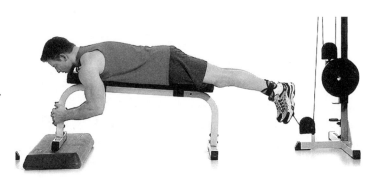

□ **FINISH:** Curl your heels as close as possible toward your rear end. Pause, then slowly return to the starting position. Keep your hips and front thighs flat on the bench throughout. (Even though this leg curl is in the hip-dominant section, your knees should be the only moving joints, ensuring you work your hamstrings without putting stress on your lower back.)

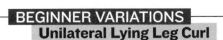

BEGINNER VARIATIONS
Unilateral Lying Leg Curl

You can do this one leg at a time so it requires only one ankle strap and makes it easier to get into position.

Towel-Assisted Lying Leg Curl

Place a rolled-up workout towel underneath your hips to provide added comfort and put your hamstrings into a more stretched-out position at the start of the movement.

Standing Hip Extension
BEGINNER LEVEL

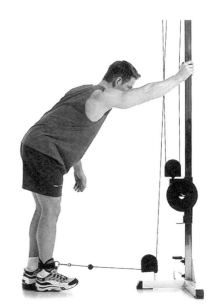

■ **START:** You'll need something thick and sturdy to stand on: a 25-pound weight plate, an aerobics step, or (last resort) a phone book. Put an ankle strap around one ankle and attach it to the low pulley. Stand facing the weight stack, about a foot in front of it (farther away if necessary to start with the cable taut), with your nonworking foot on the weight plate. Lean forward about 45 degrees from the hips, and rest your hand on something for balance (some cable machines have handles for this). Pull in your gut.

☐ **FINISH:** Pull your working leg back as far as you can without changing the angle of your torso or bending your knee. Pause, then slowly return to the starting position. Finish the set with that leg, then repeat with the other.

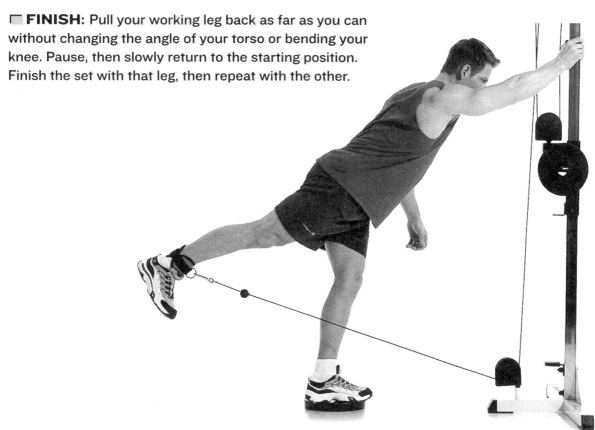

Standing Adduction
INTERMEDIATE LEVEL

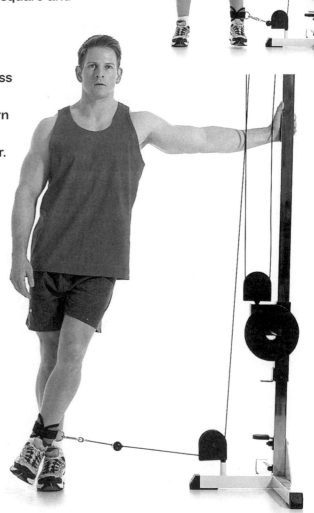

■ **START:** Put an ankle strap around one ankle and attach it to the low pulley. Stand sideways with your working foot closest to the weight stack and about a foot away from it. Hold on to the tower for balance as you lift your leg a few inches forward. Your nonworking knee should be slightly bent, and your shoulders and hips should be square and facing forward.

☐ **FINISH:** Pull your working leg across the midline of your body until it passes your other leg. Pause, then slowly return to the starting position. Finish the set with that leg, then repeat with the other.

Standing Abduction
INTERMEDIATE LEVEL

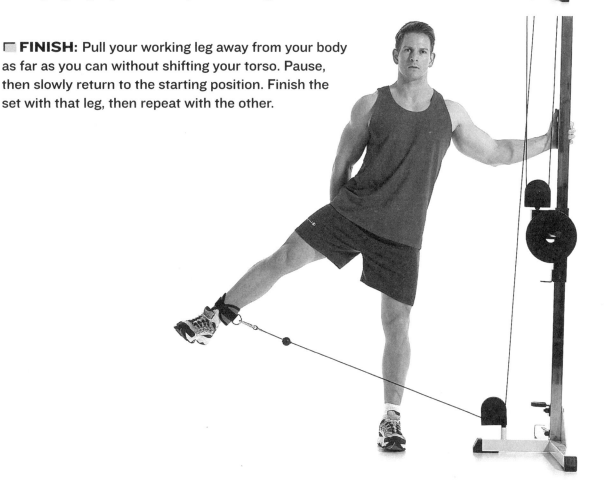

■ **START:** Same setup as for the standing adduction, but put the strap on the ankle farthest from the weight stack, and place your working leg slightly in front of your other leg.

▢ **FINISH:** Pull your working leg away from your body as far as you can without shifting your torso. Pause, then slowly return to the starting position. Finish the set with that leg, then repeat with the other.

Reverse Lunge
INTERMEDIATE LEVEL

■ **START:** Attach a stirrup handle to the low pulley. Grab the handle with your nondominant hand and stand facing the weight stack, about a foot in front of it. Your feet should be parallel and about hip-width apart. Keep your shoulders back.

▢ **FINISH:** Step back with your dominant leg and lower your body until that knee almost touches the floor and the top of your other thigh is parallel to the floor. Return to the starting position. Finish the set, then switch legs and repeat.

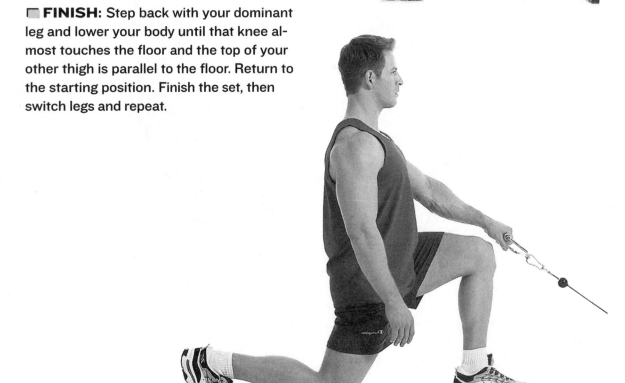

Pull-Through
ADVANCED LEVEL

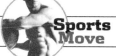

Sports Move

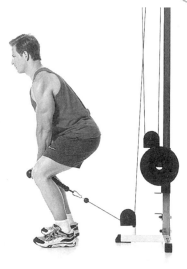

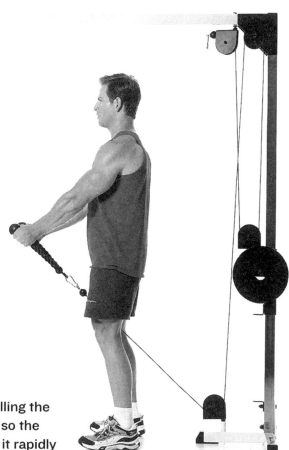

■ **START:** Attach the rope handle to the low pulley. Stand with your back to the pulley and grab the ends of the handles with your palms facing each other. Hold the handles between your legs at about knee-level. (Adjust your stance so there's tension on the cable in this position.) Set your feet even with each other and about shoulder-width apart. Bend your hips and knees, keeping your lower back flat or slightly arched.

☐ **FINISH:** Straighten your hips and knees, pulling the rope forward a foot or so. Try this slowly at first so the cable doesn't bisect your manhood, but then do it rapidly and explosively, almost as if you were jumping. This is the only exercise in this chapter that you should perform explosively. The object is to develop your rear-body muscles while improving your power for jumping and sprinting. *Warning:* This is probably the most sexually suggestive exercise you can do, so pull the curtains and be happy you're training at home, because you'll never have to do it in a public gym.

EXERCISES FOR THE CALVES

Seated Calf Raise
BEGINNER LEVEL

■ **START:** Set a bench lengthwise in front of the weight stack, and set a sturdy platform between the bench and the low pulley. Attach the straight bar to the low pulley. Grab the bar and sit up straight at the end of the bench facing the pulley. Rest your forearms on your thighs and hold the bar just above your knees. Set the balls of your feet on the platform, and lower your heels as far as you can.

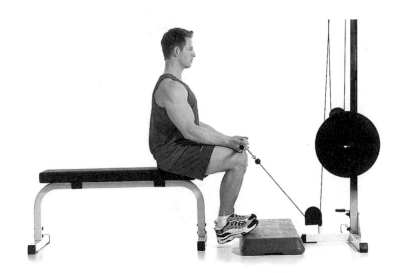

▢ **FINISH:** Push from the balls of your feet, raising your heels as high as you can. Pause, then slowly return to the starting position.

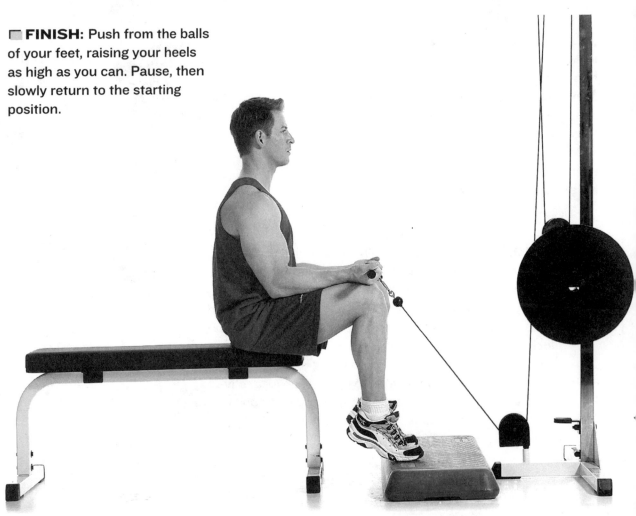

Standing Unilateral Calf Raise
INTERMEDIATE LEVEL

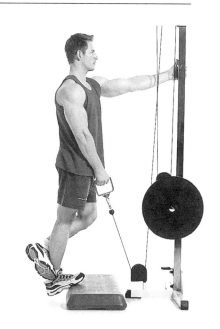

■ **START:** Position a sturdy low platform or a couple of phone books in front of the weight stack. Attach the stirrup handle to the low pulley, grab it with one hand, and place the ball of your corresponding foot squarely on the platform. Hold on to something with your free hand for balance as you lift your other foot and rest it behind the Achilles tendon of your working leg. Stand up straight, and lower your working heel as far as you can.

▢ **FINISH:** Lift your working heel as high as possible. Pause, then slowly return to the starting position. Finish the set, then switch legs and repeat.

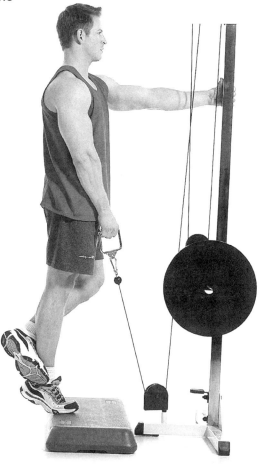

CHAPTER 10

DREAM MACHINE: A MULTISTATION HOME GYM

Without ever having done a survey, we feel confident stating that every guy who lifts weights at home has fantasized about owning one of these machines. We know we have. Who wouldn't want hardware that's safe, that lets you replicate a lot of popular health-club exercises, and that makes your home-workout space look like a clean, modern gym—as opposed to a spare bedroom with some rusted iron on the floor?

Whether you're a true beginner or an experienced exerciser, a multistation machine takes some of the intimidation and fuss out of lifting weights. It's always ready for use—no moving a barbell from floor to uprights to power rack. And it couldn't be much easier to operate. Step one: Slide a pin into the weight stack. Step two: Start lifting.

The unfortunate thing is that a multistation home gym actually limits your exercise choices. Sure, it has a cable apparatus that allows you to do most of the exercises in chapter 9, which are great for your back, abs, arms, and shoulders. When you want to work your body's bigger, more important muscles, however, you face many of the same obstacles we described in that chapter.

Take, for example, the pectoral problem. If you want to do a chest press on a machine, you've got one exercise: Sit on the seat, push out the handles, repeat for the rest of your life. Do a chest press with dumbbells or a barbell, and you've got all kinds of variations: incline, decline, close-grip, wide-grip. Granted, many multistation home gyms do offer a pec-deck apparatus, allowing you to do chest flies, which you otherwise wouldn't be able to perform at home. But this isn't much of an advantage, as flies are among our least favorite exercises—they're potentially tough on your shoulders without doing as much for your chest as barbell or dumbbell presses.

Then there's the problem of function. Most machines guide your motion to such a degree that only a very targeted muscle does the work, without much help from stabilizers or other members of your body's structural team. That's not how your body works in sports or in real life. Say, for example, you have a baby in one arm and another child crying out to be held. When you bend down to scoop up the screamer without dropping the other, you use damned-near every muscle in your body to lift the rug rats and stabilize yourself. No one muscle is isolated.

Not that sacrificing some variety and function in favor of convenience and aesthetics is bad. Not exercising at all—that's bad. Exercising exclusively on a multistation home gym is less than ideal, but far better than nothing.

Because multistations are simple to use, we won't waste space showing you how to do exercises that the machine's instruction booklet explains perfectly well. Instead, we're going to give you some ways to get more benefit from the exercises. We'd hate for you to end up using your $2,000 home gym the way we use our $2,000 home computer—by turning it into the weight-lifting equivalent of an expensive typewriter.

MIDSECTION

To repeat the obvious, the best way to work your abs, if you're a beginner, is to focus on the body-weight exercises in chapter 6. As you progress, you can make perfectly good use of your multistation gym by adding some of the cable exercises in chapter 9.

At the bottom of this page is one machine-specific exercise you can do.

Seated Cable Crunch
INTERMEDIATE LEVEL

■ **START:** Attach the straps that come with the machine to the high cable, and sit on the seat with your back to the weight stack. Hold the straps at your shoulders. If it's a single strap or a rope handle, use a neutral grip (palms facing each other); if it's two stirrup handles, use a supinated (underhand) grip.

□ **FINISH:** Most beginners just move their shoulders down. Be more effective by first pulling your belly button in toward your spine. *Then* try crunching. You'll have to use less weight and a shorter range of motion. And you'll probably feel as if someone were probing your abdominal muscles with kitchen knives. Don't worry about the sharpness of the contraction—that's what those muscles are supposed to feel like when they're really working.

CHEST AND UPPER BACK

The back exercises are no different than those in chapter 9, except the seat is more comfortable. There's a big difference with chest exercises, though. You could end up having lousy workouts, since the machine makes it easy to sit back in the seat and push out the handles without much thought to your posture. Worse, because the machine dictates your grip width, chest presses may be tough on your shoulders. You could end up with impingement syndrome, inflammation of your shoulder muscles and connective tissues that makes it hurt like hell to lift your arm. Or you could work your shoulders and triceps, rather than your chest. (Some machines have independent-action pressing arms that you have to control as you would dumbbells, which is a big improvement.)

Here's a way to guarantee that your chest works harder and your shoulders and triceps take a less important role.

BEGINNER	INTERMEDIATE	ADVANCED
CHEST	**CHEST**	**UPPER BACK**
Chest press ---------(page 275)	Pec-deck fly ----------------(page 275)	Incline lying pullover ----------(page 234)
	Unilateral pec-deck fly --------(page 275)	
UPPER BACK		
Lat pulldown ---------(page 223)	**UPPER BACK**	
Supinated lat pulldown ----------(page 224)	Wide-grip lat pulldown --------(page 224)	
Neutral-grip lat pulldown ----------(page 224)	Mixed-grip lat pulldown -------(page 224)	
Supinated cable row --(page 226)	Unilateral lat pulldown --------(page 224)	
Neutral-grip pronated cable row ----------(page 227)	Behind-the-neck lat pulldown --(page 224)	
Close-grip pronated cable row ----------(page 227)	Double pulldown --------------(page 225)	
	Pronated cable row -----------(page 227)	
	Wide-grip pronated cable row --(page 227)	
	Rope-handle pronated cable row --------------------(page 227)	
	Unilateral cable row ----------(page 228)	
	Neutral-grip unilateral cable row --------------------(page 228)	
	Supinated-grip unilateral cable row ------------------(page 228)	
	Standing unilateral high row --(page 229)	
	Bent-over row ----------------(page 230)	
	Standing pullover -------------(page 231)	
	Bent-over rear lateral raise ----(page 232)	
	Unilateral bent-over rear lateral raise -----------------(page 232)	
	Standing rear lateral raise -----(page 233)	
	Unilateral standing rear lateral raise -----------------(page 233)	
	Lying pullover ----------------(page 234)	

Chest Press
BEGINNER LEVEL

■ **START:** Adjust the seat so the pressing bar lines up with your armpits. Grab that bar with a pronated (overhand) grip and wide elbows as you sit against the backrest. Here's the trick to make the press more effective: Pinch back your shoulder blades before you start the press.

☐ **FINISH:** Push out the bar until your arms are straight but not locked. Pause, then stay in control as you bring the bar back to a few inches in front of your chest.

Pec-Deck Fly
INTERMEDIATE LEVEL

■ **START:** Sit at your machine's pec deck (also known as butterfly station) with your knees bent and your feet flat on the floor. Make sure the seat is high enough that your elbows are just below the level of your shoulders when you place your forearms and elbows behind the arm pads. Start with your upper arms in line with your torso, not behind it.

☐ **FINISH:** Pull the pads forward until they almost touch in front of you. Pause, then let them slowly return until your upper arms are again in line with your torso.

VARIATION
Unilateral Pec-Deck Fly

Same move, but do it one arm at a time, holding the seat with the other hand for balance.

SHOULDERS AND ARMS

EXERCISES FOR THE SHOULDERS

You can use your machine's cable station to do the shoulder exercises in chapter 9. The one exercise this machine adds is the shoulder press. There's no holding back here: We hate shoulder-press machines. Your shoulders are the most mobile, and thus the most vulnerable to injury, of all your joints. To take these easily destructible hinges and force them into a single range of motion is criminal.

There is, however, one way to use your machine's shoulder-press station without completely screwing with the integrity of your shoulder joints: Do a one-arm press, as described at the bottom of this page.

Unilateral Shoulder Press
BEGINNER LEVEL

■ **START:** Position yourself in the shoulder-press station (how you do this varies from machine to machine). Grab the bar with one hand, placing the other hand on your hip. Hold the bar at about jaw level, with your torso erect and your lower back in its naturally arched position.

□ **FINISH:** Press the bar overhead until your arm is straight but not locked. Allow your torso to move whichever direction feels most natural—forward, back, to the side. You shouldn't feel any pinching or jabbing inside your shoulder joint. Keep constant tension on your shoulder muscles as you lower the bar back to jaw level.

EXERCISES FOR THE BICEPS AND TRICEPS

The best biceps exercises you can do on your machine are the cable exercises in chapter 9. Your multistation does present a couple of new possibilities for your triceps. If a dip station is an optional attachment for your machine, we recommend getting one if you're an intermediate or advanced lifter. Though difficult to master, the dip is a great chest-and-triceps builder. If you're very advanced, we recommend getting both the dip apparatus and a belt for doing weighted dips.

Close-Grip Chest Press
INTERMEDIATE LEVEL

■ **START:** For this, you'll need vertical handles on your chest-press apparatus (most machines have them) and an EZ-curl cable attachment. (You can use the lat-pulldown bar, but the curved bar is easier to use.) Set the bar inside the vertical handles, position yourself in the station, and grab the bar with a narrow, overhand grip. Pull your shoulder blades together, and draw your elbows down so they're within shoulder-width apart. Start with the bar about an inch from your chest.

□ **FINISH:** Push the bar out until your arms are straight but not locked. Pause, then slowly return the bar to within an inch or so of your chest.

Dip
INTERMEDIATE LEVEL

■ **START:** Step onto the foot supports of your dip station, grabbing the ends of the handles with a neutral grip. Jump up and steady yourself. You want to start the movement with your arms straight but not locked, and your body perfectly still. You can cross your legs behind you or leave them hanging straight down. The more upright you are, the harder you work your triceps. Leaning forward shifts work to your chest and front shoulders.

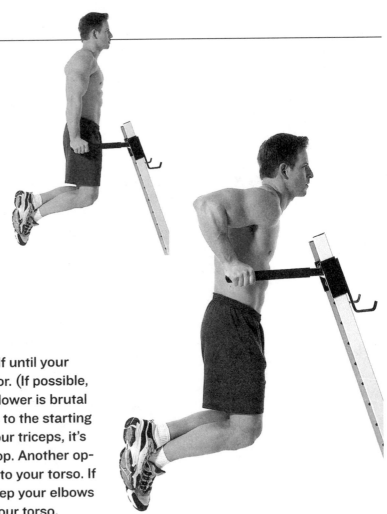

□ **FINISH:** Slowly lower yourself until your upper arms are parallel to the floor. (If possible, do this in front of a mirror; going lower is brutal to your shoulders.) Push back up to the starting position. If you're emphasizing your triceps, it's okay to lock your elbows at the top. Another option is to keep your elbows close to your torso. If you're focusing on your chest, keep your elbows unlocked or out and away from your torso.

VARIATION
Weighted Dip

Here's one of the best chest-and-triceps-building exercises you can do at home or in a gym. Wear a belt with a weight hanging from it, as shown on page 38.

LOWER BODY

Your multistation gym offers a trio of beginner-friendly lower-body options that replicate popular gym exercises. Most machines have leg-extension and leg-curl stations, and some have a leg press, too. (If the leg press is optional, you should opt for it if you're a beginner, or if you're an intermediate or advanced lifter who doesn't have free weights. If you aren't a beginner and do have free weights—particularly a barbell and a setup that allows you to do squats—skip the leg press; it just takes up space.)

Here's how to get a little more benefit from these stations.

BEGINNER	INTERMEDIATE
Leg press ------------(page 280)	Lower-feet leg press ---(page 280)
Leg extension --------(page 280)	Toes-out leg press -----(page 280)
Calf raise on leg-extension apparatus ------------(page 281)	Unilateral leg press ----(page 280)
Lying leg curl ----------(page 281)	Towel-assisted lying leg curl ---------------(page 281)
	Standing leg curl -------(page 282)
	Elevated standing leg curl --------------(page 282)

Leg Press
BEGINNER LEVEL

■ **START:** Sit back in the leg-press station with your back against the pad and your feet shoulder-width apart on the foot plate. Adjust the seat so your knees are bent slightly more than 90 degrees.

□ **FINISH:** Push the weight until your knees are straight but not locked. Pause, then return to the starting position.

INTERMEDIATE VARIATIONS
Lower-Feet Leg Press

Put more demand on the quads by placing your feet lower on the foot plate so you push off with the balls of your feet. This is a bit rougher on the knees.

Toes-Out Leg Press

If the foot plate allows, performing the exercise with your toes turned out slightly will shift demand to your inner thighs.

Unilateral Leg Press

Perform any version of this movement one leg at a time by placing just one foot on the plate.

Leg Extension
BEGINNER LEVEL

■ **START:** Sit on the leg-extension seat with the backrest adjusted so your knees line up with the rotational axis of the leg extension—if your knees are higher or lower than the axis, you risk straining them. The ankle pad should be just above the front part of your ankles, rather than at your instep or halfway up your shin.

□ **FINISH:** Extend your legs toward the ceiling in a wide arc until your legs are straight but not locked. Pause, then slowly lower.

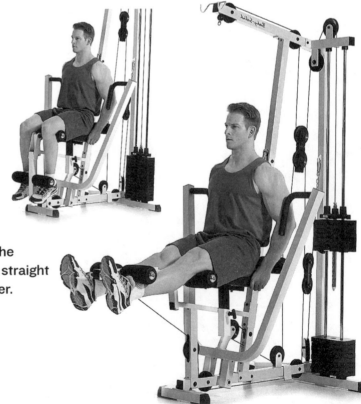

Calf Raise on Leg-Extension Apparatus
BEGINNER LEVEL

■ **START:** Stand facing the machine and slightly to one side of it. Bend one leg 90 degrees to place the ball of that foot against the leg-extension pad. If you're standing on the left side of the machine, use your right leg. Lean your hands on the machine for balance. Pull your toes toward your shin. Your nonworking leg should be slightly bent, your torso as erect as possible, and your abs pulled in.

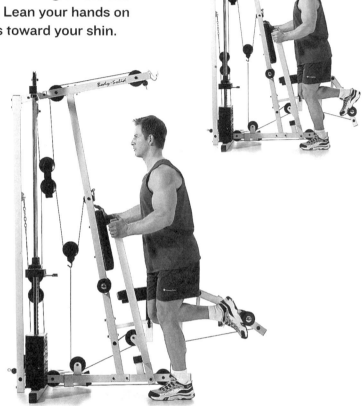

▢ **FINISH:** Push your toes back while keeping the rest of your body still. Pause, feel the contraction in your calf, then slowly return to the starting position. Finish the set, then switch legs and repeat.

Lying Leg Curl
BEGINNER LEVEL

■ **START:** Lie on the bench with your knees hanging off the back edge. Position your legs so that the part of your calves just above your Achilles tendons hits the undersides of the ankle pads.

▢ **FINISH:** Curl your lower legs up until your heels are as close to your rear end as they can get without touching it. Pause at the top before slowly lowering until your knees are almost straight.

INTERMEDIATE VARIATION
Towel-Assisted Lying Leg Curl

Place a large rolled-up bath towel beneath your hips to increase the pre-stretch on your hamstrings.

Standing Leg Curl
INTERMEDIATE LEVEL

■ **START:** Stand facing the machine and slightly to one side of it. Place one leg behind the low ankle pad and brace that knee against the knee pad. If you're standing on the left side of the machine, use your right leg. Lean your hands on the machine for balance. Your nonworking knee should be slightly bent, your torso as erect as possible, and your abs pulled in.

▢ **FINISH:** Pull your heel up toward your rear end, resting the pad on the back of your ankle and taking your heel up as high as possible. Pause, then return to the starting position. Finish the set, then switch legs and repeat.

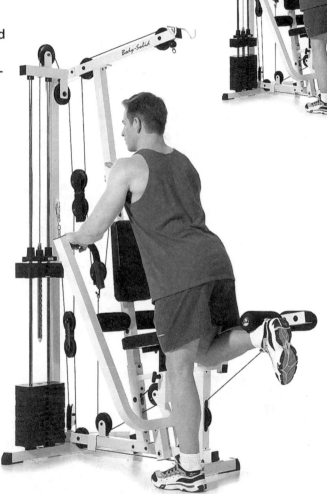

INTERMEDIATE VARIATION
Elevated Standing Leg Curl

Put your nonworking foot up on a weight plate or phone book to help keep your working ankle relaxed. The effort stays with your hams, rather than shifting to your calves.

CHAPTER 11

FOUR WORKOUT PROGRAMS FOR THE MAN WHO HAS IT ALL

By now, an obvious question has probably occurred to you: "Wouldn't I be better off with all the different types of equipment—dumbbells, barbells, and a cable apparatus, if not an entire multistation machine—instead of just one or two things?

Our response: One will suffice, if you work hard enough and creatively enough. Still, more is better. When you have it all, you can do it all. You still work your body one set at a time, but the more equipment options you have, the more interesting exercises you can do during that set. And if you want to move quickly from one exercise to the next, it helps to have a bunch of tools available to make that transition faster and simpler.

The following four workout programs show you how you could build more muscle, achieve more strength, burn more fat, or develop sports-specific power with a complete home gym. Don't worry, you don't need every workout apparatus known to man to do these programs. If you've read the preceding chapters carefully, you should be able to come up with alternatives for the stuff you don't have.

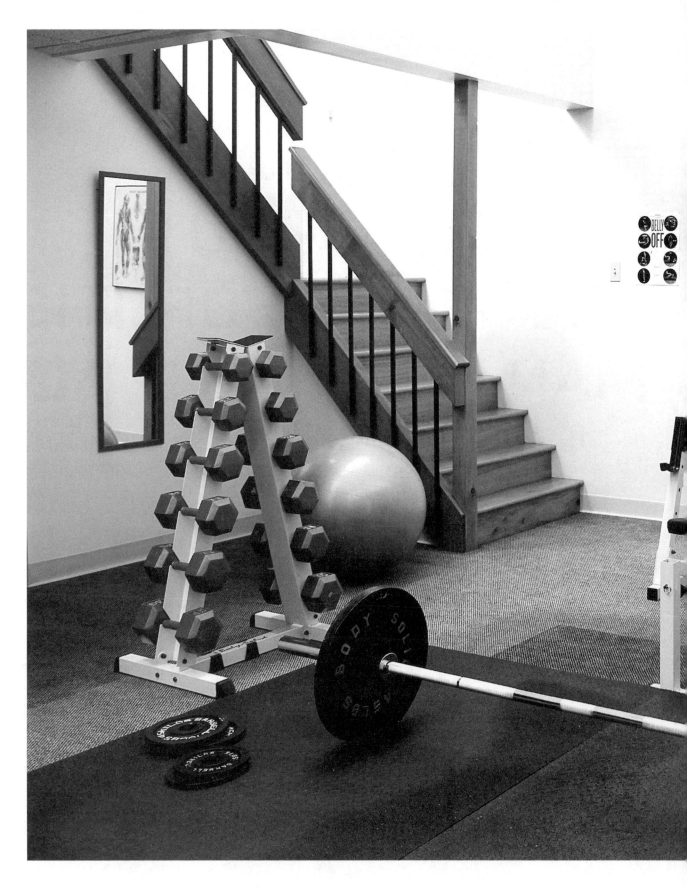

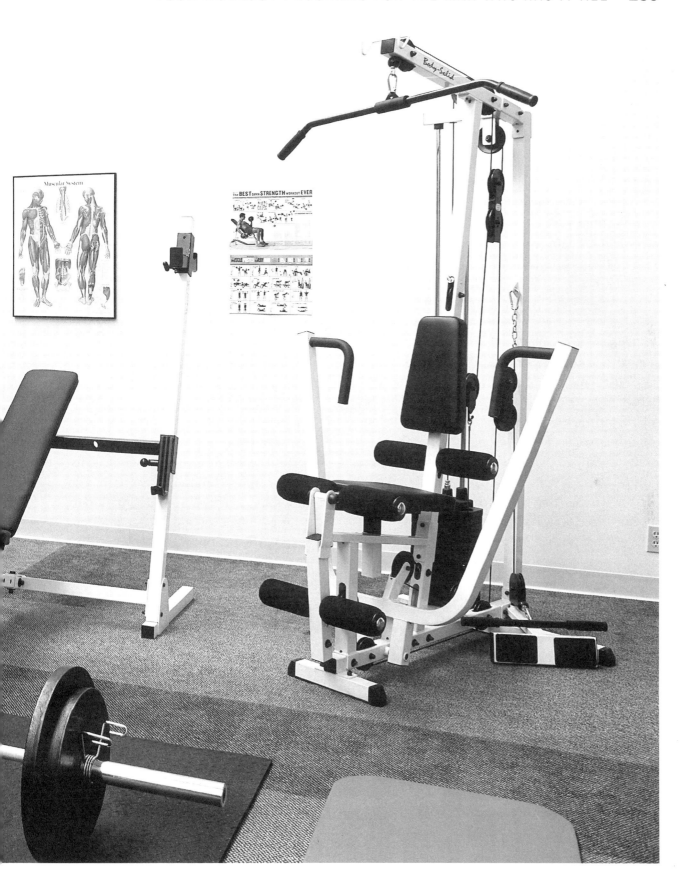

FAT-LOSS PROGRAM

If you're a chunk who's sure that a hunk resides somewhere deep beneath the remembrances of meals past, your goal is fat loss, not weight loss per se. A lower number on the scale doesn't necessarily indicate fat loss—it could just be a sign of water loss, muscle loss, or maybe even memory loss.

The purpose of the following workout is to strip fat from your frame without sacrificing any of your hard-earned, hard-working muscle. You should also see a modest bump in your aerobic capacity, since you'll be working with minimal rest between sets, thereby keeping your heart rate elevated.

Don't think you're going to do these high-rep sets with your wife's plastic-coated dumbbells. You'll lift some fairly heavy weights and alternate between upper- and lower-body exercises, so one set of muscles has a chance to recover while the other works. That maximizes the amount of muscle you gain, helping you to lose fat even faster.

You'll notice that this workout doesn't include specific exercises for mirror-friendly muscles such as biceps and triceps. To create a useful fat-burning stimulus, you need to work your biggest muscles, not just your prettiest ones. The big guys in your chest and upper back will get plenty of work thanks to the dips and rows you'll do—and all your muscles will look a hell of a lot better once you've shed their protective layer of fat.

Here's your fat-shedding mission, should you choose to accept it:

- Work out twice a week—three times if you're already very fit.

- Start by warming up with 3 to 5 minutes of a light activity that uses the large muscle groups—for example, doing jumping jacks or skipping rope.

- Each workout, go through the circuit two or three times. Following the chart below, proceed from one exercise to the next in rapid succession, pausing after each only as long as it takes to set up for the next exercise. Then do 2 to 3 minutes of cardiovascular exercise: skipping rope, treadmill running, stationary cycling—whatever you like—before repeating the circuit.

CIRCUIT WORKOUT

EXERCISE	REPS	MAIN MUSCLES WORKED	EQUIPMENT	SEE PAGE . . .
Squat	8–10	Quadriceps	Dumbbells	152
Lat pulldown	8–10	Lats	Cable	223
Stepup	10–12	Hamstrings/gluteals	Barbell	196
Incline bench press	6–8	Chest	Dumbbells	123
Split squat	8–10	Quadriceps	Cable	258
Elbow-in one-arm row	8–10	Lats	Dumbbell	130
Swiss-ball weighted crunch	10–12	Midsection	Dumbbell/Swiss ball	117
Seated military press	6–8	Shoulders	Barbell	174
Romanian deadlift	8–10	Hamstrings/gluteals	Barbell	199
Dip	6–8	Chest/triceps	Multistation	278

MUSCLE-BUILDING PROGRAM

A guy who wants to move up a shirt size must remember two exercise rules: (1) Work hard and (2) rest hard. We went over the whole yin-yang, exercise-rest relationship in chapter 1, but it's important enough to repeat: Muscles grow not during workouts but during the rest period between workouts. Exercise provides the growth stimulus, while rest provides the actual growth.

Following these two rules isn't as simple as you'd think. Some guys who think they're complying are actually transgressing three times a week. Say a guy designs a bodybuilding-style workout. He works his chest on Monday, his back on Tuesday, his legs on Wednesday, his arms on Thursday, and his shoulders on Friday. (We won't mention that he works his abs Monday through Friday.) So in reality, he's working his arms 4 days a week: He uses his triceps for chest exercises, his biceps for back exercises, and his triceps again for shoulder exercises. His arms never have time to recover, so they never grow.

There's a better way to build muscle, based on a system created by Australian strength coach Ian King, C.S.C.S. Divide your body into four functions: horizontal pushing and pulling (bench presses and rows), vertical pushing and pulling (shoulder presses and pullups), knee-dominant leg movements (squats and lunges), and hip-dominant leg movements (deadlifts and stepups). Then you put as many days as possible between workouts that rely on the same muscles. Here's how.

- Pick your 4 lifting days. Monday, Tuesday, Thursday, and Friday work best for most bodies and schedules.

- Since you'll be going heavy from the very first set, do 2 warmup sets of the first exercise each day, one with about one-third of your first-set weight, the other with two-thirds. For each of the other exercises, do at least 1 warmup set with about two-thirds of your first-set weight.

- Do supersets—consecutive sets of two different exercises, without rest (for example, a set of bench presses immediately followed by a set of bent-over rows). In the workout chart below, each superset pair is designated by a letter-number combination: You'll do a set of exercise A-1 immediately followed by a set of exercise A-2. Then rest for $1\frac{1}{2}$ to 2 minutes. Repeat that superset two more times before moving on to exercise pair B-1 and B-2.

Note that the repetition count goes up for each set of a given exercise. That means you should start with your heaviest weight and use less weight in subsequent sets. (This rep system is called a reverse pyramid, or heavy-to-light.)

WORKOUT I: HORIZONTAL PUSH/PULL

EXERCISE	SUPERSET-1 REPS	SUPERSET-2 REPS	SUPERSET-3 REPS	MAIN MUSCLES WORKED	EQUIPMENT	SEE PAGE . . .
A-1 Bench press	6	8	10	Chest	Dumbbells	122
A-2 Bent-over row	6	8	10	Lats	Dumbbells	129
B-1 Incline fly	8	10	12	Chest	Dumbbells	125
B-2 Bent-over rear lateral raise	8	10	12	Lats	Cable	232
C-1 Swiss-ball preacher curl	6	8	10	Biceps	Dumbbells/ Swiss ball	147
C-2 Overhead triceps extension	6	8	10	Triceps	Dumbbell	140

WORKOUT 2: KNEE-DOMINANT LEG EXERCISES

EXERCISE	SUPERSET-1 REPS	SUPERSET-2 REPS	SUPERSET-3 REPS	MAIN MUSCLES WORKED	EQUIPMENT	SEE PAGE . . .
A-1 Front squat	4	6	8	Quadriceps	Barbell	192
A-2 Lunge	8	10	12	Quadriceps	Dumbbells	155
B-1 Hack squat	6	8	10	Quadriceps	Barbell	193
B-2 Seated calf raise	10	12	15	Calves	Barbell	202
C-1 Standing cable crunch	10	12	15	Abs	Cable	206
C-2 Reverse crunch	10	12	15	Abs	Body weight	63

WORKOUT 3: VERTICAL PUSH/PULL

EXERCISE	SUPERSET-1 REPS	SUPERSET-2 REPS	SUPERSET-3 REPS	MAIN MUSCLES WORKED	EQUIPMENT	SEE PAGE . . .
A-1 Pullup	5	7	9	Lats	Body weight	81
A-2 Military press	5	7	9	Shoulders	Barbell	174
B-1 Upright row	8	10	12	Shoulders	Cable	236
B-2 Dip	6	8	10	Chest/triceps	Multistation or freestanding dip station	278
C-1 Hammer curl	8	10	12	Biceps	Dumbbells	148
C-2 Swiss-ball lying triceps extension	6	8	10	Triceps	Dumbbells/ Swiss ball	139

WORKOUT 4: HIP-DOMINANT LEG EXERCISES

EXERCISE	SUPERSET-1 REPS	SUPERSET-2 REPS	SUPERSET-3 REPS	MAIN MUSCLES WORKED	EQUIPMENT	SEE PAGE . . .
A-1 Deadlift	4	6	8	Hamstrings	Barbell	198
A-2 Lying leg curl	6	8	10	Hamstrings	Multistation	281
B-1 Reverse lunge	8	10	12	Hamstrings	Cable	266
B-2 Unilateral standing calf raise	8	10	12	Calves	Dumbbell	162
C-1 Hanging leg raise	8	10	12	Abs	Body weight/ chinning bar	65
C-2 Swiss-ball weighted crunch	6	8	10	Abs	Dumbbells/ Swiss ball	117

STRENGTH-BUILDING PROGRAM

When you're training for strength rather than for muscle size, you need more rest not only between workouts but also between sets *during* workouts. That's because your central nervous system needs extra recovery time. You already know that the key to muscle growth is exhausting your muscles by doing many exercise repetitions. When you train for pure strength, however, you do fewer reps with heavier weights, which doesn't fatigue your muscles as much as it taxes your nervous system.

Here's how to do a strength program.

- Schedule your three workout days per week, leaving at least a day between each. Examples: Monday, Wednesday, and Friday; or Tuesday, Thursday, and Saturday.

- Use the same warmup guidelines as for the muscle-building program.

- Alternate between two workouts: one for your upper body, one for your lower. So one week, you'll do two upper-body workouts and one lower-body. The next week, you'll do two lower-bodies and one upper.

- The upper-body workout employs supersets, with this key modification: Allow yourself a 1-minute rest each time you move from A-1 to A-2 (or B-1 to B-2, et cetera). Then rest for another minute before moving from A-2 back to A-1. Rest again for a minute or two as you move from one exercise pair to the next (from the last set of A-2 to the first set of B-1, for example).

- The lower-body workout features a technique called wave loading that stimulates your central nervous system to handle heavier lifts by increasing your weight load slightly with each of 3 sets. A second 3-set wave makes the same increases, starting with a heavier weight. So your workout might progress as follows (in pounds): 150, 155, 160 in the first 3-set wave; 155, 160, 165 in the second. You'll instinctively take longer rest periods in the second wave than in the first, for a total of 1 to 3 minutes of rest.

- When training for strength, the key is to move the weights quickly yet in a controlled manner. You'll still see significant muscle growth since some muscle fibers respond better to this type of stimulus. But the object of the routine is strength, not mass.

UPPER-BODY WORKOUT

EXERCISE	SETS	REPS	MAIN MUSCLES WORKED	EQUIPMENT	SEE PAGE . . .
A-1 Bench press	5	5	Chest	Barbell	168
A-2 Pronated bent-over row	5	5	Lats	Barbell	170
B-1 Shoulder press	5	5	Shoulders	Dumbbells	134
B-2 Pullup	5	5	Lats	Body weight	81
C-1 Weighted crunch	3	8	Abs	Dumbbells	116
C-2 Swiss ball reverse crunch	3	8	Abs	Body weight/ Swiss ball	63

LOWER-BODY WORKOUT

EXERCISE	SETS	REPS	MAIN MUSCLES WORKED	EQUIPMENT	SEE PAGE . . .
Back squat	6	5 in set 1, 4 in set 2, 3 in set 3, 5 in set 4, 4 in set 5, 3 in set 6	Quads	Barbell	191
Deadlift	6	5 in set 1, 4 in set 2, 3 in set 3, 5 in set 4, 4 in set 5, 3 in set 6	Hamstrings	Barbell	198
Swiss-ball lying hip extension/ leg curl	4	6	Hamstrings	Body weight/ Swiss ball	108
Calf raise on leg-extension apparatus	3	8	Calves	Multistation	281

SPORTS-TRAINING PROGRAM

While we realize that you may have bought this book partly to get fit for a particular sport, we can't possibly guess which sport that may be. What we can do is show you a training system that prepares you for the movements common to most sports. This program teaches your muscles to move quickly and powerfully. We concede that this type of training does produce bigger, stronger muscles. That's just gravy. What you really want out of this is power, which will help your performance in every sport this side of backgammon.

Here's what to do.

- The workouts are designated 1, 2, and 3. Do each once a week, preferably with a day of rest (or sports practice) in be-

tween. So a Monday-Wednesday-Friday or Tuesday-Thursday-Saturday schedule is best.

- Make sure you do the exercises in the order given. The general rule is that you should do explosive movements like cleans before pure-strength movements like squats and deadlifts.

- Rest for 2 to 3 minutes between sets when doing 5 sets of 5 reps, 2 minutes for 4 sets of 6 reps, and 90 seconds between sets with more than 6 repetitions. When you do supersets (again designated A-1 and A-2, et cetera), rest for a minute between the two exercises in each superset, and rest for another minute or two between one exercise pair and the next.

WORKOUT I

EXERCISE	SETS	REPS	MAIN MUSCLES WORKED	EQUIPMENT	SEE PAGE . . .
Power clean	5	5	Hamstrings/back	Barbell	200
Jump squat	5	5	Quads	Barbell	195
B-1 Swiss-ball incline chest press (alternating)	4	6	Chest	Dumbbells/ Swiss ball	123
B-2 Swiss-ball reverse pushup	4	6	Chest	Body weight/ Swiss ball	86
High woodchopper	3	8	Midsection	Cable	212

WORKOUT 2

EXERCISE	SETS	REPS	MAIN MUSCLES WORKED	EQUIPMENT	SEE PAGE . . .
A-1 Push press	5	5	Shoulders	Barbell	178
A-2 Towel pullup	5	5	Lats	Body weight	84
B-1 Bulgarian split squat	4	6	Quads	Barbell	194
B-2 Unilateral Romanian deadlift	4	6	Hamstrings	Dumbbell	159
C-1 Hanging leg raise	3	8	Midsection	Body weight/ chinning bar	65
C-2 Standing external rotation	3	10	Shoulders	Cable	242

WORKOUT 3

EXERCISE	SETS	REPS	MAIN MUSCLES WORKED	EQUIPMENT	SEE PAGE . . .
A-1 Split jump	5	5	Quads	Body weight	105
A-2 Overhead squat	5	5	Quads	Barbell	193
B-1 One-leg bent-over row (alternating)	4	6	Lats	Dumbbells	129
B-2 Dip	4	6	Chest/triceps	Multistation or freestanding dip station	278
Russian twist	3	10	Midsection	Body weight	69

CHAPTER 12

SAFE AT HOME

As luck would have it, weight lifting is one of the safest exercise activities ever invented. A study published in *Medicine and Science in Sports and Exercise* estimated that 30 percent of American men lift weights at least once a month, and only about 2 percent of those men suffer any sort of injury.

The weight-lifting injuries that do occur fall into two categories: chronic and acute. A chronic problem, also called an overuse injury, builds up over time from a variety of causes, including poor technique, too little variety in exercise selection, and muscle imbalances. Tendonitis—an overuse injury caused by damage to the connective tissues that attach muscles to bones—accounts for up to 12 percent of all weight-lifting injuries.

There's no mistaking an acute injury: Something strains or snaps, and you know it right away.

A 20-year survey of U.S. emergency rooms that looked at more severe injuries from weight lifting found some interesting trends.

- About 40 percent of injuries requiring emergency-room treatment occurred at home.
- About 80 percent of the injured lifters were men.

- Almost two-thirds of the problems were diagnosed as soft-tissue injuries (strains or sprains of muscles or connective tissues). About 28 percent were bone injuries (fractures or dislocations) or lacerations.

- Interestingly, almost one-quarter of the injuries were to a hand. No other body part came close to this rate of injury. You have to think most of the hand injuries were fractures or lacerations, although it's possible there were some sprained fingers and thumbs in the mix. This means soft-tissue injuries were spread across the rest of the body, with no one area jumping out as the place most often strained or sprained. For example, although you'd think knee injuries would be a serious threat to lifters, only about 5 percent of the ER visits were for leg injuries.

- The researchers found records of 34 fatal weight-training injuries: 33 involved free weights, 31 of them were to men, 27 involved head or neck trauma, and 22 caused death by suffocation or strangulation. You don't have to be Sherlock Holmes to figure out that many of these deaths were from bench-pressing at home without a spotter. (Larry Holmes could've guessed it right off.) The researchers didn't go into many specifics, saying only that one lifter died when a barbell fell off his homemade bench onto his neck and that "two out of three lifters who died were unsupervised at the time of injury." Lucky for you, in the next chapter we'll tell you how to avoid becoming such a sorry statistic.

Our point is this: Weight lifting is a very safe form of exercise, especially when you consider the risk-benefits ratio. (To be honest, we don't know how to calculate a risk-benefits ratio. It sounds impressive, though, and we know for certain that weight training has a lot of benefit with little risk.)

Still, one stupid move can plunge you into a world of pain. Let's take a closer look at the threats to your home weight-training safety.

TOO MUCH OF A BAD THING

Chronic overuse injuries can have any number of causes.

Maybe you're doing certain exercises too often, without giving your connective tissues enough time to recover between workouts.

Maybe your body isn't designed for the exercises you're performing. Some guys, for example, get shoulder injuries from using machines on exercises such as shoulder and chest presses. A machine forces you to lift along one circumscribed path, and if that path isn't right for your shoulder joints, they may get hurt.

Maybe you have an old athletic injury that never healed properly, so built-up scar tissue has made the muscles and connective tissues in the injured area tighter and shorter than the matching muscles on the other side of your body. For instance, if you hurt one shoulder playing football, it could have a shorter range of motion than the other. That throws off your exercise form, making it easier to reinjure yourself many years after you thought you'd recovered from the original problem.

Or maybe you have chronic strength imbalances between opposing sets of muscles. You may have strong hamstrings from running, but weak quadriceps. That could set you up for knee injuries. You could have strong pecs and front shoulders from many years of bench pressing but weak muscles in the middle of your back and your rear shoulders. That could make it easier to hurt your shoulders, since the muscles that create a forceful contraction are much stronger than the ones that have to put the brakes on that contraction to keep it from pulling your arm out of its socket.

One metaphor works for all these circumstances: Imagine that your body is a car. You know that if you drive with unbalanced or underinflated tires on one side of your car, the repercussions could be systemic—worn-out brakes, shocks, struts. The longer you let the problem linger, the worse the damage will be.

Now imagine that you have a high-performance sports car, something that goes from zero to 60 while you're pulling out of your garage. You wouldn't equip that magnificent vehicle with the same brakes you'd put in a Chrysler K car. The more powerful the accelerators, the stronger the decelerators have to be.

Balance is everything, whether you're talking about left to right or back to front. So your best protection against chronic injuries is balanced strength, balanced flexibility, and balanced muscle mass.

Balance is simple if you follow the programs in this book. Our man Mike Mejia was one of the first trainers talking about these issues, and all his programs take into account the need to balance the proportional strength and size of muscles.

WAS THAT YOUR TENDON SNAPPING, OR ARE YOU JUST GLAD TO SEE US?

From time to time, we hear about a truly gruesome weight-room injury, like a pec tearing in the middle of a maximum bench press or a biceps rolling up like a venetian blind during an 800-pound deadlift. Still, such catastrophes are rare (praise the deity of your choice here).

While it's true that heavy weights and technically complex exercises increase your risk of acute injury, it's also true that they lead to the biggest gains and make lifting interesting. We'd find it hard to get psyched for our workouts if we knew we were going to do only the safest exercises with unchallenging weights. It would be like playing basketball at a slow jog, without jumping. (That's what the game looks like when we play, but we're actually moving as fast as we can.) So the last thing we want to do is discourage you from using challenging weights and doing tough exercises.

Nor do we want to fall back on the standard fitness-book advice to "get professional instruction" on weight-lifting techniques. Yes, you can hire a personal trainer to come to your home and work with you (see chapter 18). And yes, many people who belong to gyms, where they have access to trainers, also train at home. But we suspect most of you reading this book aren't going to use either of those options.

There's a third way to learn proper technique: You probably have a video camera, right? If you have kids, you almost certainly do. And if you have sex . . . well, come on, you might use one. So tape yourself performing the complex lifts: squats, bench presses, power cleans, deadlifts. Then compare your tape to the pictures in this book. Pause it in the relevant spots, and check out your posture. Are your eyes focused straight ahead? Is your back as straight as it should be? What are your knees doing when you squat? Are your heels staying on the floor?

You can also compare your video performance to that of a lifter on one of the videotapes we'll recommend in chapter 20. If you have a digital camera, you can download your exercises onto your computer, and then compare them to Mike Mejia's form on the video demos at www.menshealth.com.

Even if you achieve the ideal exercise form, serious injuries can result from steroid use. Why do steroids have such an undesirable effect? This is just a theory, but we think that nature has installed a number of safety mechanisms throughout your musculoskeletal system that, under normal circumstances, prevent you from lifting a weight so heavy that it would tear apart your muscles or tendons. Steroids may allow you to bypass some of these physiological hall monitors. Ri-i-i-i-ip! So there's just one more reason—as if you needed it—to stay away from the juice.

CHAPTER 13

HOW YOU DOIN'?

Because your employer pays you a salary, he has a right to evaluate your performance from time to time—and you have a right to know how he thinks you're doing. We believe this same logic applies to your fitness program. You're the boss, expending time and sweat to pay for a better body. Your body is the employee, and from time to time it should report back to you. As the boss, you need to know whether your employee is getting stronger, more muscular, leaner, more flexible, or more aerobically fit. If it's not, you need to make adjustments.

Lucky for you, there are quite a few simple, inexpensive ways to measure your progress in every aspect of exercise and fitness. The following aren't clinical tests that you need a doctor or a trainer to administer. You don't have to do them consecutively, on the same day, like those physical-fitness tests you took in high school. Nor do you have to wait until the end of the fiscal year, as for your employee evaluation, when you have to justify your existence in the next year's budget. You can do one or all of them anytime you're curious about your progress.

However, we do recommend you do these tests (or at least the ones that seem most relevant to your goals) pretty early in your fitness program. Much as we hate to sound like a Hallmark graduation card, you can't know how far you've come until you know where you've been. Log your results on a chart or in a notebook—someplace where you won't forget about or lose them. Make sure you record the date. Update the numbers every month or two.

MEASURING STRENGTH

The longer you hang around the iron, the greater the chance you'll start wondering how much of the stuff you can lift. You want to test yourself, man against barbell. Our goal is to show you, the home-based ironworker, how to figure out your maximums without killing yourself.

First, the terminology: When we talk about the most weight you can lift once with good form, we usually keep it short by saying "one-rep max." Or we keep it even shorter by saying "1RM."

If you can bench-press a 200-pound barbell only once with good form, that's your 1RM for that lift. If you can't lift it once without cheating by arching your back so much that your butt comes off the bench, your 1RM is something lighter. If you can bench-press 200 twice, your 1RM is something heavier. (We'll show you how much heavier in the chart on the next page).

You do a 1RM to test yourself, to measure your strength rather than build it. If you manage to increase your 1RM, you know you've made yourself demonstrably stronger. If you're stronger, you can work with more weight on normal sets of 5 to 12 repetitions. If you work with more weight on those sets, you build more muscle in the same amount of time. With more muscle, you increase your metabolism and burn away more fat. And, if you want to, you can use your increased strength to jump higher, jack softballs farther, and leave bigger bruises on the opponents you block, check, or tackle.

A second benefit of knowing your 1RM is that it takes the guesswork out of many workout programs. Say a training program you've found in a magazine or on the Web specifically instructs you to use 60 to 70 percent of your 1RM for a designated number of reps of an exercise. Obviously, you can't do the program correctly if you don't know what number to reduce to 60 percent less weight.

Still think testing your 1RM is unnecessary? Good. Don't do it. No matter how careful you are, a one-rep max involves some risk. Don't let us talk you into doing it.

If you do want to know your 1RM, we suggest testing yourself with the following exercises.

- Bench press
- Squat
- Deadlift
- Pullup
- Military press

For safety's sake, however, we don't recommend that you actually do any repetitions at your maximum weight—especially not while alone in the darkest reaches of your basement workout room. In point of fact, the 1RM bench press is the number one cause of death during home exercise. Even if you don't drop the bar on your Adam's apple, you run the risk of pulling or tearing something. It's no use knowing how strong you are if a minute later you aren't anymore.

We suggest you test your 3RM or 5RM and then use the chart on the next page to estimate your 1RM. Though that might sound like some kind of carnival trick, a lot of researchers have done a lot of studies to come up with reliable formulas for extrapolating your 1RM. Here are the numbers from *Essentials of Strength and Conditioning,* the National Strength and Conditioning Association's textbook.

MAX REPS (RM)	1	2	3	4	5	6	7	8	9	10	12	15
% RM	100	95	93	90	87	85	83	80	77	75	67	65
SAMPLE WEIGHT (LB OR KG)	200	190	186	180	174	170	166	160	154	150	134	130

A few caveats: The fewer repetitions you do in your self-test, the better you can extrapolate your 1RM. Once you go beyond 5 reps, results will vary depending on a number of variables: your muscular endurance, your limb length (longer arms make it much harder to do a lot of bench-press reps with a given weight, for example), and perhaps even your proportion of fast-twitch (high-power) to slow-twitch (high-endurance) muscle fibers.

Safety remains an issue during a 3RM or 5RM test since you still push yourself to failure and risk dropping a loaded barbell on your sternum or squatting down with a weight you can't lift back up. Here's how to test yourself without alerting the ambulance service.

Rack it. Invest in a power rack so you have a safe place to jettison the bar if you get stuck on a max lift. For squats, set the safety bar a notch below your deepest position, so if you fail halfway up you can simply squat back down and rest the bar on the pins. Do the equivalent for the military press. For the bench press, set the pins far enough above chest level that you can get out from under an urgently racked bar.

Get help from a Pro. We realize that, despite our advice, only a small percentage of you guys reading this book will ever buy power racks. That's why we want to tell you about a machine called the ProSpot. It's expensive—about $1,295 for the home version—but worth it if you're serious about lifting at home. (You can check out the product at www.prospotfitness.com.) It features an Olympic barbell hanging from four cables, and a touch sensor embedded in the barbell to control the locking mechanism. As long as you

keep your fingers on the bar, it remains a free-weight barbell and can be used for squats, bench presses, lunges or any other bar exercise. If you get stuck on a lift, you just have to release your grasp. When either hand loses contact with the built-in sensor on the barbell, the bar instantly locks in place.

You can also use the pricier ProSpot Max model ($5,995) for negative repetitions. Say you're trying to increase your maximum bench press. One way to get used to handling heavier weights is by *lowering* heavier weights than you can lift. (We'll explain this in more detail in chapter 14.) Of course, that technique is good only if you have a spotter handy, and the spotter has to be pretty strong to be able to pull a weight that heavy off your chest. The motorized ProSpot Max eliminates the need to have a big dude hanging around by automatically pulling the bar up off your chest when you release the sensors.

Stick with safe lifts. You don't need a rack for deadlifts and pullups. Neither exercise features a loaded bar threatening to crush you. If you fail halfway through a max-weight deadlift, simply lower the bar to the floor. If you can't quite finish your last pullup, just lower yourself to the floor.

You can use dumbbells to test your bench press, although this has some obvious drawbacks. First, you can't compare your results to anyone else's, since everyone else uses a barbell. Second, it's hard to lift max-weight dumbbells to the height where you can start a repetition, since you can't rack up dumbbells on uprights as you would a barbell. Here's a trick to get around the second

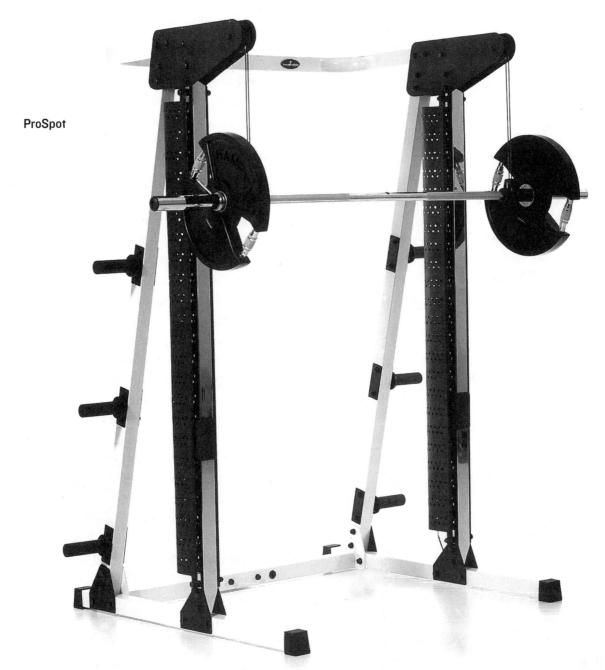

ProSpot

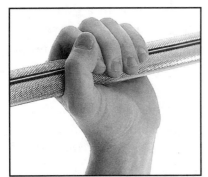

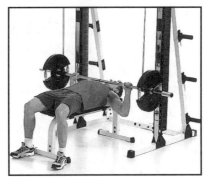

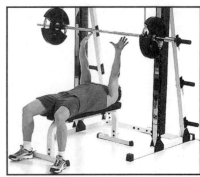

problem: Stand with the dumbbells just outside and parallel to your feet. Deadlift the weights to your thighs, move them in front of your thighs, and sit on your bench. As you lie back, kick up the weights. By the time your back hits the bench, your arms should be straight up over your chest. Set your feet on the floor, then start your repetitions.

Play the angles. If you insist on using a barbell for your maximum bench-press repetitions, set your bench at a slight angle of 10 to 15 degrees. That way, if you find yourself stuck with 225 pounds of iron on your chest, you can roll the bar down to your lap, lift your torso, then stand up and set (or drop) the weight on the floor. If your bench can't be set at such a slight angle (most home benches can't), you can set a pair of 25-pound weight plates beneath the front uprights, raising the bench an inch or so in front to facilitate your escape.

Recognize failure. This is key to avoiding injury as well as to getting at your true 1RM via your 3RM or 5RM. Failure is when you can't finish a rep. The surest sign that you've reached failure is when your form breaks down. At that point, the set is over; your last complete rep was the most you could do with that weight. If you keep trying to get the weight up after your form has failed, you invite injury. And even if you do get it up, you've got a phony max.

Count to two. You're also at failure if, despite your best effort, the weight stops moving. When that happens during a max set, give yourself 2 seconds before racking the weight. If the bar doesn't go anywhere in those 2 seconds (which will feel like an eternity), it's never going to—at least not without compromised technique or divine intervention. The former is unacceptable, and the latter is unlikely.

MEASURING MUSCULAR ENDURANCE

There's more to muscular performance than the amount of weight you can bench press or squat once. Very few of the tasks we encounter in daily life are dependent upon a single exertion lasting 3 seconds. Say you're carrying a piece of furniture up a flight of stairs, or cutting down a dead tree in your backyard. Those jobs require muscular endurance as well as strength. Here are three tests that measure your muscles' ability to perform over time or through many repetitions.

Slow squat. Stand with your feet shoulder-width apart, arms crossed in front of your chest. As slowly as you can, squat down until your thighs are parallel to the floor. Then rise back up just as slowly. If you can draw out the squat for a full 60 seconds—30 seconds to descend, another 30 seconds to rise—consider yourself in top shape.

Pushups to failure. Get down on the floor and count how many pushups you can do. You don't have to hit your chest on the floor on each pushup—instead, stop about 2 inches above the ground before you push back up. (In the military, the drill instructor puts his fist on the floor, thumb-side-up, and the recruit has to hit the fist on each pushup.) If you can do 40 pushups, you're ahead of the game.

Slow situp. The number of situps you can do in a minute gives you a good indication of your overall torso endurance and strength. There's one problem with this test: Most of us cheat like Olympic figure-skating judges when we try to do a lot of situps consecutively. For a test you can't cheat on, try the slow situp, which comes to us from Australian strength coach Ian King, C.S.C.S.

Lie on the floor with your knees bent and your feet flat on the floor. Extend your arms so they're at your sides but off the floor, palms facing down. Sit up as slowly as possible, then immediately return to the starting position, lowering yourself as slowly as you can. If you can take a full 5 seconds to sit up and another 5 seconds to lower yourself, consider your midsection very strong and fit.

MEASURING FLEXIBILITY

It's hard to find even two exercise scientists who agree about flexibility. How flexible should a guy be? Will enhanced flexibility prevent injuries? Can too much flexibility cause problems? Two things seem clear to us.

1. If you sit at a desk all day, you'll grow increasingly inflexible.

2. As you lose baseline flexibility, you lose your ability to perform life's daily tasks comfortably.

Here's a test to tell you how stiff or loose you are in your most vulnerable areas: your lower back and hamstrings.

Sit and reach. Grab a ruler (or a yardstick, if you're really tight) and sit on the floor with your legs straight in front of you. Extend your arms and hold one end of the ruler with both hands. Then keep your chest up as you lean forward at the hips, moving your hands toward your toes. Measure either how many inches your fingers go past your toes or how many inches short of your toes they end up. You're doing well if you can at least get your fingers even with your toes.

MEASURING BODY COMPOSITION

If we had to pick the number one reason guys exercise, it would be to change their body composition, or their percentage of fat versus lean tissue. The best way to measure this is with a DEXA (dual energy x-ray absorptiometry) scan that, depending on how you react to bad news, sends you into either the weight room or a spiral of depression.

Bod-Pod, an egg-shaped capsule that you sit in, uses air displacement to measure body composition and is considered nearly as accurate as a DEXA scan. Before the invention of these procedures, the gold standard was underwater weighing, which of course requires a big tank of water.

Check with your local universities and hospitals to find these services in your area.

Most people today get their fat measured with one of two low-tech devices: calipers, or a body-fat scale. A trainer or some other health professional uses calipers to pinch your skin in several (usually three or seven) locations, then plugs the numbers into a formula to calculate your body-fat percentage. The results are highly dependent on the skill and experience of the person measuring. A scale—such as the type made by Tanita—measures your body composition with a method called bioelectrical impedance. While the procedure is quicker, the results aren't considered scientifically accurate.

To show how many different results you can get from these tests, one of the editors of this book subjected himself, over the course of 1 week, to bioelectrical impedance, calipers, Bod-Pod, calipers again, and finally, DEXA. The Tanita scale showed him at a buff 12 percent body fat. The first calipers test said 17 percent, and the rest of the various tests put him at 22 to 23 percent. (Our guinea pig chose to believe the DEXA and Bod-Pod numbers, overhauled his diet and workout program and proceeded to lose about 10 pounds in 6 months.)

We tell you this to illustrate how improbable it is that the calipers or body-fat scale you can buy for home use will give you a realistic approximation of your body-fat percentage. Here are some very cheap ways to give you numbers to work with.

BMI. You've probably heard that 61 percent of the American population is overweight. Ever wonder how the government arrived at that statistic? The answer is body-mass index, or BMI. This is a crude calculation based on height and weight. Because it doesn't take into account how much of the weight is muscle, an NFL running back, for example, would be considered overweight when measured by BMI, and a linebacker or tight end might be obese, even though both athletes have very little body fat. Still, BMI can be useful for the general population, most of whom are not professional athletes named Terelle.

To figure your BMI, get a calculator and multiply your height in inches (say, 72 inches) by itself (for example, $72 \times 72 = 5,184$). Divide your weight by that number, then multiply the result by 704.5. The result is your BMI. If it's between 18.5 and 24.9, you're at low risk of major diseases. If it's not, you're considered underweight or overweight.

Waist-to-hip ratio. Here's a somewhat better way to figure out if too much of your weight is fat: Measure your waist at the narrowest point—usually your belt line. Then measure your hips at the widest point (around your buttocks), and divide your waist measurement by your hip measurement. If the result is over 1.0, you're considered "at risk" of dangerous health consequences such as heart disease. If it's under 0.9, you're considered safe. As you advance in your program, no matter your goals, your number should improve. Your hip size will grow a bit as you gain muscle, and your waist should shrink as you shed fat.

Weight. This can be the worst indicator of your progress since a tick upward on the scale isn't always bad and a downward trend isn't always as good as it looks. The weight you lose with a strict diet and cardiovascular-exercise program could include a lot of muscle, which will ultimately slow your metabolism. Conversely, a gain of a pound or two on the scale after a couple months of weight training probably means you've gained some muscle and doesn't mean you haven't lost any fat. Say you weigh 2 pounds more: That could mean you've lost 2 pounds of fat and gained 4 pounds of muscle. If you're going to use the scale to measure your progress, make sure you also track your waist size or waist-hip ratio.

Photos. Polaroids are good for more than just blackmailing your ex-girlfriend. They—or any other type of photo—can also help you track your progress. No matter how you prioritize your goals, improving your appearance probably figures in there somewhere. So document the changes in your physique. Have someone take a full-body (or at least above-the-knees) profile shot of you in your swimsuit or gym shorts. Stand in front of a bare wall for a clear view, and don't suck in or push out anything to make yourself look better or worse. Every month or two, take another shot in the exact same pose, wearing the exact same trunks or shorts. Compare the pictures to each other.

MEASURING MUSCLE MASS

Since we've already guessed that your goals include an improved appearance, we'll go further and say that bigger muscles are a large part of what you'd consider an improvement. Here are pointers for measuring the relevant sites. We recommend you measure them all if you're going to measure any. Some guys get fixated on one spot or another—usually abs and biceps—and fail to notice improvements in other areas.

Also, we recommend you take these measurements first thing in the morning, after you've gone to the bathroom but before you eat or drink anything. That's when they'll be most accurate, since you'll probably be holding the least amount of water in your skin. If you measure yourself after a workout, you include the blood you've forced into your muscles, not how big they are without the pump.

Shoulders. Stand up straight with your hands at your sides. Have a helper wrap a measuring tape around your back and across the middle parts of your shoulders before finishing at your breastbone.

Chest. Raise your arms as your helper wraps the tape around you from back to front, crossing under your shoulders and finishing at the nipple line. Lower your arms before finalizing the measurement, making sure the tape doesn't slip down your back. It should cross your shoulder blades behind you. Breathe naturally—don't inflate your chest with air to get a more Charles Atlas–like measurement.

Abdomen. Wrap the tape around your torso, making sure it crosses over your belly button. This tells you the size of your midsection at its thickest point.

Waist. This measurement reflects the narrowest point of your midsection. It's good to know both your abdomen and waist measurements, because you may see improvements in the former before the latter, and anytime you lose abdominal fat is a cause for celebration. (Just remember how you got that fat on your midsection in the first place, and celebrate accordingly.)

Hips and buttocks. Measure the widest point of your hips—around the biggest part of your butt.

Thighs. Make sure the tape goes around the largest part of each thigh.

Calves. Target the largest portion of each calf.

Forearms. Measure the thickest portion, up near each elbow. A lot of guys skip this one, preferring to judge arm girth solely by biceps size. But if this part of your arm grows, regardless of what happens above it, you know you're putting on muscle.

Upper arms. Flex and measure the meatiest part of each arm, at the biceps' peak. You can also measure your unflexed arms.

MEASURING CARDIOVASCULAR FITNESS

We're jumping ahead of ourselves a bit here, since up to this point we've barely said boo about aerobics. But even a strict iron head should see improvements in his cardio fitness as he whips himself into better shape. Here are two short, simple tests.

Step test. This one evaluates your recovery rate from a 3-minute bout of aerobic exercise. You need a platform that's about 16 inches high to step up onto. If a staircase is all you have, you'll probably need to use two of the stairs. Step up with one foot, then with the other; then step down with the first foot and then with the second, in a steady up-up-down-down cadence. Keep going for 3 minutes without resting.

Starting 5 seconds after the last step down, count your heartbeats for exactly 15 seconds by using two fingers to feel your pulse at your wrist. Multiply the total by four to get a per-minute heart rate. As your endurance improves, that rate should get lower after future step tests performed at the same pace.

One-and-a-half-mile run. Get out on a track and run, jog, walk, or crawl for a mile and a half. (On most high school and college tracks, this distance is equal to six laps.) Make sure you write down your time on the spot. If you aren't used to cardio exercise, your mind may not be clear enough to remember the number.

CHAPTER 14

IRON DEFICIENCY

You bought yourself a nice 110-pound barbell set, and within 6 months, you outgrew it. You can do all of the major exercises with the entire weight set; and on some exercises, you can lift the entire weight set with a full paint can hanging from each end of the barbell.

The easiest solution is to drive the minivan down to Muscles 'R' Us and pick up some extra weight plates. But you aren't the only one in the family who needs some heavy metal: The bill for your 12-year-old's braces is due. Until Santa puts some new iron under the tree (assuming he doesn't throw out his back carrying the weights down the chimney), you're going to have to make muscle with what you've got. Here are a few ideas.

S-L-O-W DOWN

There are times when it makes sense to lift weights fast (see the next page). Most guys do it naturally. Put on the brakes, however, and you've found a new way to challenge your muscles. Take 3 or 4 seconds for the lowering phase of each repetition. That will make any weight seem heavier to your muscles. Another benefit of slowing down is that it reduces the stress on your joints and connective tissues.

TAKE A PAUSE

Slow lifting reduces "bounce," ensuring that all the work is done by your muscles rather than by the elastic energy your muscles keep in reserve for quick bursts of power. Another way to reduce bounce is to pause for a second or two at the mid-point of the lift. For instance, hesitate in the bottom position of a squat, or leave the bar on your chest during a bench press. Each of these positions is the exercise's "sticking point"—the point where the weight seems heaviest and, therefore, where you're most likely to get stuck when attempting a maximum lift. Pausing at a sticking point will build isometric strength that'll enable you to handle heavier weights once you can finally afford to buy some.

GO REALLY FAST

Normally, we tell guys to lift slowly and in full control of the weights. Sometimes, though, it pays to go really fast. This is an advanced technique and not for the guy who thinks pectoralis major is a constellation and teres minor is the site of the Trojan War. (If you are that guy, we aren't making fun of you. A year or two from now, when you understand that the soleus has nothing to do with an eclipse, you can try speed reps for yourself, and tell us if they were worth the wait.)

We'll explain this in much more detail in chapter 15, but here's the short version: Slow reps are a great way to build muscle, but if you're lifting weights for more than muscle size—if you want to improve in a sport or boost your maximum bench press, for example—you need to develop speed as well as mass. Most athletes and competitive weight lifters today do a lot of work with light weights, pushing or pulling as quickly as possible.

PREEXHAUST YOUR STRONGEST MUSCLES

Let's say you like to start your workout with bench presses. (Not a tough guess; all you have to do is check out the lines at the bench-press stations in any gym on any Monday.) Your measly 110 pounds are not enough to challenge chest muscles that are rested and minty-fresh. So you have to do what for many guys is unthinkable: You have to tire out your muscles before you work them. Here are a couple of ways to do this.

Exhaust your chest muscles. Work them directly with chest flies or pullovers. When you get around to your beloved bench presses, the weight will feel much heavier than it is, since your pecs will be pooped.

Exhaust the muscles surrounding your chest. This means doing pullups, pulldowns, shoulder presses, rows, shrugs, or power cleans. Some of these exercises—such as the pullups—involve your chest muscles in minor ways. Shoulder presses work your triceps and the front parts of your deltoids, which also get heavy work on bench presses. When those other muscles are tired, your pectorals have to handle more of the load, with less help. Rows, shrugs, and power cleans exhaust the muscles behind your chest, weakening the base of support. And all of them make you tired, so you feel a little weaker when you get to the bench.

Other examples of pre-exhaustion are lateral raises before shoulder presses, leg extensions before squats, pullovers before lat pulldowns (the pullovers hit your chest and lats with almost equal conviction), and one-legged squats and deadlifts before traditional squats and deadlifts.

MAKE CHANGE WITH A QUARTER

Add an extra quarter-repetition to the most difficult part of a lift to make the exercise much more challenging. It works two different ways, depending on whether the exercise begins with a negative contraction (that is, with lowering the weight) or a positive contraction (raising the weight). For exercises with a negative start, add a quarter-rep to the positive portion, and vice versa.

The bench press is an example of an exercise that begins with a negative contraction. (Other examples include the squat, chest fly, and pullover.) You begin a bench press with an extra quarter-rep just as you would any bench press: Lie on the bench, hold the weight straight above your collarbone, then lower the weight to within an inch of your chest. After pausing for a second, press it up only one-quarter of the way. Lower it back down to within an inch of your chest, pause again, and press it all the way up. That's 1 repetition.

Examples of exercises that begin with a positive contraction include the lat pulldown, the row, most biceps and triceps exercises, and the pullup. To add a quarter-rep to the latter, begin normally, by hanging from the chinup bar and then pulling yourself up until your chin clears the bar. Pause, then lower yourself one-quarter of the way down. Pull yourself back up, pause again, and lower yourself all the way back down.

BLOW OUT YOUR GUNS WITH 21-REP SALUTES

The bodybuilding trick called 21s is as old as Jack LaLanne's first jockstrap, but it still works. It's especially valuable to a guy who's outgrown his weights. Say you're doing biceps curls: Do 7 repetitions through the first half of the range of motion (from the bottom to the middle), 7 reps through the second half (from the middle to the top), and then 7 through the full range. You can use it on most biceps and triceps exercises, lat pulldowns, bench presses, rows. . . virtually any upper-body exercise.

TRAIN UNILATERALLY

It seems like everything in life is done by committee these days. There's safety in numbers but also frustration that the end product is not as good as it might've been had it followed one man's vision, rather than a group's diluted version of it.

What does this have to do with your muscles?

Nothing. We just felt like ranting about the uselessness of committees.

Actually, here's the connection: Unilateral exercise—working one limb at a time—has some surprising muscle-building benefits. For starters:

It corrects strength imbalances. If you have a strength deficit—that is, if one side of your body is weaker than the other—you'll discover it here, and you can work to correct it by making your weaker side work harder.

It improves athletic performance. Sports almost never require you to simultaneously work both arms or both feet equally hard, so unilateral exercise more directly applies to athletic training.

It works more intensely. A limb working unilaterally often has more than half the strength of both limbs working together. That's because when you work a pair of limbs together, a protective mechanism called the bilateral deficit shuts down some of your motor units (combinations of nerve cells and muscle fibers) to keep you from getting hurt during the heaviest lifts. When you work with

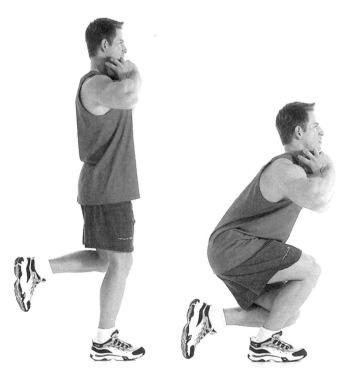

Unilateral squat

one limb at a time, however, the deficit doesn't kick in, so you can work the muscles in each limb more intensely.

So if you've maxed out the available weight on your leg curl when using both legs, try it with one leg at a time. (Start with your left leg if you're right-handed, and vice versa.) Even if you haven't maxed out, it's a good idea to work unilateral exercises into your program from time to time.

It will give you positive results from negative contractions. A physiological phenomenon that's somewhat better known than the bilateral deficit is the fact that your muscles are about 40 percent stronger when lowering a weight than when raising it. So, returning to the example of the leg curl, try lifting the weight with both legs but lowering it with one leg. That will give you a more potent muscle-building stimulus than would lowering with both legs.

It improves your balance. Unilateral exercise also changes the balance component of a movement. That's why a one-legged squat or deadlift is much harder than you'd expect—you might not be able to do these with any weight other than your own body weight. So you improve your balance and coordination as well as your strength.

BE A MAN OF THE '90S—THE 1890S

Finally, here's a way to turn that 110-pound standard barbell set you've outgrown into the most interesting training tool you've ever used. At one time or another, you've probably seen a picture of an old-time strongman wearing what look like a fig leaf and wrestling boots and hoisting fantastically huge barbells overhead with one arm. There's a lesson to be learned there—actually two, if you count the reminder that you can wear whatever the hell you want in your home gym. (Still, we don't anticipate a line of fig leaves at Abercrombie and Fitch anytime soon.) The big lesson is this: There's no rule that says you have to do unilateral

exercises with dumbbells and bilateral exercises with a barbell. You can also use your barbell for one-armed exercises and your dumbbells for traditional barbell movements.

Unilateral barbell moves. Try a "suitcase" deadlift, in which you set a barbell on the floor just outside your left ankle, grab it in the middle with your left hand, then stand up straight. The form is exactly the same as a standard deadlift, except the weight is all on one side of your body.

Another variation is a one-armed overhead shoulder press. You'll probably need two hands to lift the barbell to your left shoulder. Once it's up there, grab it in the middle with your left hand (hold it like a spear, with your palm toward your head), lean slightly to the right, and crank out a set of presses.

Finally, for really advanced guys, there's the one-armed muscle snatch. Set the barbell in front of you, against your shins, as if you were going to do a deadlift. Grab it in the middle with one hand, using an overhand grip. Then, in one motion, pull it overhead. Try to keep the bar as close to your body as you can. So the first part of a movement is like a deadlift, with the bar brushing the fronts of your legs. The next part is like a shrug and calf raise: You use your traps and calves to generate momentum with the bar. The third part is like an upright row: You pull the bar along the front of your body, with your elbow bending and your upper arms rising perpendicular to your torso. Finally, you snap the bar overhead.

It takes a lot of strength, speed, and flexibility to pull this off, and you should probably practice with a broomstick before you try it with the bar. You should definitely develop proficiency with an unweighted bar before you start adding plates. Once you've mastered it, the one-armed muscle snatch is a fun exercise with which to kick off your workouts. (Always do movements that require skill and explosive speed at the beginning of your workout.) And the muscles in your upper and middle back will let you know it's doing more than just providing amusement.

Bilateral dumbbell moves. Most guys use dumbbells with both arms at once, each arm acting independently of the other. While this is just as effective for building muscle as barbell exercises, it doesn't feel the same. Some guys forced to use dumbbells exclusively miss the sensation of exercises such as the close-grip bench press.

You can get the feeling back by holding the ends of the dumbbells together as if they formed a barbell. Try this: Set your bench at a slight incline, and hold two dumbbells together overhead. Your palms should face out, just as they would on a close-grip bench press. Then do the exercise without allowing the dumbbells to slip apart. Feel it in your chest and triceps?

You can use the same technique with pullovers and triceps extensions. Another interesting experiment is a bilateral concentration curl, holding the dumbbells together in front of you as you sit on the edge of a bench, bent over and bracing your upper arms against the insides of your knees.

There's no end to the exercises you can create, whether it's from necessity, boredom, or something else entirely.

PART 3

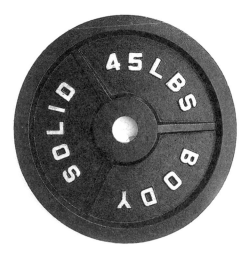

HOME, SWEAT HOME

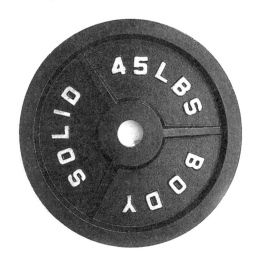

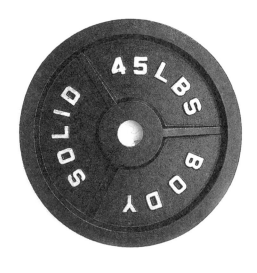

CHAPTER 15

HOME-TEAM ADVANTAGE

Most of the advice in this book is directed toward guys who work up a sweat for the same general reasons: more muscle, less fat, better health, more opportunities to critique women's tattoos.

Still, we know many guys train for the specific purpose of improving athletic performance. Even though an improved cholesterol profile is terrific, it won't help you knock a softball over the left fielder's head with the bases loaded. And while bigger biceps are nice accessories, they won't help you blow past your defender on the way to the hoop.

Many great athletes have great physiques. (If you don't believe us, ask your wife while she's watching NFL wide receivers and D-backs during the slo-mo instant replay.) Their muscles are a by-product of the type of training they do, not the reason for it. These guys don't pump up with biceps curls and lateral raises and then admire themselves in the mirror afterward. In fact, most don't pump up at all. They train with lifts that build the explosive power they need to succeed during competition. We showed you these lifts—power cleans, snatches, push presses, jump squats—in the earlier exercise chapters. Now we're going to show you how to use them to become a better athlete, as opposed to just a better physical specimen.

Before we jump into specifics, we want to say a few words about why you—if you're a guy who isn't paid to play games and who has never been asked to endorse anything sportier than his department's annual budget—might consider this type of workout.

TWITCH, TWITCH, TWITCH

Your body has three major types of muscle fibers: type-I, or slow-twitch, which are mostly used in endurance-type activities; type-IIa, which have both endurance and strength capabilities; and type-IIb, which perform quick, all-out feats of strength and power.

Most of the time, you're advised to lift weights in a slow, controlled fashion. The sustained work develops more muscle, and the controlled movements decrease your risk of injury. Unfortunately, this type of lifting mostly targets type-IIa muscle fibers, with a bit of work for the type-I fibers. The IIb fibers don't see any action at all, and plenty of research has shown that these fibers are lost when they aren't used. That means you steadily lose your ability to sprint, jump, and rip line drives into the gap.

Even if you've been lifting heavy weights for years, you may not have the ability to move those weights fast. Your body gradually loses important

functions even though it looks lean and strong. Targeting your type-IIb muscles with the following exercises will improve your agility, speed, and power so you'll not only look good but also knock 'em out on the playing field—particularly in sports involving quick reactions such as sprinting, jumping, hitting, or blocking.

A BODY BUILT FOR SHOW AND GO

The table below lists the explosive lifts we're talking about.

Here's a plan for using these weight-room exercises to improve performance on the field.

Do fast moves first. The exercises that require the most speed and coordination should come earliest in your workout. You're asking your muscles to learn new movements, and to learn to do those new movements at high speeds. That requires a fresh body and mind. The only exercises that should precede explosive weight-training exercises are explosive moves without weights, such as the plyometrics. We'll tell you about them later in this chapter.

Do few repetitions. When it comes to explosive exercises, form is everything. And form breaks down with higher repetitions. Three to five reps are the most you should attempt.

A second reason to keep your number of repetitions low is to mimic an athletic performance: In a game, you rarely repeat the same movement

EXERCISE(S)	SPORTS SKILL(S) DEVELOPED	SEE PAGE . . .
Power clean	Sprint starts, vertical jump	200
Hang clean	Checking (hockey), blocking (football), vertical jump	176
Muscle snatch	Sprint starts, shot or pass blocking (volleyball, basketball, football)	201
Push press, push jerk	Shot or pass blocking (volleyball, basketball, football)	178
Neider press	Blocking and checking (football, hockey), boxing	177
Jump squat	Vertical jump	195

multiple times. You usually have only one chance to take off and catch some air or knock down an opponent.

Use light to moderate weights. This one is counterintuitive. Normally, when you do fewer than 5 repetitions per set, you use the heaviest possible weight. The objective of these exercises, however, is to move the weight as fast as you can— remember, on the sports field, the winner is the guy who gets to the target first. You can't move a maximal weight fast, so most of the time, do explosive exercises with 40 to 60 percent of your one rep max.

Rest longer between sets. Here's another counterintuitive idea. Since you use lighter weights for fewer repetitions, you'd think you could get away with less rest. You'd be wrong. Explosive lifts take more out of your body than you think. In particular, your central nervous system goes all-out to coordinate your muscles as they work together at full speed to move an object through a fairly long trajectory.

Figure on taking a minimum of 2 minutes of rest between sets. You may even want a little more recovery time after snatches and power cleans, since they require you to move weights the greatest distances.

TRAINING CAMP

Here's a sample program to get you ready for the big homecoming game.

MONDAY

EXERCISE	SETS	REPS	SEE PAGE . . .
Power clean	3	3	200
Push jerk	3	5	178
Traveling lunge	3	8	190
Pullup	3	Max	81
Hanging leg raise	1–3	8–10	65

WEDNESDAY

EXERCISE	SETS	REPS	SEE PAGE . . .
Jump squat	3	3	195
Neider press	3	3–5	177
Snatch-grip Romanian deadlift	3	5	199
Bench press	3	8	122 or 168
One-arm row, elbow-out	3	8	130

FRIDAY

EXERCISE	SETS	REPS	SEE PAGE . . .
Muscle snatch	3	3	201
Front squat	3	5	153 or 192
Weighted dip	3	8	278
Chinup	3	Max	81
Swiss-ball weighted crunch	1–3	8–10	117

SAFE AT ANY SPEED

Since safety is one of the reasons most lifting is done slowly and with great control, it follows that high-speed, sports-specific lifting is dangerous—or at least more dangerous than the alternative. Minimize the chance of injury by following these precautions.

Warm up thoroughly. Warm muscles can rapidly accelerate and decelerate without tearing. Cold muscles can't. Warm connective tissues can maintain the integrity of your joints. Cold connective tissues can't. We recommend a minimum of 5 minutes of light activity using major muscle groups—jogging, calisthenics, jumping rope—before explosive lifts. We also recommend two or three warmup sets of the first exercise in your workouts before your "work" sets. Those warmup sets prepare not only your muscles but also your nervous system.

Stretch. Despite stretching's recent bad press, we're keeping the faith. Yes, studies of high-level athletes have shown that stretching before max-imal-effort events can reduce power production, limiting performance when it really counts. Our take: The next time you get invited to the Olympic trials, forget about stretching before the long jump. Before you power-clean heavy weights in your rec room, however, you want your muscles to be capable of a full range of motion. A world-class athlete may have that range without stretch-ing. You probably don't.

Keep your workouts low in volume. The sample workouts above include just 15 work sets. That's less than half the volume of typical body-building workouts. These exercises take more out of your body, and the more sets you do, the greater your risk of injury.

JUMP-START YOUR WORKOUTS

Plyometrics are another great training tool for ath-letes. Originally called jump training, these exer-cises allow muscles to produce maximal force as rapidly as possible. They can be as simple as skip-ping or as challenging as jumping onto boxes or hurling a medicine ball for distance. Whatever form they take, the goal is the same: to produce power by linking strength with speed.

The results you get from plyometrics come with a price. Although they don't look particularly taxing, these exercises present an all-out challenge to your muscles, joints, connective tissues, and central nervous system. Before you even consider adding them to your workouts, heed these guide-lines.

Make sure you're in decent shape. The stan-dard advice is to forget lower-body jumps until you can squat 1½ times your body weight; and to avoid upper-body plyos until you can bench-press your weight. To us, that advice seems like a Catch-22—you must be strong before you're allowed to de-velop power.

Look at kids: They don't need training to skip and jump. They do it all day, every day. It's an im-portant part of their development. Could the av-erage 40-pound kindergartner squat 60 pounds or bench 40? We doubt it.

Let's modify the standard advice and say you should build a base of strength and fitness before you turn to plyometrics. We think a solid year of strength training should do it.

Respect preexisting injuries. Make sure your injuries have healed before you do plyometrics that affect those areas. With some chronic knee and lower-back injuries, you may not be able to do plyos at all without risking further damage. (Same with wrist injuries, in the case of plyometric pushups.)

Do plyometrics first in your workouts. That means after warmups and stretching but before strength or aerobic exercises. In an ideal sit-uation, strength and aerobics should be done on one day, plyos on another, warmup and stretching every time you workout. If that's not an option, do plyos before strength and/or aero-bics work.

Rest for 2 to 3 days between plyometric work-outs. Beginners and those over age 40 may want to budget even more time for recovery. You want your muscles and connective tissues to grow stronger between workouts, and that requires full recovery from one workout to the next.

Keep reps relatively low. Try for 6 to 10 per set.

Rest for 2 to 3 minutes between sets. But stay on your feet. Stretch or walk around in be-tween sets. Don't sit and allow your muscles to stiffen.

Keep volume low. Plyometric volume is usu-ally measured in *foot contacts*, rather than in reps. The term means exactly what you think it means, although one foot landing counts as 1 contact, while two feet landing at the same time also counts as 1 contact. That's because your body—particularly your lower back—feels contact no matter how many Nikes hit the turf. Beginners should limit themselves to 60 to 80 foot contacts per workout. Advanced guys can go as high as 150 to 200, with intermediates in between.

Get off the ground. Minimize ground time and maximize air time. As soon as you land from one jump, immediately explode into the next one. Height isn't as important as speed.

Use ground that gives. Your yard is an ideal place to do plyometrics, provided you aren't in the middle of a drought. A carpeted floor can also work in a pinch.

Progress from easiest to hardest. Just as you started strength lifting with the simplest exercises—crunches, pushups, biceps curls—and then progressed to the challenging stuff in this chapter, you should also start plyos with simple standing jumps before moving onward and upward. Here are some common plyometric exercises, listed by category in order of difficulty, from easiest to hardest.

STANDING JUMPS

Hip Twist and Ankle Hop
SPORT: DOWNHILL SKIING

Stand with your feet shoulder-width apart and your upper body vertical. Hop up, twisting your hips in a 180-degree arc. As soon as you land, quickly jump again and twist in the reverse direction. Keep your upper body as still as possible; initiate the twist with your hips and legs. Do 8 to 10 reps.

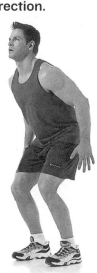

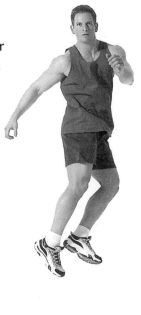

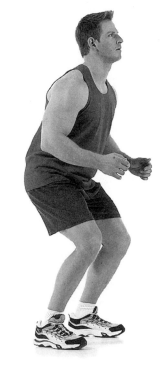

Standing Jump and Reach
SPORTS: VOLLEYBALL AND BASKETBALL

Squat slightly with your feet shoulder-width apart and your arms down at your sides. Quickly explode upward, reaching both arms overhead. Land with soft knees, then explode up again. Do 6 to 10 reps.

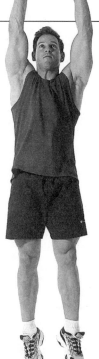

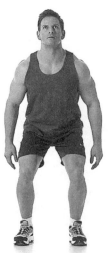

MULTIPLE HOPS AND JUMPS

Front Cone Hops
SPORTS: TENNIS AND SKIING

You'll need 6 to 10 small cones or barriers that are approximately 8 to 12 inches high. Set them in a straight line, 2 to 4 feet apart. Stand at one end of the row with your feet shoulder-width apart and your arms at your sides. Hop forward over the first barrier, swinging your arms to help with your forward momentum. Land with both feet together. Immediately repeat until you've completed the entire row of cones.

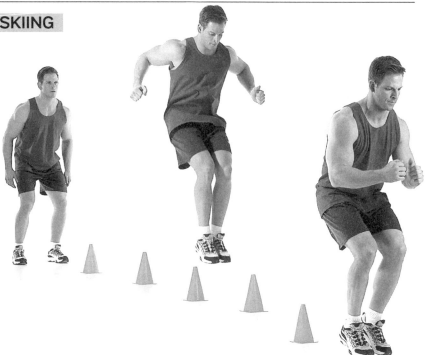

Lateral Cone Hop
SPORTS: BASKETBALL AND HOCKEY

Stand next to a cone or box that's 8 to 12 inches high, with your arms at your sides and your feet shoulder-width apart. Jump sideways over the cone and land with both feet together. Upon landing, immediately jump back over the cone. Do 8 to 10 reps.

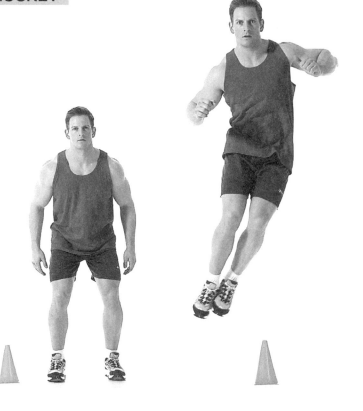

BOX JUMPS

Alternating Box Pushoffs
SPORTS: CYCLING AND SOCCER

You'll need a box that's 6 to 12 inches high. Stand with your right foot on the ground and your left on the box, with your left heel close to the edge. Push off your left foot and jump as high as possible, swinging your arms upward to help you catch more air. Switch legs in midair and land on the other side of the box with your feet reversed, your right on the box and your left on the ground. Immediately jump again. Do 4 to 6 reps with each leg. Beginners should use a lower box and stay closer to the higher end of the rep range. More advanced trainees can use a higher box for fewer reps.

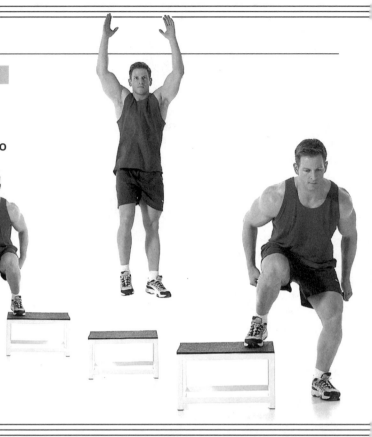

DEPTH JUMPS

Squat Depth Jump
SPORTS: CYCLING AND DIVING

You'll need a sturdy box that's 12 to 36 inches high. Stand on it in a quarter- to half-squat position, toes close to the edge. Hop off and as soon as your toes touch the ground, immediately jump again, reaching as high as possible. Do 6 to 8 reps.

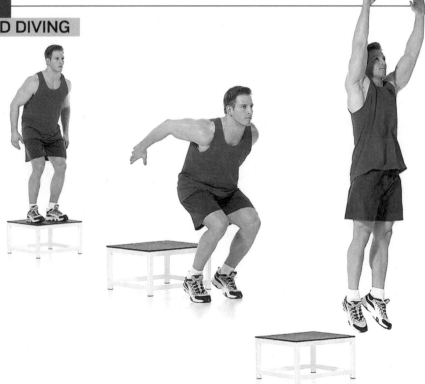

UPPER-BODY PLYOMETRICS

Plyometric Pushup
SPORTS: FOOTBALL AND HOCKEY

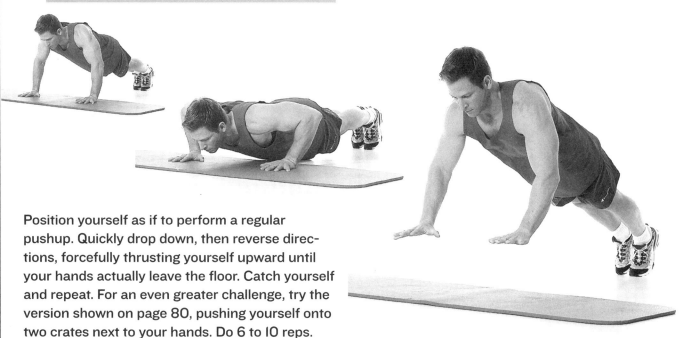

Position yourself as if to perform a regular pushup. Quickly drop down, then reverse directions, forcefully thrusting yourself upward until your hands actually leave the floor. Catch yourself and repeat. For an even greater challenge, try the version shown on page 80, pushing yourself onto two crates next to your hands. Do 6 to 10 reps.

Side Throw
SPORTS: BASEBALL AND GOLF

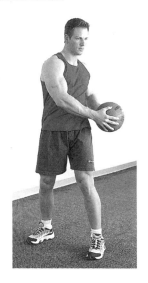

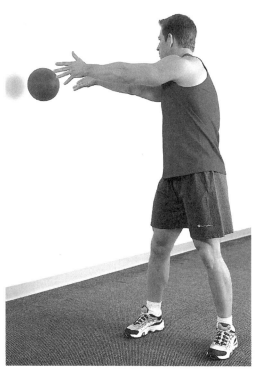

You'll need a medicine ball and a solid surface, such as a brick or concrete wall, to throw it against. (Your living room wall won't cut it— that is, unless you want a gaping hole in your drywall.) Stand about 3 feet from the wall with your feet shoulder-width apart and hold the ball on your left side. Swing it a bit farther to the left, then quickly switch directions and throw it, as hard as you can, to your right, aiming for the wall. You could also do this exercise with a partner to catch the ball and throw it back to you. Do 2 to 3 sets of 4 to 8 reps, then switch sides and repeat.

CHAPTER 16

CARDIO, THE "OLD TESTAMENT" EXERCISE

We may be a nation predicated on change, but that doesn't mean we all change at the same time. Two decades ago, the word *exercise* meant "aerobic exercise": running, cycling, swimming, rowing, cross-country skiing, aerobic dancing. Weight lifting was just something we meatheads did to compensate for feelings of sexual inadequacy.

Today, there are so many documented benefits of resistance training that many researchers and trainers are now asking a question that would've been unthinkable during the Lycra-and-leg-warmers era: Is there any real reason you *must* do traditional long, slow, steady-paced aerobic exercise?

If you ask someone speaking for the American College of Sports Medicine, he or she will tell you yes: For health and longevity, you must do a minimum of 20 minutes of steady-pace aerobic exercise three to five times per week. While the ACSM also recommends strength training and flexibility exercise, it hasn't backed down on aerobics.

We, on the other hand, think the lean, healthy lifter can live just as long and vigorous a life as the lean, healthy runner or cyclist. And we know dozens of trainers and strength coaches who don't use any traditional aerobic exercise in training their athletes and overweight clients. In fact, we talk to so many exercise professionals who share our skepticism about the benefits of aerobic exercise that we're surprised when we find ourselves arguing with someone who holds the opposite point of view. In the 1990s, we were revolutionaries. Here at the start of the 21st century, aerobics advocates seem to hold the more radical point of view.

If you like aerobic exercise, don't let us talk you out of it. We don't want to trash our brethren who enjoy running, cycling, swimming, rowing, skating, cross-country skiing, and the like. Those are all great sports and terrific forms of exercise. If, however, you do them only because you think you have to, we give you permission to switch to anaerobic exercise: weight training, sports like tennis and basketball—whatever you enjoy more and engage in consistently. We're just making an argument for guys like us, who'd rather lift than tread.

THE HEART OF THE MATTER

We'd like to back up our position with some smoking-gun research. Unfortunately, science isn't as helpful on this issue as you'd think. Lots of studies show the specific benefits of aerobic exercise on the function of the heart and lungs. But science doesn't yet know whether the big benefit of exercise—a longer life—is achievable through any type of vigorous exercise, or whether the exercise has to be aerobic.

The earliest study showing that exercise prevents heart disease was conducted on longshoremen. Dock workers who were promoted to sedentary management positions developed heart disease. This certainly demonstrated that physical activity is a powerful preventative against heart disease. It didn't necessarily make a case for aerobic exercise. After all, you wouldn't confuse a dock worker—a guy who lifts and carries heavy things all day—with a marathoner or a Tae Bo instructor.

Even though that's where the science began, "vigorous physical activity" soon became synonymous with "aerobic exercise." And that's where we take issue. If you measure your heart's functional strength by the rate per minute at which it consumes and utilizes oxygen (a calculation called VO_2 max), aerobic exercise unquestionably does your heart good. However, our understanding of heart health has grown exponentially since the aerobics movement first caught the public's attention. We now know there's more to heart health than VO_2 max. We know that strength training can reduce heart disease risk by improving blood pressure and perhaps cholesterol levels, too. And we know that stronger muscles make your heart's job easier.

WHY FAT ENDURES DESPITE ENDURANCE EXERCISE

Though heart disease is the single largest killer of American males, it's not what drives the annual post–New Year's workout craze. People are afraid of girth, not death.

Health clubs and home gyms alike are filled with men and women sweating like gladiators on stairclimbers and elliptical machines . . . and not making any progress against their stored fat. We've run out of fingers and toes counting friends and coworkers who trained for 10-Ks and half-marathons and ended up *gaining* weight, either while training or immediately after racing.

Although cardio exercise burns calories while you do it, it doesn't increase your resting metabolism, according to a 1998 study in the *American Journal of Clinical Nutrition*. In contrast, a hard weight workout can keep your metabolism elevated for 48 hours after you finish lifting. One study found that subjects who engaged in 90 minutes of strenuous resistance exercise were still burning 62 percent more calories from fat up to 16 hours after their workout. Although we'd never recommend lifting weights for 90 minutes at a time, you have to admit that's an amazing finding.

Furthermore, the very goal of weight lifting is to build more muscle, and more muscle makes you automatically burn more calories each day. Estimates of how many bonus calories you burn with extra muscle are all over the place. Some good research points to a figure between 34 and 37 calories per pound of new muscle mass per day. The equation isn't as simple as it seems—women, for example, can add muscle mass without seeing a spike in resting metabolic rate. (Bummer for our wives.) And in men, the metabolic boost seems related to increased post-workout nervous-system activity as well as increased muscle mass.

In other words, you can't just work hard for a while, add some muscle, and expect the metabolic bandwagon to roll on. The good news is, when you lift hard and lift consistently, you get metabolic benefits you couldn't get from aerobic exercise.

FORM VERSUS FUNCTION

When we argue against traditional aerobic exercise, we have to add that we like a nontraditional form of aerobic exercise called interval training. Interval exercise is more like real life (and more like strength training, for that matter) because it involves short bursts of intense work followed by periods of low-intensity movement.

We also recommend you make your interval workouts as "life specific" as possible. In life, your body relies on three energy systems, and we suggest you develop all three.

ATP-PC. These letters stand for *adenosine triphosphate-phosphocreatine*. All you need to remember is that this is your short-term energy system, used for quick bursts of all-out effort. You activate this system during sprints and maximum lifts, and in such real-life situations as pushing a car

out of a ditch or dashing across the yard to keep your toddler from wandering into the street.

Ideal activities: Running, cycling, and rope jumping.

Improve it: After a thorough moderate-intensity warmup (about 5 minutes, or until you break a light sweat), do 10-second sprints on a track or any cardio apparatus. (A "sprint" is an all-out effort.) Recover by coasting at a moderate intensity for 50 to 60 seconds. Start with 5 sprints, and build up to 10. When you're done with your sprints and recoveries, cool down with 5 more minutes at a moderate intensity.

Try this once or twice a week. If you're an absolute beginner, hold off until you've built up a fitness base.

Glycolytic pathway. You know the burning sensation you get in your muscles when you've worked them intensely for a minute or so? That's lactic acid, a waste product produced in your muscles during exercise that lasts 15 seconds to 3 minutes (although few of us can last more than a minute or two with lactic acid doing its Spanish Inquisition number on our muscle tissues). The glycolytic pathway is your intermediate energy system, bridging the gap between your ATP-PC system and your aerobic-energy system. Like the ATP-PC system, it's anaerobic, meaning your body doesn't yet use oxygen to break down fat and carbohydrates for energy.

Ideal activities: Running, cycling, rowing, swimming, and cross-country skiing.

Improve it: After a thorough warmup, go as hard as you can at a pace you can maintain for a full 30 seconds. Once the 30 seconds are up, recover by moving at a moderate pace for 60 seconds. Start with five intervals, and build up to eight. After your intervals and recoveries, cool down for 5 minutes. Do this once or twice a week.

When 30-second intervals are comfortable, increase to 45 seconds with 90 seconds of recovery. Then move up to 60-second intervals and 2 minutes of recovery. Finally, if you dare, try 90-second intervals, with 3-minute recoveries.

Aerobic. You use this system for activities lasting 2 minutes or longer. Studies have shown that you improve this system quickest when you work at varying speeds rather than one steady speed.

Ideal activities: Running (you can do jog-walk intervals if you're just starting out, or run-jog intervals if you're in pretty good shape), stair-climbing, rowing, cross-country skiing, cycling, and swimming.

Improve it: After a thorough warmup, improve your speed to one that is challenging but not so hard you can't maintain it for 2 minutes. After 2 minutes, return to a moderate pace for 2 minutes. After your intervals and recoveries, cool down for 5 minutes. Start with five intervals, and build up to eight. Try this once or twice a week.

You can increase the intervals to any length you choose. Just make sure you do intervals and recoveries at a 1-to-1 ratio.

CHAPTER 17

HOME CARDIO EQUIPMENT

Now that we've carefully explained why we hold traditional cardiovascular exercise in such low esteem, we'd like to offer some tips on how to buy treadmills. Contradictory? Sure, but our careful observation of human behavior tells us that the more strident the advice, the less people will heed it.

Take the use of treadmills, for example. Treadmill sales increased more than 400 percent in the last 12 years of the 20th century, according to the Sporting Goods Manufacturers Association's annual "Tracking the Fitness Movement" report. In 2000, Americans spent approximately $925 million on treadmills, and close to 18 million men ran or jogged that year, according to the report. These numbers indicate that indifference to our advice remains at historic levels.

On the other hand, we did recommend interval workouts in the previous chapter, and many people (we're among them) like to do intervals on equipment, rather than trust nature to give us clear weather and a dry track at the exact moment we decide to do our sprints. We also know that lots of people actually enjoy traditional cardio exercise. We don't get it, but hey, that's just us.

The following is a completely unbiased guide to buying home cardio equipment. And when we say "unbiased," we're telling the truth: Though we'd love to have some of this stuff, we wouldn't buy any of it until after we had all the strength-training equipment we needed or wanted.

NARROW YOUR CHOICES

Telling you what sort of cardio machine is best for you is like telling you whether you should prefer blondes, redheads, or brunettes. You can find studies showing that a treadmill is better than anything else for burning calories, but that doesn't matter if you prefer an exercise bike. Even though you may burn fewer calories on the bike than you would in the same amount of time on a treadmill, you come out ahead because you actually use it.

So your first job, before you buy a machine, is to ask yourself a basic, yet tough, question: "What am I most likely to use most often?" If the answer isn't obvious, follow these steps.

Stick with the basics. Never mind the wacky infomercial oddity that rocks, twists, and tills your garden. Limit your choices to machines that mimic real-life movements. You can walk or run on a treadmill, pedal on a stationary cycle, row on a rowing machine, ski on a cross-country ski machine, climb stairs on a stairclimber machine, and ellipt on an elliptical machine.

Okay, we fudged that last one. An elliptical machine uses a made-up motion that's sort of a cross between walking and skating or cross-country skiing. Studies have shown they're safe and effective for strenuous workouts, and people like to use them.

Size up your space. Though some machines fold up for more compact storage, you still need a clear area in which to use them. If your space is severely limited, consider an exercise bike, which fits easily into tight quarters. Back it against a wall and you probably need just 3 feet of width and about

4 feet from the wall out. Many guys like to do their cardiovascular exercise in front of a TV, and you have to allow a few feet for that. Even though kids can watch cartoons nose-to-screen, you probably need to keep your aging eyeballs at least 8 feet away.

Treadmills, cross-country machines, rowers, and elliptical machines take up considerably more space. Even if you push a machine into a corner, you need 6 to 7 feet lengthwise and 3 to 4 feet of depth. If you're going to watch the tube while you work out, add at least another 8 feet.

Try the ones that interest you. You may recall that chapter 4 gave detailed instructions on shopping for a multistation home gym. The most important of those guidelines bears repeating: You must try whatever it is you're thinking of buying. That means you have to wear your running shoes and sweats to the sporting goods store to give the machine a workout.

Here's a sneaky way to try several machines to see which you like best: Get a trial membership at a nearby gym. As little as a one-day pass gives you a chance to familiarize yourself with multiple machines before you attempt a purchase. The home versions of those machines will be a bit smaller and less durable, but at least you'll get an idea of whether you're a treadmill guy or an elliptor.

Just don't buy a $1,000 rowing machine if you've never rowed before. You may hate it, and you'll be stuck with a $1,000 plant stand.

Respect your previous injuries. Guys with bad knees should avoid stairclimbers. An elliptical trainer may be less jarring on the knees and lower back while exacerbating certain ankle or foot problems. Bad back? Stay away from rowers and cross-country ski machines; instead, consider a recumbent bike (a stationary bike with a bucket seat on which you sit back like Peter Fonda in *Easy Rider*).

If you want the drink holder, get the drink

holder. Many machines have optional water-bottle holders, magazine racks, and heart-rate monitors. Some may even have ashtrays and Internet-porn downloaders, for all we know. Our point is, whatever you think you want, buy it up front. Don't forgo your favorite accessory and spend the next 10 years wishing you had it. These machines aren't like cars—if you don't get the side air bags this time, you can't get them when you trade up in 5 years. If the machine you buy now doesn't last a decade, it means you didn't read this chapter carefully enough.

That's it for generalities. Here are specific tips for buying the major types of equipment.

TREADMILLS

Power source. Although nonmotorized treadmills are available, stick with a motorized tread with at least a 1.5 horsepower continuous-duty engine. Don't swoon over a machine that boasts a top speed above 12 miles per hour—to take full advantage of it, you'd have to run a sub-5-minute mile. (You may want the faster machine if you plan to do indoor sprinting workouts, however.)

Structure. Look for a model with a running surface that is at least 18 inches wide and 50 inches long so you'll have enough room to get in a good stride. If you're over 6 feet tall, look for one that's a little longer. Run at least a mile on the treadmill to make sure it fits and to see whether you like the running surface. Shock absorbency can vary quite a bit from brand to brand, so make sure the one you buy doesn't feel too squishy or hard to you.

Electronics and program options. Look for a model with preset programs that automatically change the speed and incline to simulate running on different terrains. It'll keep your workouts more interesting and challenging. An increasingly popular option is a heart-rate-controlled machine that monitors your pulse and adjusts your workout to keep you within a targeted intensity range. Your heart rate is usually monitored via a handgrip, thumb sensor, or wireless chest strap. The latter is considered the most accurate.

Price. A treadmill can cost anywhere from a few hundred bucks to $4,000. You aren't likely to find a good one for under $1,500. In the moderate-price category, try Life Fitness, Precor, and Pace-Master brands. At the high end, consider True and Landice.

ELLIPTICAL TRAINERS

Power source. You. This machine uses magnetic resistance or a flywheel. Precor's commercial version has a motor that raises or lowers the angle of incline. All machines we know of allow you to go forward or backward. Some also have arms that

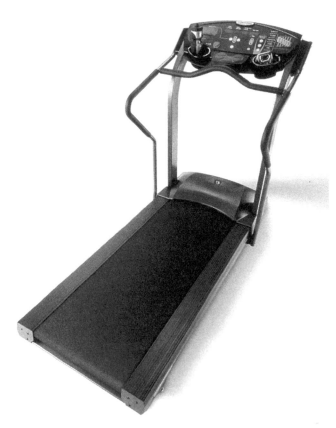

Life Fitness Treadmill T5i

you can pull back and forth to mimic a cross-country-skiing motion.

Structure. Look for a sturdy, stable machine that has a constant, smooth motion. Fit is key: Make sure the handlebars don't come too close to your body and your knees don't smack into the console. Also, try to find a machine with nonslip pedals so you'll be able to keep a consistent pace without tripping.

Electronics and program options. Although an elliptical machine can provide effective, nonimpact exercise, some guys may find it boring over the long haul. So it's best to look for a machine with preprogrammed training courses and motivating display information such as speed, distance, and resistance used. Machines that require you to turn a knob to increase resistance make it difficult to gauge progression.

Price. Elliptical machines range from $350 to $3,500. Expect to pay at least two grand for one that feels like a commercial machine. Look for Precor for a health-club-quality machine; Reebok, NordicTrack, or FitnessQuest are lower-end products.

STATIONARY BICYCLES

Power source. It's your legs against air, a flywheel, or magnetic frictionless resistance. (The last option powers the bikes in health clubs and the most expensive home models). The electronic console is battery-powered.

Structure. The key to buying a good exercise bike is fit. Make sure the bike has lots of options for adjusting the seat height and handlebar setup. If you can't find a comfortable riding position, you won't want to use it. Odds are the seat that comes with the bike will be less than comfy, so ask the salesperson to throw in an extra padded seat to seal the deal. Beyond that, the bike should feel solid and have a smooth pedal motion—even at high speeds. Also, experiment with the resistance

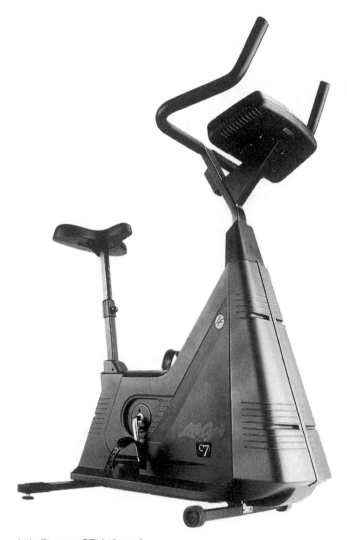

Life Fitness C7i Lifecycle

controls. Make sure they're easy to adjust. Avoid a bike that uses rubber pincers to grip the wheel—it'll feel jerky.

Electronics and program options. A basic exercise bike should have a speedometer, an odometer, and a timer so you can keep track of your workout. Of course, some high-end models offer sophisticated electronics with interval-training programs and calorie-burning information. If blinking lights and workout stats motivate you, look for something techie. Otherwise, a basic bike burns just as many calories and saves you some money, too.

Price. Exercise-bike prices go from about $200 to $2,000. You should be able to get a good-quality machine with a few bells and whistles for about $1,000. A top-of-the-line recumbent bike could sell for closer to $3,000. Top brand names are Life Fitness, Reebok, and Star Trak.

STAIRCLIMBERS

Power source. Stairclimbers are available in motorized and hydraulic models. The motorized machines are most similar to the ones in health clubs. They use chains or cables to move the steps, and they are quieter and require less maintenance than hydraulic machines that use oil- or air-filled shocks.

Structure. When you test out a stairclimber, make sure it keeps you in a good posture with your back straight and your knees behind your toes. If the machine's design makes it tough to maintain good posture, you could be setting yourself up for back and knee injuries. Also, look for a machine that has independent foot action, rather than dependent action (you push one pedal down and the other comes up). Independent models are more biomechanically correct and will give you a better workout. The movement should be quiet and smooth, and the machine should be stable with large, nonslip steps.

A second type of stairclimber is the StairMaster Stepmill. It's a treadmill-like device with revolving 8-inch steps for which you set the speed.

Electronics and program options. You can find machines with all sorts of electronic readouts, but look for one that at least provides stats on your pace, time elapsed, and distance covered so you can keep track of your progress.

Price. A low-end, piston-driven stairclimber can be had for $200. You should expect to pay more than $2,000 for a good motorized machine with the stability and smooth mechanics of the climbers you find in health clubs. And you'll pay over $3,500 for

the StairMaster Stepmill. Top brand names are StairMaster, Life Fitness, and Cat Eye.

ROWING MACHINES

Power source. Resistance can come from magnets, air, or even—in the case of the beautiful and authentic-feeling WaterRower machines—water. You'll also find inexpensive models that use piston resistance. These low-end machines tend to offer two independent rowing arms, and although they can offer an effective workout, it's not a very good simulation of actual rowing. You're better off with a wind-resistance machine, in which a flywheel creates resistance. The harder you pull, the more resistance the flywheel generates. Such a machine is more expensive, but it also provides a much more realistic rowing exercise.

Structure. Look for a solid machine with easily adjustable foot pedals, sturdy toe straps, and a seat that moves back and forth smoothly. It's important that the resistance be constant throughout the stroke. A machine with steel or aluminum parts and a chain-pulling mechanism is also a good bet since it usually lasts longer and requires minimal maintenance. The WaterRower even has a wood frame (ash, cherry, or black walnut) that can match your decor.

Electronics and program options. A quality machine usually features a computer display that shows total number of strokes, strokes per minute, and calories burned. Some high-end machines can even be linked to your home computer so you can analyze your workouts and conduct races with friends or strangers over the Internet.

Price. A quality rowing machine will set you back $750 or more. The leading brands are Concept 2, WaterRower, and Tunturi.

CROSS-COUNTRY SKI MACHINES

Power source. All you, baby.

Structure. Although ski machines are excellent

for aerobic conditioning and for burning calories, many guys find them awkward to use at first. A dependent-action machine, in which the opposing skis move equal and opposite distances on each stroke, is easiest to master. But you'll get a better workout on an independent-action ski machine because you're responsible for moving each ski back and forth.

To add an upper-body exercise component, most machines use a rope-and-pulley system. If you are tall or have extraordinarily long arms (if your friends call you Koko, for example), check to make sure the ropes are long enough. And definitely stay away from dependent-action machines that link the upper- and lower-body movements. They don't provide as effective a workout and will likely lead to boredom more quickly.

Finally, make sure the machine is stable. It's hard enough to learn how to use one of these things without worrying about doing a face-plant on your basement floor. Keep an eye out for a machine with sealed bearings; it'll require the least maintenance.

Electronics and program options. Most machines track time and distance traveled as well as calories burned.

Price. A cross-country ski machine can cost $400 to $1,500, with $700 the standard price for a decent NordicTrack machine. As for brands, NordicTrack is pretty much the entire category.

CARE AND FEEDING

No matter what type of cardio equipment you buy, you'll need to keep it clean and well-lubricated. The more you use it, the more maintenance it'll need. Diligent maintenance and cleaning should keep a quality machine in good shape for at least 10 years.

If you dread maintenance, it's best to stay away from elliptical machines and treadmills. They're considered the fussiest cardio machines.

At the other extreme, basic rowing machines and exercise bikes require the lowest-maintenance of the lot. Be forewarned: Any cheap piece of equipment is high-maintenance by design. On the bright side, cheap machines won't provide too many years of misery—they don't last long enough for that.

"FOR SALE: ONE TREADMILL. ONLY USED ONCE. SMALL DENT ON LEFT RAIL. OWNER MUST SELL TO PAY HOSPITAL BILLS."

The Sunday classifieds are filled with unwanted fitness machines looking for new owners who'll actually use them. It's not uncommon to see a quality product advertised for a fraction of what the original owner paid. Still, you know what they say about getting what you pay for. So here are a few tips to help you in your search for used cardio equipment.

Try before you buy. We know we told you this already, but our lawyers get testy if we don't say it at every opportunity. Put on your sweats, go over to the seller's house, and give the machine a spin.

Look for a solid, well-built machine. Forget about lots of techie features and gizmos. The more blinking lights, the more likely something is broken and expensive to fix.

Pay special attention to the frame. Look for any cracks, rust, and problems with the chains and bearings. Hop on to make sure the parts move smoothly and quietly. Listen for rattling and rubbing sounds, which are major red flags. A motor should sound like a motor—if it whines like your ex-wife, there's something wrong.

Comparison shop. If you aren't sure about pricing, call local stores to compare prices for similar models. It's hard to justify paying more than half the retail price, given the amount of risk you take when buying a used machine.

Get an owner's manual and a warranty. Check to see whether the warranty is transferable. If the owner doesn't have the papers, note the machine's serial number and call the manufacturer to see if the warranty can be transferred to you. The manufacturer should be able to provide an owner's manual, if that's also missing.

Check with the U.S. Consumer Product Safety Commission. Call the consumer hotline at (800) 638-2772, or log on to the Web site at www.csps.gov to make sure the manufacturer has never recalled the machine due to known defects.

Check out used-equipment stores. Or ask new-equipment retailers whether they accept used machines on consignment or as trade-ins. If they do but don't have the machine you're looking for, ask to put your name on a waiting list.

Ask health clubs whether they sell their old equipment when they upgrade. Though a gym's castoff will be well-used, a commercial-quality machine should also be more durable and well-maintained than a low-budget one.

CHAPTER 18

PERSONAL TRAINERS: YES, THEY DELIVER

Personal trainers, for better or worse, have infiltrated almost every venue of American life. Gyms are thick with them, of course. They're also invading your home, gaining entrance via . . .

Late-night infomercials. The goal of many trainers we know is to invent or endorse a gadget like the ones we'll examine in chapter 19.

Bookstores. Most fitness books are written by men or women who have trained clients—usually famous ones.

Movies, TV shows, and music videos. You think those buff stars of stage and screen get that way through discipline, strict diets, and exercise know-how? Uh-uh. Most celebs are compulsive pleasure-seekers. (Some, of course, really are disciplined athletes and exercisers, and thus disturbingly hard to mock.) When they absolutely have to look good for a role, they turn to a proven Hollywood muscle wrangler, who either cranks up their exercise, puts the clamps on their partying, pumps them full of steroids and amphetamines, or some combination thereof.

The fact that trainers are everywhere doesn't mean you have to like them or seek them out. There are times, however, when you may have a use for them. And these days, they'll come right to your home gym to help you out. Here are a few reasons why you may want to open the door and let them in.

- You have trouble starting an exercise program—your best intentions don't translate into action, and you need someone to show up regularly to put you through your paces.

- You buy some new equipment and want someone to show you how to use it efficiently and safely. Even with a book like this at their fingertips, some people prefer hands-on instruction.

- You've been exercising consistently, but you're stuck on a plateau that's short of your goals. A trainer can help you tweak your program—or create a new one—to get you moving forward again.

- You want to measure your performance, and you need someone to give you some baseline information. (Also, all the tests in chapter 13 are easier if you have someone to give you a spot, or hold the stopwatch or tape measure.)

The trick is finding a *good* trainer. It's not as easy as picking up the phone and ordering a pizza. Until someone discovers the perfect personal trainer and finds a way to clone him or her, the knowledge and experience of trainers will vary tremendously. And that doesn't even take into account personality differences. A trainer whose demeanor is that of a drill sergeant may work for the guy who needs a kick in the ass. Another guy may need a training partner, so a trainer who comes off as a buddy would help more than "Sgt. Rock." Yet another guy may prefer a female trainer who acts as more of a cheerleader. (We don't really have to explain this choice, do we?)

MIND OVER MUSCLE

Once you've decided what kind of training temperament is right for you, you still have some other qualifications to consider. First and foremost, make sure that the trainer is certified by an organization you've heard of—or, better yet, an organization we've heard of, since they're all just alphabet soup to most guys. In our experience, the three most credible organizations are the National Strength and Conditioning Association (NSCA), the American Council on Exercise (ACE), and the American College of Sports Medicine (ACSM). The NSCA offers two certifications: certified strength-and-conditioning specialist (C.S.C.S.) and certified personal trainer (N.S.C.A.-C.P.T.). The former requires a 4-year college degree (though not necessarily in an exercise-related field); the latter doesn't. Both tests require deep and broad knowledge of exercise theory and technique.

You don't need a college degree to take (or pass) the ACE or ACSM tests. Both are nonetheless demanding. For example, the success rate for first-time ACE personal trainer testees is only 65 percent.

A fourth organization we've come to trust is the International Sports Sciences Association (ISSA), which is gaining popularity and credibility. Like the other three, the ISSA has a tough certifying test and strict requirements for certification renewal.

There may be good organizations beyond those four, but we can't recommend any unequivocally.

Certification isn't the only criterion. A trainer may be good at taking tests and have one or more impressive certifications without possessing any talent for training. Conversely, someone with an academic background in exercise science—and perhaps an athletic background—may have good training instincts despite a lack of impressive certifications.

Two pieces of paper should be non-negotiable:

Every trainer should have current CPR certification from the American Heart Association as well as liability insurance.

REFERENCES

Besides showing you a résumé and the paperwork we've mentioned so far, a trainer should be willing to show you testimonials from satisfied customers. Letters of recommendation could all be B.S. that he invented in his creative-writing class, of course. So contact several of his clients. If he's good, he'll have a long list of current and former customers willing to sing his praises to you.

Your goal in contacting his clients isn't just to make sure they exist. Ask specific questions about his style and work ethic. Also ask about the results the client expected and got.

YOUR GOALS

Any trainer ahould be able to help you lose a little fat or gain a little muscle. If your goals are more distinct than that—if you want to lose a lot of fat, gain a lot of muscle, improve in a specific sport, or rehabilitate a recent injury—make sure your trainer knows how to accomplish that goal.

A trainer who knows bodybuilding inside and out may not have any idea how to improve your tennis game. And the Barbie doll who is great at motivating you with her cheerful demeanor may not have a good concept of how a guy builds the kind of muscle you want.

YOUR INJURIES AND HEALTH CONCERNS

If you have diabetes, high blood pressure, heart disease, cancer, arthritis, or any other health issue, make sure your trainer understands the problem and how to train someone with it. (ACE, to pick one example, has a special certification for trainers specializing in clients with serious health concerns.)

Another consideration is your injury history.

Most trainers know how to work with clients who have some back pain, a trick knee, or other orthopedic problems. You have to ask them about it.

PRICE

You can expect to spend anywhere from $40 to more than $150 an hour for an in-home trainer. (Most trainers will also bill you for their travel time to your home.) A trainer's price may reflect his experience and credentials—or it may not. If a trainer has worked with celebrities, you can bet he'll charge more, regardless of whether his expertise merits it.

Also, though we can't prove this, we'd bet the best-looking or best-built trainers get away with charging more than less attractive trainers with equal experience and education. That brings us to another important point: People who are good-looking were born that way. People who have great physiques might have achieved them through hard work in the gym and advanced training knowledge. Or their bodies could just as easily be the result of a garden-variety program combined with superior genetics.

SEALING THE DEAL

Once you've done your homework and selected a trainer, you have to make a few decisions that will affect how much you pay him. Most trainers have multiple rates: the highest for a single session, and progressively lower ones for longer commitments. The longer commitments usually require some advance payment. Trust us, you should have at least one session with the trainer, even if it's expensive, before you commit to a package of sessions.

If you want the trainer to design a program for you to do on your own, make sure he knows this in advance. (We've heard of people hiring trainers who refuse to give them written programs.) He may charge more for program design than for regular sessions. That can work in your favor if you put together a consulting arrangement in which he updates your program by phone or e-mail as you progress.

In the end, the quality of the trainer you end up with will reflect the amount of effort you put into hiring him. Trust your brain more than your eyes, and it could be the start of a beautiful relationship.

ASK OUR TRAINER

As helpful as a personal trainer can be, we realize that after you've bought all your exercise equipment, you may not have a lot of cash left over to pay one—no matter what he charges. So here are some common exercise questions you may have, along with answers courtesy of our favorite trainer, Mike Mejia, M.S., C.S.C.S.

You ask: I start an exercise program each January but always quit after a few months. How do I stick with it for good?

Mike says: Push yourself to do more from one workout to the next. Lift a few more pounds, do a few extra repetitions, or beat some sort of personal record. Otherwise, your fitness level plateaus, you get bored, and you quit. Similarly, you need to alter your program regularly—every 4 weeks is ideal for most guys. That means new exercises, different rep ranges, new angles.

You ask: Am I better off working out in the morning before I go to work, or at night when I get home?

Mike says: I'm partial to morning workouts. It's very liberating to know I've already met the day's greatest physical challenge so early. It gives me a heightened sense of readiness for whatever happens the rest of the day. In my experience, chronic procrastinators do best with morning workouts because if they wait until later in the day, they always come up with an excuse not to exercise.

If you have trouble getting it together before your fourth cup of java, morning workouts probably aren't for you. There's no sense in going through the motions of a halfhearted workout just to say you got it done.

Besides, you could make a good argument for evening workouts. They can be a great way to take the edge off those hard days in the salt mines. Whatever frustration and anger you've built up from dueling with coworkers or dealing with clients can power you through even the hardest workout.

Guys who are meticulous and goal-oriented do well with evening workouts. They'd rarely skip a session because, since it's on the to-do list, they have to check it off before they go to sleep.

I guess my final answer here is, do it whenever you'll give it your best effort.

You ask: If I want to do weights and cardio in the same workout, does it matter which I do first?

Mike says: It matters a great deal. Most trainers suggest arranging the exercises in order of importance to your goals. So if your primary goal is increased endurance or fat loss, they suggest you do cardio first, when your energy is highest. If your aim is to build bigger muscles, they say lift first.

While I understand this approach, I don't agree with it. In my opinion, strength training should always come first, regardless of your goals. I base this viewpoint on two facts.

1. Cardiovascular exercise—running, cycling, rowing, and so on—can hinder your efforts in the weight room. Because these activities rely heavily on your body's carbohydrate stores (the more intensely you train, the greater your need for carbohydrates as a fuel source), those stores may be at least partially depleted by the time you begin the lifting portion of your workout. And weight lifting is *entirely* dependent on carbohydrates as a fuel source.

Though your body burns fat between sets, it relies on carbohydrate energy during sets. If you've already depleted your carb supply via aerobics, you've compromised your lifting performance.

2. On the other hand, after depleting your carb reserves by lifting weights, you can still use fat for fuel during your cardio exercise. In fact, you'll probably burn *more* fat if your cardio follows weight lifting. And isn't the object of cardio exercise to burn more fat?

You ask: How much aerobic exercise can I do and still expect to build muscle?

Mike says: I've seen guys do four or five aerobic workouts per week and still manage to build muscle. These individuals are the exception, and in my experience, quite often they take advantage of a little pharmacological aid.

For the rest of us, there comes a point where aerobic exercise interferes with our efforts in the weight room. The hard part is determining exactly where that point lies. Everyone's metabolism is different; there are no universal guidelines.

The best way to find your personal point of diminishing returns is to cycle your training so that you have defined periods in which your focus is building muscle. During these cycles, scale back the aerobics to two 15 to 20 minute sessions per week, at most. Or drop them entirely. Don't worry, your heart won't shrivel up to the size of a raisin and stop pumping if you put away the running shoes for a few weeks.

Once you've increased your muscle mass, shift your focus to fat burning by reintroducing aerobics. Start with two or three weekly sessions of interval work lasting for 15 to 20 minutes at a time. (We explained intervals in chapter 16.) If you maintain strength and muscle size but don't burn fat as quickly as you'd like, you can add another session or two of aerobics.

On the other hand, if your muscle disappears faster than your fat, scale back your aerobics. Lost muscle means a slower metabolism, which makes it even harder to burn off fat.

You ask: How long should I warm up before I start my workout?

Mike says: For aerobic workouts such as cycling, running, and stairclimbing, do an easier version of your main activity. Three to 5 minutes of low-intensity activity (such as pedaling or jogging at a leisurely pace) should suffice.

Resistance training requires both a general warmup like the one I just described and a specific warmup for the muscle groups you'll target in your workout. The latter means warmup sets with anywhere from 25 to 75 percent of the weight you plan on using for your "work sets" of each exercise.

In general, heavy work sets (fewer than 8 reps) require more preparation, while moderate or light sets require less. Compound or multijoint exercises (such as squats or bench presses) require more warmup sets, while isolation or single-joint exercises (such as biceps curls or lateral raises) require fewer. And the exercises you do early in your workout require more preparation than later exercises.

Say the first exercise you're going to do in your workout is the barbell bench press (easy guess, since that's the first exercise in everyone's workout), for 2 or 3 sets of 4 to 8 repetitions. And say you're going to use 135 pounds. A single warmup set with about two-thirds of that weight—90 pounds—should work. (If you use an Olympic bar, you'd probably use 95 pounds in this example, since it's a lot easier to slap a pair of 25-pound weight plates on the 45-pound bar than it is to collect smaller plates that total exactly 90.)

On the other hand, say you're going to do 5 sets of 5 squats with 185 pounds. You should do an initial warmup set of 7 reps with 65 pounds (about one-third of your work-set weight). Then do a second set of 5 reps with 125 pounds (about two-thirds of your working weight). With even heavier weights, you could go as low as 25 percent of your work-set weight for the first of 3 warmup sets.

You ask: Why is the bench press the first exercise in everyone's workout, anyway? Do I need to perform resistance exercises in a certain order?

Mike says: Generally speaking, you should do compound or multijoint exercises that work your biggest muscle groups earliest in your workout, and do isolation or single-joint exercises for smaller muscles later. Compound exercises require the most effort, so you want to perform them when you have the most energy. You don't want to fatigue those big muscle groups before you work them. So bench presses, squats, deadlifts, dips, pullups, rows, and shoulder presses usually come before triceps exercises, biceps curls, lateral raises, and calf exercises. If, for example, you were to do triceps extensions before bench presses, you would compromise your bench-press performance—and the amount of muscle and strength you'd develop.

Of course, there are exceptions to every rule. If you're an intermediate or advanced lifter, you may stop making progress with a conventional compound-first system. During compound lifts, the smaller, assisting muscle groups run out of gas before the prime movers. In other words, during bench presses, your triceps fatigue before your pectorals and may limit the number of presses you can do. Thus, your weaker muscles prevent your stronger ones from getting the best possible workout.

You can balance things out with a technique known as preexhaustion: Start with an exercise that exhausts the big muscle group—for instance, do flies for your chest before moving on to the main-event bench presses. This ensures that your smaller, weaker muscles last just as long as your bigger, stronger ones.

You ask: How frequently should I train each muscle group?

Mike says: For years, the prevailing attitude in bodybuilding circles was that larger muscle groups (chest, lats, quads, hamstrings) should be trained twice a week, and smaller muscles (biceps, triceps, deltoids, calves, abs) three or even more times per week.

I see two problems with this model. First, frequency and intensity have an inverse relationship. The more frequently you train a muscle group, the less effort you'll be able to exert. Yet the majority of strength-training research shows that intensity is more important than volume in determining the results you get from a program. In other words, more isn't better; better is better. That's why, even in the bodybuilding world, the latest trend is toward working each muscle group—major or minor—just once a week.

The second problem is that not all of us recover at the same rate. If you are over 40, have a physically demanding job, don't sleep well, or have suboptimal dietary habits (to put it kindly), you may have more difficulty recovering from your workouts than a guy who's younger or whose lifestyle is more healthful. It's a bad idea to work muscles that haven't fully recovered. You'll use less weight or do fewer reps than in your previous workout—and either of these setbacks is completely counterproductive to your goals of getting bigger, stronger, and leaner.

How do you judge your recovery abilities? Keep a record of your workouts—a training log, in other words. (Starting on page 360, we provide a blank log for you to fill in.)

Say you work your chest on Wednesday of one week and then again the following Monday. You can compare your log entries for the two workouts to see whether you've improved, stayed the same, or regressed. If you've stayed the same, you've probably hit your chest again a day too soon. If you've regressed, you may have hit them 2 or 3 days too soon.

Sometimes, the problem is not that your chest hasn't fully recovered but that your arms are tired from another workout. Let's say that after working your chest on Wednesday, you worked your arms and shoulders on Saturday. On Monday, if your bench press is weaker than it was the previous week, the problem may not be your chest—it could be that your triceps and shoulders are still exhausted from Saturday's workout.

That's why I rarely recommend entire workouts for smaller muscles such as arms and shoulders. Training triceps and shoulders with your chest, and biceps with your back, makes it easier to gauge your total recovery.

You ask: What about my abdominals? Can I work them every day?

Mike says: You certainly can, but why would you want to? First of all, despite what they tell you on those late-night infomercials, no amount of abdominal work by itself is going to miraculously burn fat from your midsection—or anywhere else on your body. The only way to accomplish that is to consume fewer calories than you burn each day, and engage in a regular resistance-training program, with the occasional bout of aerobic work thrown in for good measure. Yeah, I know that's not what they say in those ads for the AbDemolisher. Trust me, it's in the fine print.

An equally important point: Genetics determines where fat is deposited on your body as well as where it disappears when you start working it off. On most men, deep abdominal fat—the stuff underneath your muscles, also called visceral fat—moves first. Subcutaneous fat, which lies between your muscles and skin and prevents your six-pack from showing, gets worked off in a genetically determined pattern. So you may lose the fat on your neck before you lose your love handles.

Fat burning, though, is only half the equation. The other half is muscle building. Your abdominals are made of skeletal muscle, just like your pecs, lats, quads, and biceps. You wouldn't dream of working those other muscles on a daily basis, would you? (If you would, reread the opening chapters of this book.) Your abs aren't any different. If you want to make them bigger, you have to give them a growth stimulus—in other words, hard exercise against resistance—followed by time to repair themselves and grow bigger and stronger.

A confounding variable is the fact that your abs have a role in promoting proper posture and stabilizing your spine. So they need some endurance capabilities. In that sense, they're sort of like your legs: They need to be able to hold you upright and keep you moving. At the same time, they need strength and power for those times when you're trying to drive a softball over the fence at the company picnic, or protect your back as you carry that keg up the back stairwell to your dorm room.

My suggestion is to cycle your ab training, just as you would training for any other muscle group. Begin by working your abs four or five times a week, focusing primarily on high-rep endurance work with exercises like bicycles, crunches, and vacuums. After 2 to 3 weeks of that, switch to more challenging exercises that don't allow for as many reps, such as incline reverse crunches, barbell rollouts, and cable crunches. Finally, work your way up to the type of exercises that really help build strength and power, such as hanging leg raises, cable woodchoppers, and Swiss-ball weighted crunches. Each segment of training should last 2 to 3 weeks, although the muscle- and strength-building workouts lend themselves more to 3 weeks of 3-days-a-week training.

Then, after about a week's respite from ab training, you can switch back to an endurance program and start over again. Soon, you'll have a strong, powerful abdominal wall that will keep you protected from injury. And if you lay off the Budweiser, people will notice it.

You ask: Is it better to perform the exercises in this book fast or slowly?

Mike says: Yes.

As a fitness professional, my automatic response is to say "slowly." The majority of lifters perform exercises with poor technique. Though lifting weights quickly does not make their form worse, it does increase the likelihood of injury.

Another issue is efficacy. While fast lifts are acknowledged by most as a useful tool for sports-specific training, most of us know from experience that slower lifting speeds are better for producing muscle growth. When you eliminate momentum from your lifts, your muscles stay under tension longer, which provides a greater growth stimulus than ballistic lifts in which muscles contract more powerfully and release tension in a couple of seconds.

Slow, controlled lifting is a fine and useful practice. Some guys, though, have taken it off the deep end. The prime example is the Superslow Exercise Guild (no connection to the Lollipop Guild—these guys actually exist). Members of this organization believe that you should lift weights at a set cadence—usually 10 seconds up, 5 seconds down. They perform every exercise this way, every workout. We'll give them points for safety—it's impossible to hurt yourself training like this. (They also use machines, further increasing the safety factor.) The problem with this technique is that the strength you build is specific to the speed at which you build it. If you lift slowly, your body learns to move better only at that slow pace.

Slow-speed lifting is a good idea in two circumstances: Beginners who lift slowly learn proper form, keep control of the weights, and avoid injury. Advanced lifters who switch to slow lifts and more time under tension may see gains in muscle size. (This remains theoretical; no studies I know of show that advanced lifters make more gains with slower lifts. Anecdotally, it's worked for me and other guys I know.)

The opposite seems to be true as well. If experienced lifters used to working at deliberate speeds begin to lift weights quickly, they'll probably make gains in size and strength. During strength cycles, you can lift near-maximal loads as fast as possible (the weight still moves slowly, though your muscles try as hard as they can to move it quickly).

The faster you lift, the more risk you take. With risk comes some reward, in that you may see new muscle growth and will certainly see improvements in strength and power. The latter gains can apply to sports or just enable you to handle heavier loads when you return to lifting at conventional speeds.

You ask: How many sets should I do, and how long should I rest in between them?

Mike says: The number of sets you do is determined by the number of repetitions you perform. Reps are determined by the amount of weight you want to use. And weight depends on—you guessed it—your goals.

If you're training for strength, you have to use weights that are close to your maximums. You can't do many repetitions with loads that heavy, so you have to do more sets to get a noticeable training effect. For instance, you might do 5 sets of 5 reps, or 8 sets of 3, or perhaps even 10 sets of 1.

On the other hand, if you're more interested in bodybuilding-type workouts for packing on muscle, you use lighter weights and do 8 to 12 reps per set, most of the time. You don't need to do many sets per exercise—just 2 or 3, usually. (Of course, they have to be good sets that take your muscles to fatigue.) Any more than that is overkill, unless you're on steroids. And if you are on steroids, you don't need my training advice. Go ahead and do 20 sets of everything—and don't come crying to me when your testicles shrink to the size of rabbit pellets.

Finally, if you're doing extremely high reps—15 to 25 per set—for muscular endurance, you shouldn't do more than 2 sets per exercise. If you don't get all the possible benefits from that, use more weight.

The amount of rest you take between each of these sets is inversely related to the number of reps you perform. For low-rep, high-load sets, rest for at least 2 minutes before going again. This allows your muscles and central nervous system to recuperate. When using more moderate loads for conventional muscle-building sets of 8 to 12 reps, take 1 to 2 minutes of rest between sets. And believe it or not, you can get away with as little as 30 seconds between sets when you're lifting light weights for high reps.

So, to review, heavy weights = low reps, which = high sets, which = lots of rest. Light loads = high reps, which = fewer sets, which = less rest. See, I told you it was simple.

You ask: How do I, as a beginner, know how much weight I should use?

Mike says: Select a weight that you can lift 12 to 20 times. This weight may seem too light, and it probably is too light to build serious muscle. Building muscle, however, is not your object right out of the gate. You first need to strengthen your connective tissues and improve your muscular endurance. Just as important, you must master the basic exercises. Heavier weight could strain your tendons and ligaments, and possibly prevent you from developing good form.

You ask: How often, and by how much, should I increase the amount of weight I use?

Mike says: As often as you can, as long as you do it systematically—while keeping your ego in check. At the gym, it's not uncommon for me to see a guy struggle to complete his reps with a particular weight, finish with terrible form, then slap another 20 pounds on the bar for his next set. I stand there thinking, "He was using too much weight on that last set—why is he even attempting a heavier weight?"

Ego aside, a lot of guys increase weight too fast just because they can. Beginners quickly realize they can bump up by enormous percentages workout after workout. They may not realize that while their muscles are ready to handle more weight, their connective tissues aren't. So they end up with chronic, nagging injuries to their shoulders, knees, elbows, and, worst of all, lower back.

You can avoid this with disciplined protocols for increasing weight. If you're a beginner, restrict your increases to 10 percent per exercise per week. For example, if you can lift 80 pounds, next week move up to about 88 pounds, then 97 pounds, then 107 pounds, and so on. If a weight feels too light, make the exercise harder by working slower or doing more reps or taking less time between sets or exercises.

If you're a more advanced exerciser (that is, if you've been training for at least 6 months), increase by no more than 5 percent a week. This increases the physiological stimulus of the exercise without creating an overwhelming challenge that impedes your progress. It also gives your connective tissues a chance to adapt to the new loads.

On some exercises, it's hard to increase just 5 or 10 percent. If you're using 20-pound dumbbells and the next heaviest pair is 25s, that's a 25 percent increase. So I recommend the PlateMates described in chapter 4. If you attach a $1\frac{1}{4}$-pound PlateMate to that 20-pound dumbbell, you increase by just over 5 percent. Add a $2\frac{1}{2}$-pound PlateMate to the 20-pounder, and you go up a little more than 10 percent. That's close enough for comfort.

You ask: How often should I change my program?

Mike says: The short answer is, as fast as you adapt to it. The ultimate goal of any training program is to improve your physical tolerance to the exercise stimulus, thus inducing a training effect. In other words, you make some sort of physiological adaptation—you get bigger or stronger, improve your endurance or speed, et cetera.

The tricky part is figuring out how long this process takes. If you abandon a program too soon, you may not get all the possible benefits before moving on to a less-beneficial program. Stay with a program too long, and you'll inevitably stop making gains. More lifters make the second mistake than the first, staying with a workout long after it's stopped producing any new benefits. A minority of guys are skittish enough to jump from program to program without ever seeing the results they should be getting.

You can't reliably know when to switch unless you keep detailed training logs. When you no longer see improvements from one workout to the next, it's time to shake things up.

Even a training log won't help you if you change your program every time you work out, in an attempt to keep your exercise habit mentally stimulating. Though some trainers recommend this strategy, seeking variety for the sake of variety makes it nearly impossible to gauge your progress. You can chart physical changes, such as the size of your waist or breadth of your chest. But if you don't see improvements, you have no way to figure out what you're doing wrong.

On the other hand, if you set up a program to systematically increase your strength and work capacity, you know you're making improvements that will lead to changes in your physique. If you try to gain strength or increase exercise volume and can't, you know there's something wrong with your program.

You ask: I've noticed some differences in strength from one side of my body to the other. Can I—and should I—correct this?

Mike says: Most people have a dominant side that is stronger yet less flexible than the nondominant side. This could lead to injuries down the road. Thankfully, the problem is easily fixed.

The best solution is to work unilaterally with dumbbells, your body weight, or perhaps cables.

First fix: Do unilateral exercises with your nondominant side first, then repeat the set with your dominant side. Don't do more reps with the dominant limb, even though you could. Your nondominant limb will eventually catch up the other one, and from there you can develop strength bilaterally.

Second fix: Start with your dominant side and force your other side to catch up. For instance, with your dominant arm, do 10 reps with a 30-pound dumbbell. With your nondominant arm, do just 6 reps. Rest for a few seconds, then crank out 1 or 2 more reps on your nondominant side. Repeat until you complete 10 reps. This forces your weaker limb to catch up to the stronger one without holding the stronger one back. Use this technique until you can do the same number of reps on each side without pausing to complete the final few on your nondominant side. Then alternate the arm you start each exercise with, to make sure both are capable of the same workload.

Third fix: You can also do more sets with your nondominant arm, using either of the techniques just described.

You ask: What are supersets, and why should I do them?

Mike says: A superset simply refers to two different exercises performed in rapid succession. Exactly which exercises you choose depends on your individual training goals. A standard superset pairs exercises that work opposing muscle groups—

bench presses and rows, for example, or biceps curls and triceps extensions. This forces one muscle to relax while the other works, enabling you to handle slightly more weight than normal and to push harder than usual on subsequent sets.

A compound set is a type of superset in which you pair two exercises for the same muscle group. For instance, you perform a set of bench presses to the point of fatigue, then move immediately to a set of flies. Although your chest could no longer perform the pressing motion, by switching to flies you can extend the set and make the muscle group work harder than usual.

Finally, you can also perform supersets by pairing completely unrelated muscle groups. Say, for example, that after doing a set of shoulder presses, you immediately move on to a set of calf raises. While this doesn't add any particular benefit to either set of muscles, it does save time. The first muscle group recovers while you work the second, yet you move the whole time.

No matter which type of superset you do, however, your overall speed has less to do with saving time than with your training goals. If you're interested in improving muscular endurance and getting a conditioning effect, you can proceed immediately from one exercise to the other until you've performed the desired number of sets for each. If you want more strength and size, on the other hand, you're probably better off resting for between 30 and 60 seconds after each exercise.

You ask: What is failure, and should I seek it on all my sets?

Mike says: First, let's distinguish between failure and fatigue. When you get to the end of a set and your muscles are so tired you can't do another rep without compromising form, you are fatigued. Failure is when you push your body after it's fatigued, doing partial repetitions, "cheat" reps (you break form and allow other muscles to help

lift the weight a couple more times), "forced" reps (a training partner helps you do the extra reps), or "breakdown" or "drop" sets (when you hit fatigue, you decrease the amount of weight you're lifting and keep going until you hit fatigue again, then decrease the weight one more time).

Bodybuilders have been doing high-intensity techniques such as forced reps and drop sets for eons. That doesn't necessarily mean that you should use them.

I think these techniques can sometimes help to accelerate gains in size and strength. I also think that repeated or prolonged use of them is counterproductive. They place tremendous stress on your joints and connective tissue, and they take a toll on your central nervous system, too, requiring you to take a lot longer to recover from workouts. As if that weren't enough, consider that consistently pushing yourself to the absolute brink can not only increase your risk of injury but also depress your immune function, leaving you less energetic and more susceptible to illness and infection.

There's nothing wrong—and something right—with occasionally pushing yourself beyond your limits, as long as you observe safety precautions. Warm up thoroughly, have a spotter on hand if there's a chance you'll get stuck under the bar, and make sure your body is ready for the challenge (don't try to reach failure while still sore from another workout, for example, or while recovering from an illness). Still, it isn't necessary to work to failure all the time—and doing it even some of the time is risky. It's easier than you think to go too far and set your training back weeks, if not months.

You ask: Is muscle soreness really a sign of a good workout?

Mike says: Most guys who've been training for a while come to expect soreness, and trust it. That tight, slightly achy feeling a day or two after a good workout tells us we gave our muscles a good growth stimulus. The exact mechanisms that cause post-workout soreness aren't completely understood, although the main culprit seems to be the normal training-induced muscle damage that prompts new muscle growth during recovery.

If the damage is too severe, however, your body can't repair itself properly, and you make no progress. This is the case when you're too sore to perform your next workout with the same intensity you used in the one that made you sore in the first place. I should add here that training sore muscles isn't a good idea. It only creates more damage, and it could make your muscles smaller and weaker.

The best way to keep soreness to a minimum is to make reasonable increases in the amount of weight you use from one workout to the next, as described in chapter 14. Also, avoid adding a lot of sets to a workout. Build up your sets gradually. And when you try a new exercise or return to one you haven't used in a while, take it easy. Use less weight than you think you should, and limit yourself to 2 or 3 sets.

You ask: How can I tell whether I'm overtraining?

Mike says: Obviously, the first sign is those continually sore, aching muscles and joints. Constant soreness means you aren't giving yourself enough recovery time. Another bad sign is a chronic, dull ache in your knees, shoulders, or lower back.

Another symptom of overtraining is a disappointing performance—you can't lift as much or do as many reps or complete your workout in the usual amount of time. All these signal that your body is tapped out and needs a rest.

Other clues include difficulty sleeping, a loss of appetite, irritability, and even suppressed immune function. So if you're a chronically sore, irritable insomniac who gets frequent colds and never seems to make any training progress, do yourself and your family a favor: Take a week off from training every 8 to 10 weeks.

You ask: How long will it take before I start to see results from my program?

Mike says: For years, the party line given by most fitness professionals has been "4 to 6 weeks." Indeed, it can often take at least that long before you start to see any tangible results. You may notice changes sooner if you work hard and if your body is naturally responsive.

Response time also depends on the type of results you're looking for. You could see changes in strength and flexibility after one or two workouts. You also might notice a change in tone early in the process. *Tone* is perhaps the most misused term in the entire exercise universe. Short for *tonus*, it means the amount of tension in your muscles. Most exercisers, and even a lot of trainers, mistakenly refer to "muscle tone" when they're really talking about fat-to-muscle ratio—the less fat you have, the leaner you are, and the more "toned" your appearance.

Real changes in body composition—such as a lower ratio of fat to muscle—take longer. They're also more dependent on effort and genetics. Some guys start losing fat almost immediately after starting a program, and within 4 weeks they may have noticeably more muscle. For other guys, the same changes could take months.

CHAPTER 19

AS SEEN ON TV: INFOMERCIAL MACHINES

How come so many of the machines advertised on Saturday-morning infomercials sound like something that should come in a plain brown wrapper? Soloflex. Ab-Doer. French Fitness Tickler.

Okay, we made up that last one. As for the first two . . . well, the words *Yeah, baby!* come to mind.

These devices—with or without sexy names—fall into a perpetually bewildering category of exercise equipment. For lack of an established generic term, let's call them alternative-resistance products.

Some of them are completely legitimate—once you get used to them, they should help you build solid muscle. Others aren't worth a nickel. What they all have in common is good-to-great marketing.

Here's a closer look at the major players in the alt-res category, why they may be attractive options if you lack space for or can't afford the equipment featured in chapter 4, and what you can expect from each.

BATTLE OF THE BANDS

The biggest players in the alt-res universe, Soloflex and Bowflex, use rubber or plastic to provide resistance. While these raw materials are fine for auto parts and birth-control apparatuses, we have a hard time believing they could be useful tools for building muscle.

We realize that rubber bands are used for light resistance in physical-therapy and rehabilitation settings. We've seen aerobics classes in which rubber bands (in a full palette of stimulating colors) add a light resistance component to the stepping and stomping and whatever else women do in those sessions. And we'll even concede that a sufficiently thick hunk of rubber could provide a challenging form of resistance for your muscles.

Just because it could, does that mean it does? We don't know. On the other hand, we can think of lots of reasons why working with rubber bands is a bad idea over the long haul. First, rubber is stiffer—and harder to move—when a room is cold, and more pliable in a warmer room. So your "strength" would artificially rise or fall depending on the ambient temperature of your workout space.

Second, rubber gets stretched out over time. A well-used chunk of rubber most likely provides much less resistance than a new slab.

Since we're so skeptical, we searched exercise-science databases for studies confirming the muscle-building effects of alt-res products such as Soloflex and Bowflex. We found exactly one, from 1990. In this 12-week study, three groups of female athletes each trained on a different type of resistance equipment: free weights, Nautilus, and Soloflex. (We couldn't find any studies on Bowflex.) The athletes lost about the same amount of fat with all three types of equipment. They also gained the same amount of strength, with one exception: Those who used the Soloflex gained less strength on the leg press than the others did.

A claim you'll find on the Web sites of the most popular machines is that they prevent injuries, avoid aggravating existing injuries, or some variation on that theme. Again, we couldn't find any research substantiating these claims. The only reason we could think of for why such a machine would be safer than any other weight machine is that it's less effective. If it were as challenging to muscles as an iron-based machine, it would have exactly the same potential for producing injury. In fact, given the awkwardness of some of the exercises you perform on these machines, we suspect the potential for injury would be greater, not less.

So we're left with our initial impressions of these machines and some opinions we've formed during our travels in the health-and-fitness industry.

Soloflex. The "Soloflex guy" was one of the first symbols of the buff-male aesthetic that took hold in the 1980s and early '90s. Yet we don't know whether it's possible to build a body like his with a machine as simple as the one popularized by his shirtless torso.

The Soloflex machine features a set of rubber bands representing various weights—5 to 100 pounds. You slip these bands on the apparatus, and lift the bar. You can also slip free weights over the bar, making it theoretically possible to pile up to 900 pounds of resistance on it. You need 4 feet by 4 feet of space in which to work out.

The Soloflex Web site shows a couple dozen exercises, some of which (the chest press, in particular) look like potentially decent muscle builders, and some of which look silly. You can see that the model can't get a full range of motion on the leg press and bent-over row, and the squats look awful. On other exercises, the model leans in or leans back to points we'd never recommend on the free-weight or cable version of the movement.

One point in its favor is that the Soloflex allows you to do body-weight exercises, including pullups, dips, and ab movements.

The problem we have with the Soloflex is the same problem we have with a Smith machine: The bar only goes up and down, so you work your muscles in only one plane of motion. Granted, one plane of motion beats the hell out of none. Even so, for the money you'd pay for Soloflex (more than $1,500), we think you'd want all possible planes.

Bowflex. The Bowflex relies on a series of bendable plastic rods to create resistance. Unlike with Soloflex, you move in multiple planes of motion, as you would with a cable machine. Your movements also have more of a true weight-lifting "feel." You'll notice a difference, although not as big a difference as with the Soloflex.

Prices range from about $700 to $2,000. The space requirements are 6 feet by 9 feet to work out with the Bowflex Ultimate model, and $2\frac{1}{2}$ by 4 feet to store the machine when it's folded up. The sizes of other models vary.

A final word about Bowflex and Soloflex: Be very careful about buying either of these machines used. Unless you're very familiar with the device, you won't know whether it works properly. With a new machine, you can trust that it functions correctly and that any awkwardness you feel is part of the learning curve.

OUR BODIES, OUR WEIGHT STACKS

Another type of alt-res device uses body weight, cleverly leveraged. The most popular and best product we know of in this category is the Total Gym, a sliding bench with cables that allows you to do dozens of exercises with your body weight as resistance. (As with Soloflex, you can add weight plates, which you'll certainly need to do to get enough resistance on exercises like the leg press.)

Total Gym has its roots in physical-therapy settings, and it functionally resembles the Reformer, a piece of equipment used in Pilates. (In fact, for $300 you can add Pilates-enabling equipment to certain Total Gym models.)

What we like best about Total Gym is that it allows exercise in all planes of movement. The range of motion resembles that of cable exercises. There's a learning curve to the exercises, since you wouldn't naturally choose to do most of these movements while lying on a bench and pulling on a handle attached to a cable. Despite that, we give it high marks because it's functional and portable.

The price is between $1,000 and $1,500. The necessary space amounts to 10 by 2 feet in which to work out, and $3\frac{1}{2}$ by 2 to store the machine.

"AND IF YOU CALL NOW, WE'LL THROW IN THESE BICEPS, ABSOLUTELY FREE!"

The infomercial industry produces an estimated $1 billion in sales each year, and get-fit-quick products are among the most popular offerings. Sometimes—as in the case of the aforementioned products—you really can build muscle with the product being hawked. Other times, you'd be better off flipping to the Playboy channel and working on those wrist flexors. Here are some of the ways you can tell the good from the bad.

Learn to speak the language. Infomercials typically load up their sales pitches with a lot of jargon that sounds scientific but really isn't. This usually precedes a promise of astounding results in a very short time frame. Stop us if you've heard this one: If it sounds too good to be true, it probably is.

A sure sign of B.S. is a promise that the product will reduce fat in a select area of your physique—midsection, thighs, and butt are the usual places, though we suppose someone could invent the Jowlmaster 3000, with the promise of a slimmer face in 3 weeks or your money back. While it's true that visceral fat—the deadly stuff around your organs and beneath your midsection muscles—disappears quickly with exercise, when you're talking about subcutaneous fat—the nonlethal but unsightly tissue between your muscles and skin—your genetics determine where it stays and where it goes. Even a good, consistent diet-and-workout program might thin your face as it leaves you with stubborn love handles. Liposuction is the only way to remove fat from a predetermined area.

Remember: "Satisfaction guaranteed" doesn't include postage. With infomercial products that are "not found in any store," you can't try before you buy. Despite a "30-day risk-free trial offer," most of the time you have to pay for all shipping and handling. That could mean between $50 and $100—each way. And good luck getting the thing back in the original packing materials.

Don't trust the experts. Remember when Orson Welles, near the end of his life, did commercials for a brand of wine that was, to put it delicately, not a favorite of connoisseurs? Did he do those endorsements because he wanted the world to know about a great wine that had been unfairly overlooked by the editors of *Wine Spectator*? Hell, no. He was looking for the biggest paychecks he could get for the least amount of work.

Now consider what motivates a fitness expert to appear in an infomercial. Let's say he's spent a few years in the trenches—getting debauched celebrities in shape for movies, lecturing bored undergraduates, attempting to train powerful executives who regard exercise as only slightly less despicable than their alimony payments.

He figures he's paid his dues, and he's ready to cash in. Whatever got him excited about fitness in the first place is long gone, replaced by a desire to make more money for less work. A successful infomercial is the exercise-industry version of the lottery. When your number hits, you never again have to wake up at 5:00 in the morning to work with people you don't like. And you may just wake up in a new vacation home on St. Bart's.

These guys know their credibility is eternally compromised as soon as they're introduced with the words *But don't take our word for it. Here's fitness expert. . . .* They may not know that Orson Welles said, "You make your name on the way up and your money on the way down." They sure understand the idea, though.

Beware of "studies." Considering that infomercial fitness experts aren't credible, the studies they cite aren't necessarily reliable, either. Researchers can find so many ways to cook data that it's a wonder none of them appear on *Iron Chef*. It is possible that a cited study is legit. It's just as possible that it's a complete crock.

Your strategy: Distrust them all, and let Google sort them out. If an Internet search turns up compelling evidence that the study is legit, fine. If it doesn't, you've saved yourself four easy payments.

WHEN SCIENCE MEETS SNAKE OIL

Sometimes legitimate scientists are hired by magazines, consumer-watchdog organizations, or nonprofit exercise associations to look into the claims made on infomercials. Here are the results of studies of three infomercial products.

Ab-Doer

What it is: A machine with a small bench on which you sit to grip shoulder-high handlebars and rotate your torso in various directions.

The claim: "A flat, firm stomach the easy way. . . . Flattens your stomach in just minutes a day."

Results of a study at California State University, Northridge: Ab-Doer exercise is no better, and sometimes worse, than a traditional crunch.

Time Works

What it is: This exercise machine combines a lower-body stepping movement with a side-to-side torso twist.

The claim: "Full-body fitness in just 4 minutes a day."

Results of a study at Appalachian State University in Boone, North Carolina: The exercise program doesn't provide enough stimuli for fitness improvement.

Electrical Muscle Stimulation

What it is: A device that stimulates the muscles with electrical current via small padded electrodes affixed to the skin.

The claim: Build muscle without any effort. Just sit on the couch, hook up to the machine, and watch your muscles grow.

Results of a study at the University of Wisconsin, La Crosse: Electrical muscle stimulation is ineffective, time-consuming, and—at times—even painful.

CHAPTER 20

WATCH LIST: OUR FAVORITE EXERCISE VIDEOS

There aren't many workout videos produced for the visible-plumbing population—for good reason. Males buy just 2 to 3 percent of the hundreds of thousands of exercise videos sold each year by Collage Video, the leading purveyor in the field. This statistic seems pretty easy to explain. Women, in our experience, are comfortable with step-by-step exercise instruction. Guys prefer to pick up a few general pointers and wing it from there.

There are some practical issues, too. It's a lot easier, physically, for a 5-foot-4 woman to exercise in front of a television set. A 6-foot man needs to stand farther away from the TV to get a clear view and avoid neck strain. He also needs to clear more room in front of him to accommodate his longer arms and legs.

That said, we know that some guys do like to work out to videos. And we acknowledge that some of the videos out there are worth the effort to find them and set up a space to use them. The best ones are motivating, give you new routines, and teach you new exercises, or at least better form on the exercises you already know.

WORKING OUT TO A VIDEO

If you've never taken group-exercise classes (and we assume you haven't), it takes a while to get the hang of exercise videos. The only thing that keeps you from feeling like a complete imbecile is the fact no one can see you flailing around. Here are a couple of things to keep in mind while you thrash around the rec room.

- Try to mirror the instructor's moves, since he's facing you. When he moves to his left, you move to your right. Good leaders will cue you correctly (saying "left" when he means your left, not his).

- It's not cheating to use the pause button. Don't get frustrated if you can't do a choreographed kickboxing, step, yoga, or aerobic routine on your first attempt. Pause, rewind, and try again. Some of the best videos change moves quickly because once you learn them, you'll get bored with too much repetition. They assume you'll stop and repeat multiple times while you're learning.

- When you're learning an aerobic or step routine, skip the arm movements entirely and concentrate on the footwork. You can add the arms later, change them so they feel natural to you, or skip them forever. (They're mainly for show anyway—unless you hold weights in your hands, they don't add much to the workout.) Anytime you have trouble with the steps, just jog in place or, if you're using a step, do your basic up-up-down-down until you either catch the new step or the instructor switches to a more manageable move.

- If you're following a kickboxing video and you're having trouble coordinating punches and kicks, concentrate on one or the other, then switch the next time you do the workout. Or concentrate on your upper body for 10 minutes, rewind, do the same 10 minutes of the workout while concentrating on your lower body, then rewind again and try both. You don't have to finish the tape to benefit from the workout.

- If you're working out to a cardio or step video with a female leader, you may need to make some modifications. Since women are generally smaller and shorter-limbed, they tend to move faster. You may find that you flail your arms and don't land your feet fully. Feel free to slow down, even if it means your timing isn't on the beat of the music. (Turn down the volume so that doesn't bother you.) Or do the moves in half-time (take two beats for one movement).

WORKOUT VIDEOS THAT WORK FOR GUYS

Don't bother looking for workout tapes or DVDs at your local video store—or any other mainstream retailer, for that matter. You'll end up choosing from among Richard Simmons, Denise Austin, or whichever knocked-up starlet decided to cash in on her pregnancy by making a prenatal-workout video.

The public library is no better. It probably has some old Jane Fonda tapes (and we don't mean *Barbarella*), a couple of pregnancy workouts, and maybe some yoga with taffy-limbed women in pastel leotards, accompanied by music that would put Enya to sleep.

Here are the best sources for workout videos.

- Collage Video has been selling workout videos exclusively since 1987. You can read customer comments and order online at www.collagevideo.com, or phone

(800) 433-6769 to get advice from a consultant who has actually done the workouts and can help you find a video to suit your needs and preferences. At the time we called, 4 of their 12 consultants were male, and the catalogue included more than 370 titles.

- Amazon.com (www.amazon.com) has an extensive workout-video collection, with both editorial and reader reviews. If you want to browse workout videos, click "video," then "fitness." You'll see several categories to choose from, such as "kickboxing," "weight training," "body parts" (not the ones you're thinking of, trust us), and so on. If you know which video title or exercise leader you want, select "VHS" or "DVD" in the "product" box, then search for the video's or leader's name.

Although some female workout leaders use slow, controlled moves that emphasize muscle more than choreography, you'll probably be more comfortable starting out with a guy leader. (Richard Simmons is technically a male, but you wouldn't describe him as a *guy*. A guy is someone you want to have a beer with, not someone your wife would look to for tips on keeping her legs smooth and silky.)

When you read reviews from Amazon or Collage, look for words like *athletic, strength,* and *weights*; and avoid terms such as *buns, tone, tummy,* and, of course, *easy* and *light*.

Better yet, choose from the guy-friendly list below. We focused on series and leaders, since new titles are added frequently to successful series.

The videos designated "Beginner/Intermediate" are for regular guys and are designed as beginning-to-end workouts. Many of the ones under the "Advanced" heading were created for personal trainers, physical therapists, and strength coaches.

Some depict workouts, meant to be followed in real time. Most are collections of exercises and training techniques. You can use them to gather ideas for your own workouts or learn better form. You can't just pop them in, follow along, and expect to get a workout. Some of the instructions fly by pretty fast, in more technical language than you're probably used to.

Still, we include them because we've learned a lot from them, and we think our most advanced, adventurous readers will appreciate the information they offer.

BEGINNER-TO-INTERMEDIATE LEVEL

Tae-Bo. Martial artist and B-movie action star Billy Blanks invented Tae-Bo as a tough mix of kickboxing and aerobic conditioning. If you're new to this format, start with one of the basic workouts in the series so you learn the fundamentals. You won't feel your testosterone level drop when you do these workouts. They rate zero on the wimpiness scale.

Cardio Athletic Kickbox. Eversley Forte leads these high-intensity workouts designed for intermediate to advanced exercisers. This is heavy-duty cardio, with good instruction from Forte. Choose from *Cardio Athletic Kickbox, Cardio Athletic Kickbox Instructor Series I,* and *Cardio Athletic Kickbox II*.

Scott Helvenston. Former Navy SEAL instructor Helvenston leads two series of military-style calisthenics workouts: *Navy SEAL Training Camp* (eight videos) and *True-Fit Training* (three videos). Three levels are demonstrated; no equipment is needed.

Men of Steel. This series started strong but proved uneven (as you can tell by reading customer reviews on Amazon.com.) The original *Abs of Steel* video, featuring Kurt Brungardt, gets the highest marks. Another winner is *Abs and Chest of Steel* with Michael Perron.

Gilad Janklowicz. Janklowicz has been offering simple, idiot-proof cardio-workout videos in a Hawaiian setting forever. (He also stars in some titles in the *Men of Steel* series.) If you want straightforward cardio with no dancing or flinging arms, and you don't feel like a complete nimrod when pretending to work out on the beach, this is your man.

Gin Miller. We're torn about including the original Step Reebok gal here. If you can deal with group-exercise aerobics, Miller's videos are the most guy-friendly of the step videos—lots of stepping, no dancing. The step and Swiss-ball workouts are tough, requiring strength, stamina, and even a degree of athleticism.

Rodney Yee. Yee has made more than a dozen yoga-workout videos, many for beginners, a few for intermediates and athletes. Some are inexpensively priced 20-minute workouts. Yee manages to make yoga look like a reasonable thing to do with your time, which is quite an impressive accomplishment.

ADVANCED LEVEL

Paul Chek. You already know how much we like Swiss-ball exercises. Unfortunately, it never occurred to us to design entire programs around them. It did occur to Chek, one of the world's foremost proponents of Swiss-ball exercise. Some of his videos are actual workouts; others (such as the *Strong 'n' Stable Swiss-Ball Weight Training* series) illustrate moments from a variety of possible workouts. If you can't find them through Amazon or Collage, check out www.paulchekseminars.com.

Advanced Strength Training. The three tapes in this series from Human Kinetics show you different takes on the subject. *High-Intensity Training* features the somewhat controversial idea that you get the best results by performing 1 set of each exercise in your routine to failure. (We say it's controversial because we don't agree

with it. But, hey, peaches aren't the only fruit.) *High-Volume Training* focuses on multiple-set routines, such as those we advocate in this book. *Keys to Superior Strength* steps away from the focus on building muscle to look at training for muscular performance. You can buy them singly or as a set. Each video teaches concepts and techniques, and shows a whole workout with several variations, but just a few repetitions, of each exercise. You can either learn a new routine to do later or keep the remote on your weight bench so you can pause the video to complete each set while you work out.

Bryan Kest's Power Yoga **series.** Kest looks like he could walk into a bar and walk out with any woman he wanted . . . with the blessing of whatever guy she happened to be with before he got there. He comes off as half Mick Jagger, half Jedi—either of which is rare enough in a yogi. The workouts, which you do along with Kest, are demanding (intermediate-to-advanced level). You can buy them as singles or as a set.

Juan Carlos Santana. Santana is a trainer's trainer—whenever there's a convention of athletic trainers and strength coaches, chances are you'll see the dynamic Santana giving lectures and seminars. At his Web site, www.opsfit.com, you'll find his video series. These aren't follow-along workouts; they're mostly designed to help trainers work with athletes or clients under a variety of circumstances. We're huge fans of his two-part series *The Essence of Dumbbell Training.* His two-part series for exercise bands and cable machines includes more than 80 exercises. And his two-part Swiss-ball series may be the best of the bunch.

Ian King, C.S.C.S. You've seen King's name a few times in this book; like Santana, he's a strength coach who's admired by other trainers for his unique programs and for his ability to explain them simply and clearly. Most of his videos (you'll find more than a dozen at www.kingsports.net) are geared toward trainers. There aren't any fancy production values in these videos. All you get is King explaining and demonstrating exercises, techniques, and training systems. For many of us, that's as good as it gets.

VIDEOS FOR CARDIO MACHINES

When you do cardio at the gym, you usually find yourself in front of a bank of TV screens tuned to *SportsCenter* and *Crossfire*. At home, you can do better. Many videos are designed for home exercisers on treadmills or exercise bikes, allowing you to pretend you're pedaling or trekking through cool scenery rather than going nowhere in your basement. Here are a couple of interesting choices.

Video Cycle. Each video in this series takes you biking through a different location, such as the Grand Tetons, Hawaii, British Columbia, or the Oregon Coast. No instructor—you just ride and watch the scenery whir by.

Video Stride. You run or walk on your treadmill and watch mountains, country roads, or villages in places such as Switzerland, Hawaii, or the Canadian Rockies.

SAMPLE WORKOUTS AND TRAINING LOGS

The following are sample 4-week workouts from chapters 6 through 10. We've filled in the first few columns of each log to suggest exercises, sets, and repetitions. In the last few columns, you fill in the amount of weight you used and the actual number of repetitions you performed.

You can write on these pages—hey, it's your book—or photocopy the logs to keep your book pristine. (But please, do us a favor and at least sweat on the paper a little bit. There's nothing more depressing to us than an unused workout book. Ours are thrashed, and we're proud of that fact.)

4-WEEK BODY-WEIGHT WORKOUT

EQUIPMENT REQUIRED

- Chinning bar
- Sturdy chair or bench
- Milk jugs, soup cans, and other household objects discussed in chapters 3 and 6

STRENGTHS

- Such a workout is great for general conditioning and increasing muscular endurance.
- Pullups and chinups are among the best exercises for upper-back strength and muscular development.
- You can do a wide variety of interesting, effective abdominal exercises without specialized workout equipment.

WEAKNESSES

- It's very difficult to build lower-body muscle and strength without weights.
- Beginners won't be able to do pullups and chinups, and thus will have a hard time building upper-back muscles.
- There are very few effective arm and shoulder exercises you can do using nothing but body weight—chinups and chair dips are good exercises, but there aren't many other options.

BEGINNER LEVEL

Perform this workout 2 or 3 times a week. Each workout, try to increase either the number of repetitions you do or the amount of resistance you use. When you can do all the suggested repetitions of an exercise, refer to chapter 6 for ways to make the exercise more challenging.

BEGINNER BODY-WEIGHT WEEK 1

MUSCLES	EXERCISE	Sets	Target Reps	WORKOUT 1 Weight	Reps	WORKOUT 2 Weight	Reps	WORKOUT 3 Weight	Reps
Transverse abdominis	Vacuum	Set 1	6-10*						
Lower abs	Reverse crunch	Set 1	10-15						
Upper abs	Crunch	Set 1	10-15						
Obliques	Oblique crunch	Set 1	10-15						
Lower back	Prone Superman	Set 1	10-15						
Lower body	Split squat	Set 1	12-15						
Chest, front shoulders, triceps	Pushup	Set 1	10-15						
Upper back	Assisted pullup	Set 1	10-15						
Shoulders	Lateral raise	Set 1	10-15						
Upper back	One-arm row, elbow in	Set 1	10-15						
Biceps	Self-resisted biceps curl†	Set 1	10-15‡						
Calves	Unilateral calf raise†	Set 1	10-15‡						

* Hold for 20 to 30 seconds per repetition † Optional ‡Each side

BEGINNER BODY-WEIGHT WEEK 2

MUSCLES	EXERCISE	Sets	Target Reps	WORKOUT 1 Weight	Reps	WORKOUT 2 Weight	Reps	WORKOUT 3 Weight	Reps
Transverse abdominis	Vacuum	Set 1	6-10*						
Lower abs	Reverse crunch	Set 1	10-15						
Upper abs	Crunch	Set 1	10-15						
Obliques	Oblique crunch	Set 1	10-15						
Lower back	Prone Superman	Set 1	10-15						
Lower body	Split squat	Set 1	12-15						
Chest, front shoulders, triceps	Pushup	Set 1	10-15						
Upper back	Assisted pullup	Set 1	10-15						
Shoulders	Lateral raise	Set 1	10-15						
Upper back	One-arm row, elbow in	Set 1	10-15						
Biceps	Self-resisted biceps curl†	Set 1	10-15‡						
Calves	Unilateral calf raise†	Set 1	10-15‡						

* Hold for 20 to 30 seconds per repetition † Optional ‡Each side

BEGINNER BODY-WEIGHT WEEK 3

MUSCLES	EXERCISE	Sets	Target Reps	WORKOUT 1		WORKOUT 2		WORKOUT 3	
				Weight	Reps	Weight	Reps	Weight	Reps
Transverse abdominis	Vacuum	Set 1	6–10*						
Lower abs	Reverse crunch	Set 1	10–15						
Upper abs	Crunch	Set 1	10–15						
Obliques	Oblique crunch	Set 1	10–15						
Lower back	Prone Superman	Set 1	10–15						
Lower body	Split squat	Set 1	12–15						
Chest, front shoulders, triceps	Pushup	Set 1	10–15						
Upper back	Assisted pullup	Set 1	10–15						
Shoulders	Lateral raise	Set 1	10–15						
Upper back	One-arm row, elbow in	Set 1	10–15						
Biceps	Self-resisted biceps curl†	Set 1	10–15‡						
Calves	Unilateral calf raise†	Set 1	10–15‡						

* Hold for 20 to 30 seconds per repetition † Optional ‡ Each side

BEGINNER BODY-WEIGHT WEEK 4

MUSCLES	EXERCISE	Sets	Target Reps	WORKOUT 1		WORKOUT 2		WORKOUT 3	
				Weight	Reps	Weight	Reps	Weight	Reps
Transverse abdominis	Vacuum	Set 1	6–10*						
Lower abs	Reverse crunch	Set 1	10–15						
Upper abs	Crunch	Set 1	10–15						
Obliques	Oblique crunch	Set 1	10–15						
Lower back	Prone Superman	Set 1	10–15						
Lower body	Split squat	Set 1	12–15						
Chest, front shoulders, triceps	Pushup	Set 1	10–15						
Upper back	Assisted pullup	Set 1	10–15						
Shoulders	Lateral raise	Set 1	10–15						
Upper back	One-arm row, elbow in	Set 1	10–15						
Biceps	Self-resisted biceps curl†	Set 1	10–15‡						
Calves	Unilateral calf raise†	Set 1	10–15‡						

* Hold for 20 to 30 seconds per repetition † Optional ‡ Each side

INTERMEDIATE LEVEL

This is called a split routine, meaning you divide your muscle groups in half and work them on separate days. Workout A hits midsection and lower-body muscles. Workout B hits upper-body muscles.

We recommend that you do a total of three workouts per week, alternating between Workouts A and B. So the first week you might do A on Monday, B on Tuesday, and A on Friday; then do B the following Monday, and so on. In that case, you do each workout six times in 4 weeks.

If you want to work out four times a week, you can do A on Monday, B on Tuesday, A again on Thursday, and B on Friday. In that case, we recommend following this program for 3 weeks instead of 4. So you still do each workout six times before changing your program.

INTERMEDIATE BODY-WEIGHT WORKOUT A: MIDSECTION AND LOWER BODY

MUSCLES	EXERCISE	Sets	Target Reps	WORKOUT 1 Weight	Reps	WORKOUT 2 Weight	Reps	WORKOUT 3 Weight	Reps	WORKOUT 4 Weight	Reps	WORKOUT 5 Weight	Reps	WORKOUT 6 Weight	Reps
Transverse abdominis	Bridge	Set 1	1*	—	Sec:	—	Sec:	—	Sec:	—	Sec:	—	Sec:	—	Sec:
Lower abs	Pulse-up	Set 1	8–10												
		Set 2	8–10												
		Set 3‡	8–10												
Upper abs	Towel crunch	Set 1	8–10												
		Set 2	8–10												
		Set 3‡	8–10												
Obliques	Crunch with lateral flexion	Set 1	8–10†												
		Set 2	8–10†												
		Set 3‡	8–10†												
Obliques (rotational movement)	Russian twist	Set 1	8–10												
		Set 2	8–10												
		Set 3‡	8–10												
Lower back	Bird dog	Set 1	8–10												
		Set 2	8–10												
		Set 3‡	8–10												
Glutes, hamstrings	Lying hip extension	Set 1	8–10												
		Set 2	8–10												
		Set 3‡	8–10												
Entire lower body	Bulgarian split squat	Set 1	8–10												
		Set 2	8–10												
		Set 3‡	8–10												
Lower back, glutes, hamstrings	Reverse hyperextension	Set 1	8–10												
		Set 2	8–10												
		Set 3‡	8–10												
Calves	Seated calf raise§	Set 1	8–10												
		Set 2	8–10												
		Set 3‡	8–10												

* Hold for as long as you can, up to 60 seconds   † Each side   ‡ Optional set   § Optional exercise

INTERMEDIATE BODY-WEIGHT WORKOUT B: UPPER BODY

MUSCLES	EXERCISE	Sets	Target Reps	WORKOUT 1		WORKOUT 2		WORKOUT 3		WORKOUT 4		WORKOUT 5		WORKOUT 6	
				Weight	Reps	Weight	Reps	Weight	Reps	Weight	Reps	Weight	Reps	Weight	Reps
Upper back	Wide-grip pullup	Set 1	*												
Upper back	Pullup	Set 1	*												
Upper back, biceps	Chinup	Set 1	Max												
Upper chest, shoulders, triceps	Pushup with elevated feet	Set 1	8–10												
Chest, shoulders, triceps	Pushup with stacked feet	Set 1	8–10												
Chest, shoulders, triceps	Chair dip	Set 1	8–10												
Upper back, rear shoulders	Prone reverse fly	Set 1	8–10												
		Set 2	8–10												
		Set 3	8–10												
Shoulders	External rotation	Set 1	8–10												
		Set 2	8–10												
		Set 3	8–10												

* Stop 1 repetition short of what you think is your maximum

ADVANCED LEVEL

Here's a tough collection of exercises that challenge your strength, balance, coordination, and muscular endurance. You can use this as a stand-alone workout you perform two or three times a week, or as a program you do once a week as an adjunct to any other type of workout you do, at home or in a gym.

ADVANCED BODY-WEIGHT WEEK 1

MUSCLES	EXERCISE	Sets	Target Reps	WORKOUT 1		WORKOUT 2		WORKOUT 3	
				Weight	Reps	Weight	Reps	Weight	Reps
Upper back, biceps	One-arm chinup	Set 1	Max*						
Upper back	Towel pullup	Set 1	Max						
Upper back, biceps	Chinup	Set 1	Max						
Chest, shoulders, triceps	Plyometric pushup	Set 1	Max						
Chest	Towel fly	Set 1	Max						
Chest, shoulders, triceps, abdominals	Walking pushup		Max						
Shoulders, triceps	Pike pushup	Set 1	Max						
Lower body (knee-dominant)	One-leg squat	Set 1	8–10*						
Lower body (knee-dominant)	Split jump	Set 1	8–10*						
Lower body (hip-dominant)	King deadlift	Set 1	8–10*						
Lower body (hip-dominant)	Swiss-ball lying hip extension/leg curl	Set 1	8–10						
Abdominals	Situp	Set 1	Max						

* Each side

ADVANCED BODY-WEIGHT WEEK 2

MUSCLES	EXERCISE	Sets	Target Reps	WORKOUT 1		WORKOUT 2		WORKOUT 3	
				Weight	Reps	Weight	Reps	Weight	Reps
Upper back, biceps	One-arm chinup	Set 1	Max*						
Upper back	Towel pullup	Set 1	Max						
Upper back, biceps	Chinup	Set 1	Max						
Chest, shoulders, triceps	Plyometric pushup	Set 1	Max						
Chest	Towel fly	Set 1	Max						
Chest, shoulders, triceps, abdominals	Walking pushup		Max						
Shoulders, triceps	Pike pushup	Set 1	Max						
Lower body (knee-dominant)	One-leg squat	Set 1	8–10*						
Lower body (knee-dominant)	Split jump	Set 1	8–10*						
Lower body (hip-dominant)	King deadlift	Set 1	8–10*						
Lower body (hip-dominant)	Swiss-ball lying hip extension/leg curl	Set 1	8–10						
Abdominals	Situp	Set 1	Max						

* Each side

ADVANCED BODY-WEIGHT WEEK 3

MUSCLES	EXERCISE	Sets	Target Reps	WORKOUT 1		WORKOUT 2		WORKOUT 3	
				Weight	Reps	Weight	Reps	Weight	Reps
Upper back, biceps	One-arm chinup	Set 1	Max*						
Upper back	Towel pullup	Set 1	Max						
Upper back, biceps	Chinup	Set 1	Max						
Chest, shoulders, triceps	Plyometric pushup	Set 1	Max						
Chest	Towel fly	Set 1	Max						
Chest, shoulders, triceps, abdominals	Walking pushup	Set 1	Max						
Shoulders, triceps	Pike pushup	Set 1	Max						
Lower body (knee-dominant)	One-leg squat	Set 1	8–10*						
Lower body (knee-dominant)	Split jump	Set 1	8–10*						
Lower body (hip-dominant)	King deadlift	Set 1	8–10*						
Lower body (hip-dominant)	Swiss-ball lying hip extension/leg curl	Set 1	8–10						
Abdominals	Situp	Set 1	Max						

* Each side

ADVANCED BODY-WEIGHT WEEK 4

MUSCLES	EXERCISE	Sets	Target Reps	WORKOUT 1		WORKOUT 2		WORKOUT 3	
				Weight	Reps	Weight	Reps	Weight	Reps
Upper back, biceps	One-arm chinup	Set 1	Max*						
Upper back	Towel pullup	Set 1	Max						
Upper back, biceps	Chinup	Set 1	Max						
Chest, shoulders, triceps	Plyometric pushup	Set 1	Max						
Chest	Towel fly	Set 1	Max						
Chest, shoulders, triceps, abdominals	Walking pushup	Set 1	Max						
Shoulders, triceps	Pike pushup	Set 1	Max						
Lower body (knee-dominant)	One-leg squat	Set 1	8–10*						
Lower body (knee-dominant)	Split jump	Set 1	8–10*						
Lower body (hip-dominant)	King deadlift	Set 1	8–10*						
Lower body (hip-dominant)	Swiss-ball lying hip extension/leg curl	Set 1	8–10						
Abdominals	Situp	Set 1	Max						

* Each side

4-WEEK DUMBBELL WORKOUT

EQUIPMENT REQUIRED

- Dumbbells
- Adjustable bench
- Swiss ball

STRENGTHS

- Dumbbells are (in our opinion) the best tools for building upper-body muscle. They offer the most variety and the greatest ranges of motion.
- Although barbells are better for building maximal strength, dumbbells are much easier on the shoulder and elbow joints.
- Dumbbells provide the most versatility for imitating athletic moves and developing sport-specific workouts.

WEAKNESSES

- It's hard to use dumbbells to develop maximal strength—it's expensive to buy fixed dumbbells at the heaviest weights, and it's impractical to pile plates onto dumbbell handles. Most of us don't have enough 10-pound plates to create, say, a pair of 80-pound dumbbells. And if we use bigger plates, such as 25-pounders, the dumbbells are unwieldy on many exercises.
- It's awkward to move the heaviest dumbbells into position for exercises such as bench presses.
- It's difficult to develop serious lower-body muscle using dumbbells alone. Heavy squats and deadlifts are out of the question, and even on lunges your grip may give out before you've worked your leg muscles intensely enough.

BEGINNER LEVEL

Perform this workout two or three times a week. Each workout, try to increase either the number of repetitions or the amount of resistance. You'll see that most of the exercises give you the option of performing a second set. If you decide to do 2 sets, you have three possible ways to work.

Circuits. Do a single set of all the exercises in this workout, then go back and do a second set of all the exercises. In other words, do two circuits.

A warmup set and a work set. Do the first set as a warmup, using half to two-thirds of the weight you would normally use for the exercise. Rest for 30 to 60 seconds, then do a work set with the normal weight.

Two work sets. As you get closer to the intermediate level, you can do 2 sets with the normal weight on each exercise. When you do multiple sets, we recommend you stop the sets short of failure. That is, don't push your muscles to the absolute limit on either set—especially the first set.

When you can do all the suggested repetitions of an exercise, increase the weight.

BEGINNER DUMBBELL WEEK I

MUSCLES	EXERCISE	Sets	Target Reps	WORKOUT I		WORKOUT 2		WORKOUT 3	
				Weight	Reps	Weight	Reps	Weight	Reps
Lower abs	Reverse crunch	Set 1	10–15						
Upper abs	Crunch	Set 1	10–15						
Lower back	Prone Superman	Set 1	10–15						
Lower body	Sumo squat	Set 1	12–15						
		Set 2†	12–15						
Chest, front shoulders, triceps	Bench press	Set 1	10–15						
		Set 2†	10–15						
Lower body	Reverse lunge	Set 1	12–15						
		Set 2†	12–15						
Upper back	Pullover	Set 1	10–15						
		Set 2†	10–15						
Shoulders, triceps	Shoulder press	Set 1	10–15						
		Set 2†	10–15						
Upper back, biceps	Bent-over row	Set 1	10–15						
		Set 2†	10–15						
Shoulders, traps	Upright row	Set 1	10–15						
		Set 2†	10–15						
Shoulders	Side-lying external rotation	Set 1	10–15*						
Triceps	Lying triceps extension	Set 1	10–15*						
Biceps	Seated concentration curl	Set 1	10–15*						
Calves	Seated calf raise	Set 1	12–15						

* Each arm   † Optional set

BEGINNER DUMBBELL WEEK 2

MUSCLES	EXERCISE	Sets	Target Reps	WORKOUT 1 Weight	Reps	WORKOUT 2 Weight	Reps	WORKOUT 3 Weight	Reps
Lower abs	Reverse crunch	Set 1	10–15						
Upper abs	Crunch	Set 1	10–15						
Lower back	Prone Superman	Set 1	10–15						
Lower body	Sumo squat	Set 1	12–15						
		Set 2†	12–15						
Chest, front shoulders, triceps	Bench press	Set 1	10–15						
		Set 2†	10–15						
Lower body	Reverse lunge	Set 1	12–15						
		Set 2†	12–15						
Upper back	Pullover	Set 1	10–15						
		Set 2†	10–15						
Shoulders, triceps	Shoulder press	Set 1	10–15						
		Set 2†	10–15						
Upper back, biceps	Bent-over row	Set 1	10–15						
		Set 2†	10–15						
Shoulders, traps	Upright row	Set 1	10–15						
		Set 2†	10–15						
Shoulders	Side-lying external rotation	Set 1	10–15*						
Triceps	Lying triceps extension	Set 1	10–15*						
Biceps	Seated concentration curl	Set 1	10–15*						
Calves	Seated calf raise	Set 1	12–15						

* Each arm   † Optional set

BEGINNER DUMBBELL WEEK 3

MUSCLES	EXERCISE	Sets	Target Reps	WORKOUT 1 Weight	Reps	WORKOUT 2 Weight	Reps	WORKOUT 3 Weight	Reps
Lower abs	Reverse crunch	Set 1	10–15						
Upper abs	Crunch	Set 1	10–15						
Lower back	Prone Superman	Set 1	10–15						
Lower body	Sumo squat	Set 1	12–15						
		Set 2†	12–15						
Chest, front shoulders, triceps	Bench press	Set 1	10–15						
		Set 2†	10–15						
Lower body	Reverse lunge	Set 1	12–15						
		Set 2†	12–15						
Upper back	Pullover	Set 1	10–15						
		Set 2†	10–15						
Shoulders, triceps	Shoulder press	Set 1	10–15						
		Set 2†	10–15						
Upper back, biceps	Bent-over row	Set 1	10–15						
		Set 2†	10–15						
Shoulders, traps	Upright row	Set 1	10–15						
		Set 2†	10–15						
Shoulders	Side-lying external rotation	Set 1	10–15*						
Triceps	Lying triceps extension	Set 1	10–15*						
Biceps	Seated concentration curl	Set 1	10–15*						
Calves	Seated calf raise	Set 1	12–15						

* Each arm   † Optional set

BEGINNER DUMBBELL WEEK 4

MUSCLES	EXERCISE	Sets	Target Reps	WORKOUT 1		WORKOUT 2		WORKOUT 3	
				Weight	Reps	Weight	Reps	Weight	Reps
Lower abs	Reverse crunch	Set 1	10–15						
Upper abs	Crunch	Set 1	10–15						
Lower back	Prone Superman	Set 1	10–15						
Lower body	Sumo squat	Set 1	12–15						
		Set 2†	12–15						
Chest, front shoulders, triceps	Bench press	Set 1	10–15						
		Set 2†	10–15						
Lower body	Reverse lunge	Set 1	12–15						
		Set 2†	12–15						
Upper back	Pullover	Set 1	10–15						
		Set 2†	10–15						
Shoulders, triceps	Shoulder press	Set 1	10–15						
		Set 2†	10–15						
Upper back, biceps	Bent-over row	Set 1	10–15						
		Set 2†	10–15						
Shoulders, traps	Upright row	Set 1	10–15						
		Set 2†	10–15						
Shoulders	Side-lying external rotation	Set 1	10–15*						
Triceps	Lying triceps extension	Set 1	10–15*						
Biceps	Seated concentration curl	Set 1	10–15*						
Calves	Seated calf raise	Set 1	12–15						

* Each arm   † Optional set

INTERMEDIATE LEVEL

This program is called a split routine, meaning you divide your muscle groups and work them on separate days. Workout A hits your chest and upper back, Workout B targets your midsection and lower-body muscles, and Workout C goes after your shoulders and arms.

We recommend that you do each workout once a week for 4 weeks. After 4 weeks, make some adjustments to your routine: change exercises, decrease the number of repetitions while increasing weights, etcetera. Or try the advanced workout for 4 weeks.

INTERMEDIATE DUMBBELL WORKOUT A: CHEST AND UPPER BACK

MUSCLES	EXERCISE	Sets	Target Reps	WEEK 1 Weight	Reps	WEEK 2 Weight	Reps	WEEK 3 Weight	Reps	WEEK 4 Weight	Reps
Chest, shoulders, triceps	Incline bench press	Set 1	6–10								
		Set 2	6–10								
		Set 3*	6–10								
Upper back	Pronated bent-over row	Set 1	6–10								
		Set 2	6–10								
		Set 3*	6–10								
Chest, shoulders, triceps	Piston-style bench press	Set 1	6–10								
		Set 2*	6–10								
Upper back	Piston-style bent-over row	Set 1	6–10								
		Set 2*	6–10								
Chest	Swiss-ball fly	Set 1	6–10								
		Set 2*	6–10								
Upper back	Pullup or EZ-bar pullover†	Set 1	6–10								
		Set 2	6–10								
		Set 3*	6–10								
		Set 4*	6–10								
Rear shoulders, rotator cuffs	Supinated seated reverse fly	Set 1	6–10								
		Set 2*	6–10								

* Optional set † You can use the pullover as a warmup exercise for pullups

INTERMEDIATE DUMBBELL WORKOUT B: MIDSECTION AND LOWER BODY

MUSCLES	EXERCISE	Sets	Target Reps	WEEK 1 Weight	WEEK 1 Reps	WEEK 2 Weight	WEEK 2 Reps	WEEK 3 Weight	WEEK 3 Reps	WEEK 4 Weight	WEEK 4 Reps
Rectus abdominis	Weighted crunch	Set 1	8–12								
		Set 2	8–12								
		Set 3*	8–12								
Obliques	Reverse woodchopper	Set 1	8–12†								
		Set 2	8–12†								
		Set 3*	8–12†								
Lower body (knee-dominant)	Lunge	Set 1	8–12†								
		Set 2	8–12†								
		Set 3*	8–12†								
Lower body (knee dominant)	Front squat	Set 1	8–12								
		Set 2	8–12								
		Set 3*	8–12								
Hamstrings	Decline leg curl	Set 1	8–12								
		Set 2	8–12								
		Set 3*	8–12								
Lower back, gluteals, hamstrings	Romanian deadlift	Set 1	8–12								
		Set 2	8–12								
		Set 3*	8–12								
Lower back, gluteals, hamstrings	Back extension	Set 1	8–12								
		Set 2	8–12								
		Set 3*	8–12								
Calves	Unilateral standing calf raise	Set 1	8–12†								
		Set 2*	8–12†								
Calves	Seated calf raise	Set 1	8–12†								
		Set 2*	8–12†								

* Optional set   † Each side

INTERMEDIATE DUMBBELL WORKOUT C: SHOULDERS AND ARMS

MUSCLES	EXERCISE	Sets	Target Reps	WEEK 1 Weight	Reps	WEEK 2 Weight	Reps	WEEK 3 Weight	Reps	WEEK 4 Weight	Reps
Shoulders, triceps	Rotation press	Set 1	6–10								
		Set 2	6–10								
		Set 3*	6–10								
Shoulders, traps	Alternating upright row	Set 1	6–10								
		Set 2	6–10								
		Set 3*	6–10								
External rotators	Standing scarecrow	Set 1	6–10								
		Set 2*	6–10								
Chest, shoulders, triceps	Close-grip bench press	Set 1	6–10								
		Set 2*	6–10								
Triceps	Overhead triceps extension	Set 1	6–10								
		Set 2*	6–10								
Biceps	Incline curl	Set 1	6–10								
		Set 2	6–10								
		Set 3*	6–10								
		Set 4*	6–10								
Biceps	Piston-style hammer curl	Set 1	6–10								
		Set 2*	6–10								

* Optional set

ADVANCED LEVEL

This workout is an interesting continuation of the intermediate routine. You can begin with it if you think you're ready, but we recommend you use the intermediate routine as a sort of running start to this program. The big switch is that you'll hit most muscle groups in each workout, instead of targeting them in separate workouts.

ADVANCED DUMBBELL WORKOUT A

MUSCLES	EXERCISE	Sets	Target Reps	WEEK 1		WEEK 2		WEEK 3		WEEK 4	
				Weight	Reps	Weight	Reps	Weight	Reps	Weight	Reps
Lower body (hip-dominant), upper back	Power clean	Set 1	3–5								
		Set 2	3–5								
		Set 3	3–5								
		Set 4	3–5								
		Set 5	3–5								
Shoulders	Standing piston-style shoulder press	Set 1	6–10								
		Set 2	6–10								
		Set 3*	6–10								
Upper back	One-leg bent-over row	Set 1	6–10								
		Set 2	6–10								
		Set 3*	6–10								
Lower body (knee-dominant)	45-degree traveling lunge	Set 1	6–10								
		Set 2	6–10								
		Set 3*	6–10								
Abdominals	Swiss-ball Russian twist	Set 1	6–10								
		Set 2*	6–10								

* Optional set

ADVANCED DUMBBELL WORKOUT B

MUSCLES	EXERCISE	Sets	Target Reps	WEEK 1		WEEK 2		WEEK 3		WEEK 4	
				Weight	Reps	Weight	Reps	Weight	Reps	Weight	Reps
Chest, upper back	T pushup	Set 1	4–6*								
		Set 2	4–6*								
		Set 3	4–6*								
		Set 4	4–6*								
		Set 5	4–6*								
Lower body (knee-dominant)	Unilateral squat	Set 1	6–12*								
		Set 2	6–12*								
		Set 3†	6–12*								
Chest, triceps	Alternating bench press	Set 1	6–10*								
		Set 2	6–10*								
		Set 3†	6–10*								
Lower body (hip dominant)	Good morning	Set 1	8–12								
		Set 2†	8–12								
Abdominals	Long-arm weighted crunch	Set 1	8–12								
		Set 2†	8–12								
Biceps	Incline Zottman curl	Set 1	6–10								
		Set 2†	6–10								
Biceps	45-degree prone curl	Set 1	6–10								
		Set 2†	6–10								

* Each side   † Optional set

ADVANCED DUMBBELL WORKOUT C

MUSCLES	EXERCISE	Sets	Target Reps	WEEK 1		WEEK 2		WEEK 3		WEEK 4	
				Weight	Reps	Weight	Reps	Weight	Reps	Weight	Reps
Upper back, shoulders	Hang clean	Set 1	4–6								
		Set 2	4–6								
		Set 3	4–6								
		Set 4	4–6								
Upper back, chest	Alternating pullover	Set 1	6–10*								
		Set 2†	6–10*								
Upper traps	Overhead shrug	Set 1	4–6								
		Set 2†	4–6								
External rotators	Prone scarecrow	Set 1	6–10								
		Set 2†	6–10								
Chest	Swiss-ball fly	Set 1	6–10								
		Set 2†	6–10								
Triceps	Unilateral overhead extension with lean	Set 1	6–10*								
		Set 2†	6–10*								
Triceps	Bilateral kickback	Set 1	6–10								
		Set 2†	6–10*								
Calves	Explosive calf jump	Set 1	10–15								
		Set 2	10–15								
		Set 3†	10–15								

* Each side   † Optional set

4-WEEK BARBELL WORKOUT

EQUIPMENT REQUIRED

- Barbell
- EZ-curl bar
- Bench with uprights for bench presses and squats, or power rack
- Chinning bar

STRENGTHS

- For increasing your overall strength and power, nothing beats the barbell.
- Ask any trainer or strength coach the two best exercises for overall muscle mass, and chances are he'll say, "Squat and deadlift." No other apparatuses—dumbbells, cables, or machine—will ever come close to matching the muscle-building effects of these two barbell exercises.

WEAKNESSES

- Barbells can be very tough on joints. Strain on elbow and wrist joints can be alleviated by using curl bars. And strain on knee joints during squats and lunges can be eliminated with good form. But if barbell exercises hurt your shoulder joints, there isn't much relief, other than switching to dumbbells.
- You can have strength imbalances—one arm or leg stronger than the other—and not know it if you work with nothing but barbells. Research has shown that this problem takes care of itself over time, but for beginners, these strength imbalances can make barbell exercise awkward.

BEGINNER LEVEL

Perform this workout two or three times a week. Each workout, try to increase either the number of repetitions or the amount of resistance. When you can do all the suggested repetitions of an exercise with good form, increase the weight.

You'll note that the workout gives you a choice of doing either 1 or 2 sets of most exercises. However, that doesn't mean you *should* do 2 sets, especially if you're an absolute beginner. Research shows beginners get about the same results with 1 set as they do with multiple sets. We suggest sticking to 1 set until you learn the exercises and start to see results.

At that point, you'll probably want to challenge yourself with an extra set of some exercises. Even then, however, we don't want to see you doing an extra set of all of the exercises. Just pick a few, and make sure you keep them in balance. If you do 2 sets of bench presses, do 2 sets of reverse pushups.

Focus your multiset efforts on the big-muscle exercises: squats, stepups, presses, rows. The smaller muscles—biceps, triceps, calves—not only get worked during the big-muscle exercises but also grow just as well with 1 set as they would with 2 or 3.

Note that the exercises are performed in a different sequence in alternating weeks. That gives you a different training stimulus—one week you'll do your bench presses when you're fresh, and the next week you'll do them when you're thrashed. The change will keep your muscles guessing, and thus developing faster.

BEGINNER BARBELL WEEK 1

MUSCLES	EXERCISE	Sets	Target Reps	WORKOUT 1		WORKOUT 2		WORKOUT 3	
				Weight	Reps	Weight	Reps	Weight	Reps
Transverse abdominis	Vacuum	Set 1	6–10*						
Lower abs	Reverse crunch	Set 1	10–15						
Upper abs	Crunch	Set 1	10–15						
Obliques	Oblique crunch	Set 1	10–15						
Lower back	Prone Superman	Set 1	10–15						
Chest, front shoulders, triceps	Bench press	Set 1	8–10						
		Set 2†	8–10						
Upper back	Reverse pushup	Set 1	8–10						
		Set 2†	8–10						
Shoulders, triceps	Military press	Set 1	8–10						
		Set 2†	8–10						
Shoulders, traps	Upright row	Set 1	8–10						
		Set 2†	8–10						
Triceps	Lying triceps extension	Set 1	8–10						
Biceps	Standing curl	Set 1	8–10						
Lower body (hip-dominant)	Stepup	Set 1	10–12						
		Set 2†	10–12						
Lower body (knee-dominant)	Split squat‡	Set 1	10–12						
		Set 2†	10–12						
Calves	Seated calf raise	Set 1	10–12						

* Hold for 20–30 seconds per repetition   † Optional set   ‡ Start with the body-weight version, and when you can do 12 reps with each leg, add resistance. First, add just the bar, then when you can do 12 reps with each leg, add weight plates

BEGINNER BARBELL WEEK 2

MUSCLES	EXERCISE	Sets	Target Reps	WORKOUT 1		WORKOUT 2		WORKOUT 3	
				Weight	Reps	Weight	Reps	Weight	Reps
Transverse abdominis	Vacuum	Set 1	6–10*						
Lower abs	Reverse crunch	Set 1	10–15						
Upper abs	Crunch	Set 1	10–15						
Obliques	Oblique crunch	Set 1	10–15						
Lower back	Prone Superman	Set 1	10–15						
Lower body (knee-dominant)	Split squat†	Set 1	10–12						
		Set 2‡	10–12						
Lower body (hip-dominant)	Stepup	Set 1	10–12						
		Set 2‡	10–12						
Shoulders, traps	Upright row	Set 1	8–10						
		Set 2‡	8–10						
Shoulders, triceps	Military press	Set 1	8–10						
		Set 2‡	8–10						
Chest, front shoulders, triceps	Bench press	Set 1	8–10						
		Set 2‡	8–10						
Upper back	Reverse pushup	Set 1	8–10						
		Set 2‡	8–10						
Triceps	Lying triceps extension	Set 1	8–10						
Biceps	Standing curl	Set 1	8–10						
Calves	Seated calf raise	Set 1	10–12						

* Hold for 20–30 seconds per repetition   † Start with the body-weight version, and when you can do 12 reps with each leg, add resistance. First, add just the bar, then when you can do 12 reps with each leg, add weight plates   ‡ Optional set

BEGINNER BARBELL WEEK 3

MUSCLES	EXERCISE	Sets	Target Reps	WORKOUT 1		WORKOUT 2		WORKOUT 3	
				Weight	Reps	Weight	Reps	Weight	Reps
Transverse abdominis	Vacuum	Set 1	6–10*						
Lower abs	Reverse crunch	Set 1	10–15						
Upper abs	Crunch	Set 1	10–15						
Obliques	Oblique crunch	Set 1	10–15						
Lower back	Prone Superman	Set 1	10–15						
Chest, front shoulders, triceps	Bench press	Set 1	8–10						
		Set 2†	8–10						
Upper back	Reverse pushup	Set 1	8–10						
		Set 2†	8–10						
Shoulders, triceps	Military press	Set 1	8–10						
		Set 2†	8–10						
Shoulders, traps	Upright row	Set 1	8–10						
		Set 2†	8–10						
Triceps	Lying triceps extension	Set 1	8–10						
Biceps	Standing curl	Set 1	8–10						
Lower body (hip-dominant)	Stepup	Set 1	10–12						
		Set 2†	10–12						
Lower body (knee-dominant)	Split squat‡	Set 1	10–12						
		Set 2†	10–12						
Calves	Seated calf raise	Set 1	10–12						

* Hold for 20–30 seconds per repetition   † Optional set   ‡ Start with the body-weight version, and when you can do 12 reps with each leg, add resistance. First, add just the bar, then when you can do 12 reps with each leg, add weight plates

BEGINNER BARBELL WEEK 4

MUSCLES	EXERCISE	Sets	Target Reps	WORKOUT 1 Weight	Reps	WORKOUT 2 Weight	Reps	WORKOUT 3 Weight	Reps
Transverse abdominis	Vacuum	Set 1	6–10*						
Lower abs	Reverse crunch	Set 1	10–15						
Upper abs	Crunch	Set 1	10–15						
Obliques	Oblique crunch	Set 1	10–15						
Lower back	Prone Superman	Set 1	10–15						
Lower body (hip-dominant)	Split squat†	Set 1	10–12						
		Set 2‡	10–12						
Lower body (hip-dominant)	Stepup	Set 1	10–12						
		Set 2‡	10–12						
Shoulders, traps	Upright row	Set 1	8–10						
		Set 2‡	8–10						
Shoulders, triceps	Military press	Set 1	8–10						
		Set 2‡	8–10						
Chest, front shoulders, triceps	Bench press	Set 1	8–10						
		Set 2‡	8–10						
Upper back	Reverse pushup	Set 1	8–10						
		Set 2‡	8–10						
Triceps	Lying triceps extension	Set 1	8–10						
Biceps	Standing curl	Set 1	8–10						
Calves	Seated calf raise	Set 1	10–12						

* Hold for 20–30 seconds per repetition   † Start with the body-weight version, and when you can do 12 reps with each leg, add resistance. First, add just the bar, then when you can do 12 reps with each leg, add weight plates   ‡ Optional set

INTERMEDIATE LEVEL

This is called a split routine, meaning you divide your muscle groups and work them on separate days. In this case, you'll do three different workouts. Workout A hits chest and upper back. Workout B goes after midsection and lower-body muscles. And Workout C focuses on shoulders, traps, and arms.

We recommend that you limit yourself to three workouts a week. Barbell exercises are tougher on your joints than body-weight, dumbbell, or cable exercises, and,

in our experience, you need more time to recover from them.

These workouts give you a wide range of sets and repetitions. We recommend you do 2 warmup sets and 2 work sets of each exercise. Use perhaps one-third of your work-set weight on the first warmup set, and two-thirds on the second warmup. You can also use a little more weight on the second work set than you used on the first.

INTERMEDIATE BARBELL WORKOUT A: CHEST AND UPPER BACK

MUSCLES	EXERCISE	Sets	Target Reps	WEEK 1		WEEK 2		WEEK 3		WEEK 4	
				Weight	Reps	Weight	Reps	Weight	Reps	Weight	Reps
Chest, shoulders, triceps	Incline bench press	Set 1	6–10								
		Set 2	6–10								
		Set 3*	6–10								
		Set 4*	6–10								
Upper back, biceps	Supinated bent-over row	Set 1	6–10								
		Set 2	6–10								
		Set 3*	6–10								
		Set 4*	6–10								
Chest, shoulders, triceps	Close-grip bench press	Set 1	6–10								
		Set 2	6–10								
		Set 3*	6–10								
		Set 4*	6–10								
Upper back	Pullup or EZ-bar pullover†	Set 1	6–10								
		Set 2	6–10								
		Set 3*	6–10								
		Set 4*	6–10								

* Optional set   † You can use the pullover as a warmup exercise for pullups

INTERMEDIATE BARBELL WORKOUT B: MIDSECTION AND LOWER BODY

MUSCLES	EXERCISE	Sets	Target Reps	WEEK 1 Weight	Reps	WEEK 2 Weight	Reps	WEEK 3 Weight	Reps	WEEK 4 Weight	Reps
Abdominals	Barbell rollout	Set 1	8–12								
		Set 2*	8–12								
Obliques	Full-contact twist	Set 1	8–12†								
		Set 2*	8–12†								
Lower body (knee-dominant)	Back squat	Set 1	8–10								
		Set 2	8–10								
		Set 3*	8–10								
		Set 4*	8–10								
Lower body (hip-dominant)	Deadlift	Set 1	8–10								
		Set 2	8–10								
		Set 3*	8–10								
		Set 4*	8–10								
Lower-body (knee-dominant)	Lunge	Set 1	8–10								
		Set 2	8–10								
		Set 3*	8–10								
		Set 4*	8–10								
Lower body (hip-dominant)	Romanian deadlift	Set 1	8–10								
		Set 2	8–10								
		Set 3*	8–10								
		Set 4*	8–10								

* Optional set † Each side

INTERMEDIATE BARBELL WORKOUT C: SHOULDERS, TRAPS, AND ARMS

MUSCLES	EXERCISE	Sets	Target Reps	WEEK 1 Weight	Reps	WEEK 2 Weight	Reps	WEEK 3 Weight	Reps	WEEK 4 Weight	Reps
Traps, shoulders, arms	Hang clean	Set 1	4–6								
		Set 2	4–6								
		Set 3*	4–6								
Shoulders, traps, triceps	Behind-the-neck press	Set 1	6–10								
		Set 2	6–10								
		Set 3*	6–10								
Triceps	French press	Set 1	6–10								
		Set 2	6–10								
Biceps	Reverse curl	Set 1	6–10								
		Set 2	6–10								

* Optional set

ADVANCED LEVEL

This workout not only introduces some challenging new exercises but also pulls you back to full-body workouts. You'll work most of your major muscle groups in each of the three workouts. We recommend you do the intermediate routine before attempting this program, even if you're already an advanced lifter.

ADVANCED BARBELL WORKOUT A

MUSCLES	EXERCISE	Sets	Target Reps	WEEK 1 Weight	Reps	WEEK 2 Weight	Reps	WEEK 3 Weight	Reps	WEEK 4 Weight	Reps
Lower body (hip-dominant), upper back	Power clean	Set 1	3–5								
		Set 2	3–5								
		Set 3	3–5								
		Set 4	3–5								
		Set 5	3–5								
Shoulders, triceps	Push press	Set 1	3–5								
		Set 2	3–5								
		Set 3*	3–5								
Lower body (knee-dominant)	Front squat	Set 1	4–6								
		Set 2	4–6								
		Set 3*	4–6								
Lower body (hip-dominant)	Deadlift	Set 1	2–4†								
		Set 2	2–4†								
		Set 3	2–4†								
		Set 4	2–4†								
		Set 5	2–4†								
		Set 6	2–4†								
		Set 7*	2–4†								
		Set 8*	2–4†								
Abdominals	Situp	Set 1	5–10								
		Set 2	5–10								
		Set 3	5–10								

* Optional set   † Upon completion of each rep, set the weight on the floor, regrip the bar, and reset your body for the lift; in other words, each set is really a collection of 3 to 5 single deadlifts, rather than steady-speed repetitions. This allows you to use a heavier weight and still focus on form on each rep

ADVANCED BARBELL WORKOUT B

MUSCLES	EXERCISE	Sets	Target Reps	WEEK 1		WEEK 2		WEEK 3		WEEK 4	
				Weight	Reps	Weight	Reps	Weight	Reps	Weight	Reps
Lower body (knee-dominant)	Back squat	Set 1	5								
		Set 2	5								
		Set 3	5								
		Set 4	5								
		Set 5	5								
Chest, shoulders, triceps	Bench press	Set 1	3*								
		Set 2	3*								
		Set 3	3*								
		Set 4	3*								
		Set 5	3*								
Upper back, biceps	T-bar row	Set 1	6–8								
		Set 2	6–8								
		Set 3	6–8								
Shoulders, external rotators	Cuban press	Set 1	4–6								
		Set 2†	4–6								
Lower body (hip-dominant)	Good morning	Set 1	8–10								
		Set 2	8–10								
		Set 3†	8–10								
Obliques	Oblique V-up	Set 1	8–10‡								
		Set 2	8–10‡								
		Set 3†	8–10‡								

* Rack the weight after each rep, sit up, take a deep breath, and then completely reset your body and grip for the next rep; in other words, a "set" consists of 3 single reps, allowing you to use a heavier weight and focus on form each rep   † Optional set   ‡ Each side

ADVANCED BARBELL WORKOUT C

MUSCLES	EXERCISE	Sets	Target Reps	WEEK 1 Weight	WEEK 1 Reps	WEEK 2 Weight	WEEK 2 Reps	WEEK 3 Weight	WEEK 3 Reps	WEEK 4 Weight	WEEK 4 Reps
Lower body (hip-dominant), upper back	Muscle snatch	Set 1	2–4*								
		Set 2	2–4*								
		Set 3	2–4*								
Upper back, chest, triceps	Pullover	Set 1	5–8								
		Set 2	5–8								
		Set 3†	5–8								
Triceps	Incline lying triceps extension	Set 1	6–8								
		Set 2	6–8								
		Set 3	6–8								
		Set 4†	6–8								
		Set 5†	6–8								
Triceps	Close-grip bench press	Set 1	4–6								
		Set 2	4–6								
		Set 3†	4–6								
Biceps	Prone 45-degree curl	Set 1	6–8								
		Set 2	6–8								
		Set 3†	6–8								
		Set 4†	6–8								
Calves	Standing calf raise	Set 1	6–10								
		Set 2	6–10								
		Set 3†	6–10								

* As with deadlifts in Workout A, set the weight on the floor upon completion of each rep, and reset your body and grip   † Optional set

4-WEEK CABLE WORKOUT

EQUIPMENT REQUIRED

- Cable station
- Variety of attachments: stirrup handle, rope handles, long straight bar (usually used for lat pulldowns), short straight bar (for curls), ankle straps
- Bench
- Swiss ball (for advanced routine only)
- Dumbbell or other weighted object that can be held in one hand (for advanced routine only)

STRENGTHS

- Cable machines are safe and fun—even the most heavy-duty barbell-heads use cables for several exercises, when they have access to them.
- Cables foster great upper-back and shoulder development because they let you maintain tension on these muscles as you raise and lower the weights; they also allow you to hold contracted positions longer than you're able to with free weights.
- You can do unusual and effective abdominal exercises.

WEAKNESSES

- You won't develop much pure strength and power.
- It's very tough to give your chest and lower-body muscles a good muscle-building stimulus with cables alone.
- Cable arm exercises are good complements to dumbbell and barbell exercises, but you probably won't see great arm-muscle development with cable exercises alone.

BEGINNER LEVEL

Perform this workout two or three times a week. Each workout, try to increase either the number of repetitions or the amount of resistance. When you can do all the suggested repetitions of an exercise, refer to chapter 14 for ways to make the exercise more challenging.

BEGINNER CABLE WEEK 1

MUSCLES	EXERCISE	Sets	Target Reps	WORKOUT 1		WORKOUT 2		WORKOUT 3	
				Weight	Reps	Weight	Reps	Weight	Reps
Transverse abdominis	Vacuum	Set 1	6–10*						
Lower abs	Reverse crunch	Set 1	10–15						
Upper abs	Crunch	Set 1	10–15						
Obliques	Oblique crunch	Set 1	10–15						
Lower back	Prone Superman	Set 1	10–15						
Chest	Unilateral high-cable fly	Set 1	10–12						
		Set 2†	10–12						
Chest, front shoulders, triceps	Pushup	Set 1	10–12						
		Set 2†	10–12						
Upper back	Lat pulldown	Set 1	10–12						
		Set 2†	10–12						
Upper back	Supinated row	Set 1	10–12						
		Set 2†	10–12						
Shoulders, traps	Upright row	Set 1	10–15						
		Set 2†	10–15						
Shoulders	Lateral raise	Set 1	10–15‡						
Shoulders	External rotation	Set 1	10–15‡						
Biceps	Standing curl	Set 1	10–15‡						
Triceps	Pushdown	Set 1	10–15						
Lower-body (knee-dominant)	Split squat	Set 1	12–15						
		Set 2†	12–15						
Hamstrings	Lying leg curl	Set 1	12–15						
		Set 2†	12–15						
Lower-body (hip-dominant)	Standing hip extension	Set 1	12–15‡						

* Hold for 20–30 seconds per repetition   † Optional set   ‡ Each side

BEGINNER CABLE WEEK 2

MUSCLES	EXERCISE	Sets	Target Reps	WORKOUT 1		WORKOUT 2		WORKOUT 3	
				Weight	Reps	Weight	Reps	Weight	Reps
Transverse abdominis	Vacuum	Set 1	6–10*						
Lower abs	Reverse crunch	Set 1	10–15						
Upper abs	Crunch	Set 1	10–15						
Obliques	Oblique crunch	Set 1	10–15						
Lower back	Prone Superman	Set 1	10–15						
Chest	Unilateral high-cable fly	Set 1	10–12						
		Set 2†	10–12						
Chest, front shoulders, triceps	Pushup	Set 1	10–12						
		Set 2†	10–12						
Upper back	Lat pulldown	Set 1	10–12						
		Set 2†	10–12						
Upper back	Supinated row	Set 1	10–12						
		Set 2†	10–12						
Shoulders, traps	Upright row	Set 1	10–15						
		Set 2†	10–15						
Shoulders	Lateral raise	Set 1	10–15‡						
Shoulders	External rotation	Set 1	10–15‡						
Biceps	Standing curl	Set 1	10–15‡						
Triceps	Pushdown	Set 1	10–15						
Lower-body (knee-dominant)	Split squat	Set 1	12–15						
		Set 2†	12–15						
Hamstrings	Lying leg curl	Set 1	12–15						
		Set 2†	12–15						
Lower-body (hip-dominant)	Standing hip extension	Set 1	12–15‡						

* Hold for 20–30 seconds per repetition   † Optional set   ‡ Each side

BEGINNER CABLE WEEK 3

MUSCLES	EXERCISE	Sets	Target Reps	WORKOUT 1		WORKOUT 2		WORKOUT 3	
				Weight	Reps	Weight	Reps	Weight	Reps
Transverse abdominis	Vacuum	Set 1	6–10*						
Lower abs	Reverse crunch	Set 1	10–15						
Upper abs	Crunch	Set 1	10–15						
Obliques	Oblique crunch	Set 1	10–15						
Lower back	Prone Superman	Set 1	10–15						
Chest	Unilateral high-cable fly	Set 1	10–12						
		Set 2†	10–12						
Chest, front shoulders, triceps	Pushup	Set 1	10–12						
		Set 2†	10–12						
Upper back	Lat pulldown	Set 1	10–12						
		Set 2†	10–12						
Upper back	Supinated row	Set 1	10–12						
		Set 2†	10–12						
Shoulders, traps	Upright row	Set 1	10–15						
		Set 2†	10–15						
Shoulders	Lateral raise	Set 1	10–15‡						
Shoulders	External rotation	Set 1	10–15‡						
Biceps	Standing curl	Set 1	10–15‡						
Triceps	Pushdown	Set 1	10–15						
Lower-body (knee-dominant)	Split squat	Set 1	12–15						
		Set 2†	12–15						
Hamstrings	Lying leg curl	Set 1	12–15						
		Set 2†	12–15						
Lower-body (hip-dominant)	Standing hip extension	Set 1	12–15‡						

* Hold for 20–30 seconds per repetition   † Optional set   ‡ Each side

BEGINNER CABLE WEEK 4

MUSCLES	EXERCISE	Sets	Target Reps	WORKOUT 1 Weight	WORKOUT 1 Reps	WORKOUT 2 Weight	WORKOUT 2 Reps	WORKOUT 3 Weight	WORKOUT 3 Reps
Transverse abdominis	Vacuum	Set 1	6–10*						
Lower abs	Reverse crunch	Set 1	10–15						
Upper abs	Crunch	Set 1	10–15						
Obliques	Oblique crunch	Set 1	10–15						
Lower back	Prone Superman	Set 1	10–15						
Chest	Unilateral high-cable fly	Set 1	10–12						
		Set 2†	10–12						
Chest, front shoulders, triceps	Pushup	Set 1	10–12						
		Set 2†	10–12						
Upper back	Lat pulldown	Set 1	10–12						
		Set 2†	10–12						
Upper back	Supinated row	Set 1	10–12						
		Set 2†	10–12						
Shoulders, traps	Upright row	Set 1	10–15						
		Set 2†	10–15						
Shoulders	Lateral raise	Set 1	10–15‡						
Shoulders	External rotation	Set 1	10–15‡						
Biceps	Standing curl	Set 1	10–15‡						
Triceps	Pushdown	Set 1	10–15						
Lower-body (knee-dominant)	Split squat	Set 1	12–15						
		Set 2†	12–15						
Hamstrings	Lying leg curl	Set 1	12–15						
Lower-body (hip-dominant)	Standing hip extension	Set 1	12–15‡						

* Hold for 20–30 seconds per repetition † Optional set ‡ Each side

INTERMEDIATE LEVEL

This is called a split routine, meaning you divide your muscle groups in half and work them on separate days. Workout A hits chest and back. Workout B goes after abdominal and lower-body muscles. Workout C focuses on shoulders and arms. You'll note that these workouts contain body-weight exercises to make up for the lack of effective cable exercises for certain muscle groups.

We recommend that you do each workout once a week for 4 weeks.

INTERMEDIATE CABLE WORKOUT A: CHEST AND BACK

MUSCLES	EXERCISE	Sets	Target Reps	WEEK 1			WEEK 2			WEEK 3			WEEK 4		
				Weight	Reps		Weight	Reps		Weight	Reps		Weight	Reps	
Upper chest, shoulders, triceps	Pushup with elevated feet	Set 1	8–10												
		Set 2	8–10												
		Set 3*	8–10												
Lower chest	Unilateral low-cable fly	Set 1	8–10†												
		Set 2	8–10†												
		Set 3*	8–10†												
Upper back	Wide-grip lat pulldown	Set 1	8–10												
		Set 2	8–10												
		Set 3*	8–10												
Upper back	Bent-over row	Set 1	8–10												
		Set 2	8–10												
		Set 3*	8–10												
Rear shoulders	Unilateral bent-over rear lateral raise	Set 1	8–10†												
		Set 2	8–10†												
		Set 3*	8–10†												

* Optional set   † Each side

INTERMEDIATE CABLE WORKOUT B: ABDOMINALS AND LOWER BODY

MUSCLES	EXERCISE	Sets	Target Reps	WEEK 1		WEEK 2		WEEK 3		WEEK 4	
				Weight	Reps	Weight	Reps	Weight	Reps	Weight	Reps
Rectus abdominis	Kneeling cable crunch	Set 1	10–12								
		Set 2	10–12								
		Set 3*	10–12								
Obliques	Standing oblique crunch	Set 1	10–12†								
		Set 2	10–12†								
		Set 3*	10–12†								
Lower body (knee-dominant)	Bulgarian split squat (body weight only)	Set 1	10–12†								
		Set 2	10–12†								
		Set 3*	10–12†								
Lower body (knee-dominant)	Lunge	Set 1	10–12†								
		Set 2	10–12†								
		Set 3*	10–12†								
Lower body (hip-dominant)	Reverse lunge	Set 1	10–12†								
		Set 2	10–12†								
		Set 3*	10–12†								
Inner thighs	Standing adduction	Set 1	10–12†								
Outer thighs	Standing abduction	Set 1	10–12†								
Calves	Standing unilateral calf raise	Set 1	10–12†								
		Set 2	10–12†								
		Set 3*	10–12†								
Calves	Seated calf raise	Set 1	10–12								
		Set 2	10–12								
		Set 3*	10–12								

* Optional set   † Each side

INTERMEDIATE CABLE WORKOUT C: SHOULDERS AND ARMS

MUSCLES	EXERCISE	Sets	Target Reps	WEEK 1 Weight	WEEK 1 Reps	WEEK 2 Weight	WEEK 2 Reps	WEEK 3 Weight	WEEK 3 Reps	WEEK 4 Weight	WEEK 4 Reps
Shoulders, traps	Upright row	Set 1	8–10								
		Set 2	8–10								
		Set 3*	8–10								
Shoulders	Lean-away lateral raise	Set 1	8–10†								
		Set 2	8–10†								
		Set 3*	8–10†								
External rotators	Standing external rotation	Set 1	8–10								
		Set 2	8–10								
		Set 3*	8–10								
Triceps	Lying triceps extension	Set 1	8–10								
		Set 2	8–10								
		Set 3*	8–10								
Triceps	Rope pushdown	Set 1	8–10								
		Set 2	8–10								
		Set 3*	8–10								
Biceps	Reverse-grip standing curl	Set 1	8–10								
		Set 2	8–10								
		Set 3*	8–10								
Biceps	Lying curl	Set 1	8–10								
		Set 2	8–10								
		Set 3*	8–10								

* Optional set   † Each side.

ADVANCED LEVEL

This workout not only introduces some challenging new exercises but also pulls you back to full-body workouts. You'll work most of your major muscle groups in each of the three workouts. We recommend you do the intermediate routine before attempting this program, even if you're already an advanced lifter.

ADVANCED CABLE WORKOUT A

MUSCLES	EXERCISE	Sets	Target Reps	WEEK 1 Weight	WEEK 1 Reps	WEEK 2 Weight	WEEK 2 Reps	WEEK 3 Weight	WEEK 3 Reps	WEEK 4 Weight	WEEK 4 Reps
Upper back	Behind-neck lat pulldown	Set 1	6–10								
		Set 2	6–10								
		Set 3	6–10								
		Set 4	6–10								
		Set 5	6–10								
Upper back, chest, triceps	Pullover	Set 1	6–10								
		Set 2	6–10								
		Set 3*	6–10								
Chest	Unilateral Swiss-ball fly	Set 1	8–10†								
		Set 2	8–10†								
		Set 3*	8–10†								
Triceps	Swiss-ball overhead extension	Set 1	6–10								
		Set 2	6–10								
		Set 3*	6–10								
Triceps	Unilateral crossover pushdown	Set 1	6–10†								
		Set 2	6–10†								
		Set 3*	6–10†								
Lower body (knee-dominant)	Bulgarian split squat	Set 1	8–10†								
		Set 2	8–10†								
		Set 3*	8–10†								
Hamstrings	Lying leg curl	Set 1	8–10								
		Set 2	8–10								
		Set 3*	8–10								

* Optional set   †Each side

ADVANCED CABLE WORKOUT B

MUSCLES	EXERCISE	Sets	Target Reps	WEEK 1		WEEK 2		WEEK 3		WEEK 4	
				Weight	Reps	Weight	Reps	Weight	Reps	Weight	Reps
Lower body (hip-dominant)	Pull-through	Set 1	8–10								
		Set 2	8–10								
		Set 3	8–10								
		Set 4	8–10								
		Set 5	8–10								
Shoulders, triceps	Unilateral seated shoulder press	Set 1	6–10†								
		Set 2	6–10†								
		Set 3*	6–10†								
Lower body (knee-dominant)	Diagonal rotation squat	Set 1	8–10†								
		Set 2	8–10†								
		Set 3*	8–10†								
Front shoulders, lower traps	Front raise	Set 1	6–10								
		Set 2	6–10								
		Set 3*	6–10								
Rear shoulders, external rotators	Standing sideways external rotation	Set 1	6–10†								
		Set 2	6–10†								
		Set 3*	6–10†								
Obliques, lower back	Low woodchopper	Set 1	8–10†								
		Set 2	8–10†								
		Set 3*	8–10†								

* Optional set   † Each side

ADVANCED CABLE WORKOUT C

MUSCLES	EXERCISE	Sets	Target Reps	WEEK 1		WEEK 2		WEEK 3		WEEK 4	
				Weight	Reps	Weight	Reps	Weight	Reps	Weight	Reps
Upper back	Seated wide-grip pronated row	Set 1	6–10								
		Set 2	6–10								
		Set 3	6–10								
		Set 4	6–10								
		Set 5	6–10								
Upper back, rear shoulders	Seated row to neck	Set 1	6–10								
		Set 2	6–10								
		Set 3*	6–10								
Upper back, chest	Incline lying pullover	Set 1	6–10								
		Set 2	6–10								
		Set 3*	6–10								
Biceps	Swiss-ball preacher curl	Set 1	6–10								
		Set 2	6–10								
		Set 3*	6–10								
Biceps	Unilateral crucifix curl	Set 1	6–10†								
		Set 2	6–10†								
		Set 3*	6–10†								
Abdominals	Kneeling three-way cable crunch	Set 1	4–6‡								
		Set 2	4–6‡								
		Set 3*	4–6‡								

* Optional set   † Each side   ‡ Each direction (center, to left, to right)

4-WEEK MULTISTATION-GYM WORKOUT

EQUIPMENT REQUIRED

- Multistation home gym that includes: stirrup handle, rope handles, long straight bar (for lat pulldowns), short straight bar (for curls), ankle straps. Your home machine must allow you to do leg extensions and leg curls; leg presses; dips; chest presses and flies; weighted ab crunches; and shoulder presses, in addition to all the cable exercises in chapter 10.
- This workout also requires an exercise bench and/or a Swiss ball.
- The advanced workout requires a belt from which to hang weights for weighted dips.

STRENGTHS

- It's absolutely the most beginner-friendly of all home-exercise options.
- It's as safe as exercise can get—and fun, too.
- Options like chest presses, flies, and dips mean very good chest and triceps development.
- The cable station offers great upper-back and shoulder options, letting you maintain tension on these muscles and hold positions longer than with free weights.

WEAKNESSES

- Your strength development is limited by the size of the weight stack.
- Even with the leg-press attachment, it's hard for intermediate and advanced exercisers to get good lower-body development.
- You can do a lot of biceps exercises with the cables, but you'll probably find it's hard to develop really good biceps size and strength without free weights.

BEGINNER LEVEL

Perform this workout two or three times a week. Each workout, try to increase either the number of repetitions or the amount of resistance. When you can do all the suggested repetitions of an exercise, refer to chapter 14 for ways to make the exercise more challenging.

BEGINNER MULTISTATION WEEK I

MUSCLES	EXERCISE	Sets	Target Reps	WORKOUT 1		WORKOUT 2		WORKOUT 3	
				Weight	Reps	Weight	Reps	Weight	Reps
Transverse abdominis	Vacuum	Set 1	6–10*						
Lower abs	Reverse crunch	Set 1	10–15						
Upper abs	Crunch	Set 1	10–15						
Obliques	Oblique crunch	Set 1	10–15						
Lower back	Prone Superman	Set 1	10–15						
Chest, front shoulders, triceps	Chest press	Set 1	10–12						
		Set 2†	10–12						
Chest	Pec-deck fly	Set 1	10–12						
		Set 2†	10–12						
Upper back	Lat pulldown	Set 1	10–12						
		Set 2†	10–12						
Upper back	Supinated row	Set 1	10–12						
		Set 2†	10–12						
Shoulders, triceps	Shoulder press	Set 1	10–12						
		Set 2†	10–12						
Shoulders, traps	Upright row	Set 1	10–15						
Shoulders	External rotation	Set 1	10–15‡						
Biceps	Standing curl	Set 1	10–15						
Triceps	Pushdown	Set 1	10–15						
Lower-body (knee-dominant)	Leg press	Set 1	12–15						
		Set 2†	12–15						
Hamstrings	Leg curl	Set 1	12–15						
		Set 2†	12–15						
Calves	Calf raise on leg-extension apparatus	Set 1	12–15‡						

* Hold for 20–30 seconds per repetition   † Optional set   ‡ Each side

BEGINNER MULTISTATION WEEK 2

MUSCLES	EXERCISE	Sets	Target Reps	WORKOUT 1 Weight	WORKOUT 1 Reps	WORKOUT 2 Weight	WORKOUT 2 Reps	WORKOUT 3 Weight	WORKOUT 3 Reps
Transverse abdominis	Vacuum	Set 1	6–10*						
Lower abs	Reverse crunch	Set 1	10–15						
Upper abs	Crunch	Set 1	10–15						
Obliques	Oblique crunch	Set 1	10–15						
Lower back	Prone Superman	Set 1	10–15						
Chest, front shoulders, triceps	Chest press	Set 1	10–12						
		Set 2†	10–12						
Chest	Pec-deck fly	Set 1	10–12						
		Set 2†	10–12						
Upper back	Lat pulldown	Set 1	10–12						
		Set 2†	10–12						
Upper back	Supinated row	Set 1	10–12						
		Set 2†	10–12						
Shoulders, triceps	Shoulder press	Set 1	10–12						
		Set 2†	10–12						
Shoulders, traps	Upright row	Set 1	10–15						
Shoulders	External rotation	Set 1	10–15‡						
Biceps	Standing curl	Set 1	10–15						
Triceps	Pushdown	Set 1	10–15						
Lower-body (knee-dominant)	Leg press	Set 1	12–15						
		Set 2†	12–15						
Hamstrings	Leg curl	Set 1	12–15						
		Set 2†	12–15						
Calves	Calf raise on leg-press apparatus	Set 1	12–15‡						

* Hold for 20–30 seconds per repetition   † Optional set   ‡ Each side

BEGINNER MULTISTATION WEEK 3

MUSCLES	EXERCISE	Sets	Target Reps	WORKOUT 1		WORKOUT 2		WORKOUT 3	
				Weight	Reps	Weight	Reps	Weight	Reps
Transverse abdominis	Vacuum	Set 1	6–10*						
Lower abs	Reverse crunch	Set 1	10–15						
Upper abs	Crunch	Set 1	10–15						
Obliques	Oblique crunch	Set 1	10–15						
Lower back	Prone Superman	Set 1	10–15						
Chest, front shoulders, triceps	Chest press	Set 1	10–12						
		Set 2†	10–12						
Chest	Pec-deck fly	Set 1	10–12						
		Set 2†	10–12						
Upper back	Lat pulldown	Set 1	10–12						
		Set 2†	10–12						
Upper back	Supinated row	Set 1	10–12						
		Set 2†	10–12						
Shoulders, triceps	Shoulder press	Set 1	10–12						
		Set 2†	10–12						
Shoulders, traps	Upright row	Set 1	10–15						
Shoulders	External rotation	Set 1	10–15‡						
Biceps	Standing curl	Set 1	10–15						
Triceps	Pushdown	Set 1	10–15						
Lower-body (knee-dominant)	Leg press	Set 1	12–15						
		Set 2†	12–15						
Hamstrings	Leg curl	Set 1	12–15						
		Set 2†	12–15						
Calves	Calf raise on leg-press apparatus	Set 1	12–15‡						

* Hold for 20–30 seconds per repetition　† Optional set　‡ Each side

BEGINNER MULTISTATION WEEK 4

MUSCLES	EXERCISE	Sets	Target Reps	WORKOUT 1			WORKOUT 2			WORKOUT 3		
				Weight	Reps		Weight	Reps		Weight	Reps	
Transverse abdominis	Vacuum	Set 1	6–10*									
Lower abs	Reverse crunch	Set 1	10–15									
Upper abs	Crunch	Set 1	10–15									
Obliques	Oblique crunch	Set 1	10–15									
Lower back	Prone Superman	Set 1	10–15									
Chest, front shoulders, triceps	Chest press	Set 1	10–12									
		Set 2†	10–12									
Chest	Pec-deck fly	Set 1	10–12									
		Set 2†	10–12									
Upper back	Lat pulldown	Set 1	10–12									
		Set 2†	10–12									
Upper back	Supinated row	Set 1	10–12									
		Set 2†	10–12									
Shoulders, triceps	Shoulder press	Set 1	10–12									
		Set 2†	10–12									
Shoulders, traps	Upright row	Set 1	10–15									
Shoulders	External rotation	Set 1	10–15‡									
Biceps	Standing curl	Set 1	10–15									
Triceps	Pushdown	Set 1	10–15									
Lower-body (knee-dominant)	Leg press	Set 1	12–15									
		Set 2†	12–15									
Hamstrings	Leg curl	Set 1	12–15									
		Set 2†	12–15									
Calves	Calf raise on leg-press apparatus	Set 1	12–15‡									

* Hold for 20–30 seconds per repetition　　† Optional set　　‡ Each side

INTERMEDIATE LEVEL

This is called a split routine, meaning you divide your muscle groups and work them on separate days. Workout A hits chest and back. Workout B goes after ab-dominal and lower-body muscles. Workout C focuses on shoulders and arms. We recommend that you do each workout once a week for 4 weeks.

INTERMEDIATE MULTISTATION WORKOUT A: CHEST AND BACK

MUSCLES	EXERCISE	Sets	Target Reps	WEEK 1 Weight	Reps	WEEK 2 Weight	Reps	WEEK 3 Weight	Reps	WEEK 4 Weight	Reps
Chest, shoulders, triceps	Dip	Set 1	8–10								
		Set 2	8–10								
		Set 3*	8–10								
Chest	Unilateral pec-deck fly	Set 1	8–10†								
		Set 2	8–10†								
		Set 3*	8–10†								
Upper back	Wide-grip lat pulldown	Set 1	8–10								
		Set 2	8–10								
		Set 3*	8–10								
Upper back	Bent-over supinated row	Set 1	8–10								
		Set 2	8–10								
		Set 3*	8–10								
Rear shoulders	Unilateral bent-over rear lateral raise	Set 1	8–10†								
		Set 2	8–10†								
		Set 3*	8–10†								

* Optional set   † Each side

INTERMEDIATE MULTISTATION WORKOUT B: ABDOMINALS AND LOWER BODY

MUSCLES	EXERCISE	Sets	Target Reps	WEEK 1		WEEK 2		WEEK 3		WEEK 4	
				Weight	Reps	Weight	Reps	Weight	Reps	Weight	Reps
Rectus abdominis	Seated cable crunch	Set 1	10–12								
		Set 2	10–12								
		Set 3*	10–12								
Obliques	Standing oblique crunch	Set 1	10–12†								
		Set 2	10–12†								
		Set 3*	10–12†								
Lower body (knee-dominant)	Toes-out leg press	Set 1	10–12								
		Set 2	10–12								
		Set 3*	10–12								
Hamstrings	Elevated standing leg curl	Set 1	10–12†								
		Set 2	10–12†								
		Set 3*	10–12†								
Lower body (hip-dominant)	Reverse lunge (cable)	Set 1	10–12†								
		Set 2	10–12†								
		Set 3*	10–12†								
Inner thighs	Standing adduction	Set 1	10–12†								
Outer thighs	Standing abduction	Set 1	10–12†								
Calves	Unilateral calf raise on leg-extension apparatus	Set 1	10–12†								
		Set 2	10–12†								
		Set 3*	10–12†								
Calves	Seated calf raise (cable)	Set 1	10–12								
		Set 2	10–12								
		Set 3*	10–12								

* Optional set   † Each side

INTERMEDIATE MULTISTATION WORKOUT C: SHOULDERS AND ARMS

MUSCLES	EXERCISE	Sets	Target Reps	WEEK 1		WEEK 2		WEEK 3		WEEK 4	
				Weight	Reps	Weight	Reps	Weight	Reps	Weight	Reps
Shoulders, traps	Upright row	Set 1	8–10								
		Set 2	8–10								
		Set 3*	8–10								
Shoulders	Lean-away lateral raise	Set 1	8–10†								
		Set 2	8–10†								
		Set 3*	8–10†								
External rotators	Standing external rotation	Set 1	8–10†								
		Set 2	8–10†								
		Set 3*	8–10†								
Triceps	Close-grip bench press	Set 1	8–10								
		Set 2	8–10								
		Set 3*	8–10								
Triceps	Rope pushdown	Set 1	8–10								
		Set 2	8–10								
		Set 3*	8–10								
Biceps	Reverse-grip standing curl	Set 1	8–10								
		Set 2	8–10								
		Set 3*	8–10								
Biceps	Lying curl	Set 1	8–10								
		Set 2	8–10								
		Set 3*	8–10								

* Optional set   † Each side

ADVANCED LEVEL

This workout not only introduces some challenging new exercises but also pulls you back to full-body workouts. You'll work most of your major muscle groups in each of the three workouts. We recommend you do the intermediate routine before attempting this program, even if you're already an advanced lifter.

ADVANCED MULTISTATION WORKOUT A

MUSCLES	EXERCISE	Sets	Target Reps	WEEK 1 Weight	Reps	WEEK 2 Weight	Reps	WEEK 3 Weight	Reps	WEEK 4 Weight	Reps
Upper back	Behind-neck lat pulldown	Set 1	6–10								
		Set 2	6–10								
		Set 3	6–10								
		Set 4	6–10								
		Set 5	6–10								
Upper back, chest, triceps	Pullover	Set 1	6–10								
		Set 2	6–10								
		Set 3*	6–10								
Chest	Unilateral chest press	Set 1	4–6†								
		Set 2	4–6†								
		Set 3*	4–6†								
Triceps	Swiss-ball overhead extension	Set 1	6–10								
		Set 2	6–10								
		Set 3*	6–10								
Triceps	Unilateral crossover pushdown	Set 1	6–10†								
		Set 2	6–10†								
		Set 3*	6–10†								
Lower body (knee-dominant)	Unilateral leg press	Set 1	8–10†								
		Set 2	8–10†								
		Set 3*	8–10†								
Hamstrings	Leg curl	Set 1	8–10								
		Set 2	8–10								
		Set 3*	8–10								

* Optional set   † Each side

ADVANCED MULTISTATION WORKOUT B

MUSCLES	EXERCISE	Sets	Target Reps	WEEK 1		WEEK 2		WEEK 3		WEEK 4	
				Weight	Reps	Weight	Reps	Weight	Reps	Weight	Reps
Lower body (hip-dominant)	Pull-through	Set 1	8–10								
		Set 2	8–10								
		Set 3	8–10								
		Set 4	8–10								
		Set 5	8–10								
Chest	Swiss-ball incline unilateral cable fly	Set 1	6–10†								
		Set 2	6–10†								
		Set 3*	6–10†								
Front shoulders, lower traps	Front raise	Set 1	6–10								
		Set 2	6–10								
		Set 3*	6–10								
Lower body (hip-dominant)	Lower-feet leg press	Set 1	8–10†								
		Set 2	8–10†								
		Set 3*	8–10†								
Rear shoulders, external rotators	Standing sideways external rotation	Set 1	6–10†								
		Set 2	6–10†								
		Set 3*	6–10†								
Obliques, lower back	Low woodchopper	Set 1	8–10†								
		Set 2	8–10†								
		Set 3*	8–10†								

* Optional set   † Each side

ADVANCED MULTISTATION WORKOUT C

MUSCLES	EXERCISE	Sets	Target Reps	WEEK 1 Weight	Reps	WEEK 2 Weight	Reps	WEEK 3 Weight	Reps	WEEK 4 Weight	Reps
Upper back	Seated wide-grip pronated row	Set 1	6–10								
		Set 2	6–10								
		Set 3	6–10								
		Set 4	6–10								
		Set 5	6–10								
Chest, shoulders, triceps	Weighted dip	Set 1	4–6								
		Set 2	4–6								
		Set 3*	4–6								
Upper back, rear shoulders	Seated row to neck	Set 1	6–10								
		Set 2	6–10								
		Set 3*	6–10								
Biceps	Swiss-ball preacher curl	Set 1	6–10								
		Set 2	6–10								
		Set 3*	6–10								
Biceps	Unilateral crucifix curl	Set 1	6–10†								
		Set 2	6–10†								
		Set 3*	6–10†								
Abdominals	Kneeling three-way cable crunch	Set 1	4–6‡								
		Set 2	4–6‡								
		Set 3*	4–6‡								

* Optional set   † Each side   ‡ Each direction (center, to left, to right)

4-WEEK ALL-EQUIPMENT WORKOUT

EQUIPMENT REQUIRED

- Multistation home gym that includes a cable station with the following attachments: stirrup handle, rope handles, long straight bar, short straight bar, ankle straps
- Olympic barbell and EZ-curl bar
- Bench with uprights for bench presses and squats, or power rack
- Dumbbells
- Chinning bar

STRENGTHS

- You have it all—the ideal equipment for every purpose.

WEAKNESSES

- Your friends don't know enough about exercise to be jealous of your setup.

BEGINNER LEVEL

Perform this workout two or three times a week. Each workout, try to increase either the number of repetitions or the amount of resistance. When you can do all the suggested repetitions of an exercise with good form, increase the weight.

You'll note that the workout gives you a choice of doing either 1 or 2 sets of most exercises. However, that doesn't mean you *should* do 2 sets, especially if you're an absolute beginner. Research shows beginners get about the same results with 1 set as they do with multiple sets. We suggest sticking to 1 set until you learn the exercises and start to see results.

At that point, you'll probably want to challenge yourself with an extra set of some exercises. Even then, however, we don't want to see you doing an extra set of all of them. Just pick a few, and make sure you keep them in balance. If you do 2 sets of bench presses, do 2 sets of reverse pushups.

Focus your multiset efforts on the big-muscle exercises: squats, stepups, presses, rows. The smaller muscles—biceps, triceps, calves—not only get worked during the big-muscle exercises but also grow just as well with 1 set as they would with 2 or 3.

Note that the exercises are performed in a different sequence in alternating weeks. That gives you a different training stimulus—one week you'll do your bench presses when you're fresh, and the next week you'll do them when you're thrashed. The change will keep your muscles guessing, and thus developing faster.

BEGINNER ALL-EQUIPMENT WEEK 1				WORKOUT 1		WORKOUT 2		WORKOUT 3	
MUSCLES	EXERCISE	Sets	Target Reps	Weight	Reps	Weight	Reps	Weight	Reps
Transverse abdominis	Vacuum	Set 1	6–10*						
Lower abs	Reverse crunch	Set 1	10–15						
Upper abs	Crunch	Set 1	10–15						
Obliques	Oblique crunch	Set 1	10–15						
Lower back	Prone superman	Set 1	10–15						
Chest, front shoulders, triceps	Chest press (machine)	Set 1	8–10						
		Set 2†	8–10						
Upper back	Lat pulldown	Set 1	8–10						
		Set 2†	8–10						
Shoulders, triceps	Dumbbell shoulder press	Set 1	8–10						
		Set 2†	8–10						
Shoulders, traps	Barbell upright row	Set 1	8–10						
		Set 2†	8–10						
Triceps	Pushdown	Set 1	8–10						
Biceps	Seated concentration curl	Set 1	8–10						
Lower body (hip-dominant)	Stepup‡	Set 1	10–12						
		Set 2†	10–12						
Lower body (knee-dominant)	Split squat‡	Set 1	10–12						
		Set 2†	10–12						
Calves	Seated calf raise (barbell or dumbbells)	Set 1	10–12						

* Hold for 20–30 seconds per repetition   † Optional set   ‡ Start with the body-weight version, and when you can do 12 reps with each leg, add a barbell or dumbbells

BEGINNER ALL-EQUIPMENT WEEK 2

MUSCLES	EXERCISE	Sets	Target Reps	WORKOUT 1 Weight	WORKOUT 1 Reps	WORKOUT 2 Weight	WORKOUT 2 Reps	WORKOUT 3 Weight	WORKOUT 3 Reps
Transverse abdominis	Vacuum	Set 1	6–10*						
Lower abs	Reverse crunch	Set 1	10–15						
Upper abs	Crunch	Set 1	10–15						
Obliques	Oblique crunch	Set 1	10–15						
Lower back	Prone superman	Set 1	10–15						
Lower body (knee-dominant)	Split squat‡	Set 1	10–12						
		Set 2†	10–12						
Lower body (hip-dominant)	Stepup‡	Set 1	10–12						
		Set 2†	10–12						
Shoulders, traps	Barbell upright row	Set 1	8–10						
		Set 2†	8–10						
Shoulders, triceps	Dumbbell shoulder press	Set 1	8–10						
		Set 2†	8–10						
Chest, front shoulders, triceps	Chest press (machine)	Set 1	8–10						
		Set 2†	8–10						
Upper back	Lat pulldown	Set 1	8–10						
		Set 2†	8–10						
Triceps	Pushdown	Set 1	8–10						
Biceps	Seated concentration curl	Set 1	8–10						
Calves	Seated calf raise	Set 1	10–12						

* Hold for 20–30 seconds per repetition   † Optional set   ‡ Start with the body-weight version, and when you can do 12 reps with each leg, add a barbell or dumbbells

BEGINNER ALL-EQUIPMENT WEEK 3

MUSCLES	EXERCISE	Sets	Target Reps	WORKOUT 1 Weight	Reps	WORKOUT 2 Weight	Reps	WORKOUT 3 Weight	Reps
Transverse abdominis	Vacuum	Set 1	6–10*						
Lower abs	Reverse crunch	Set 1	10–15						
Upper abs	Crunch	Set 1	10–15						
Obliques	Oblique crunch	Set 1	10–15						
Lower back	Prone superman	Set 1	10–15						
Chest, front shoulders, triceps	Chest press (machine)	Set 1	8–10						
		Set 2†	8–10						
Upper back	Lat pulldown	Set 1	8–10						
		Set 2†	8–10						
Shoulders, triceps	Dumbbell shoulder press	Set 1	8–10						
		Set 2†	8–10						
Shoulders, traps	Barbell upright row	Set 1	8–10						
		Set 2†	8–10						
Triceps	Pushdown	Set 1	8–10						
Biceps	Seated concentration curl	Set 1	8–10						
Lower body (hip-dominant)	Stepup‡	Set 1	10–12						
		Set 2†	10–12						
Lower body (knee-dominant)	Split squat‡	Set 1	10–12						
		Set 2†	10–12						
Calves	Seated calf raise	Set 1	10–12						

* Hold for 20–30 seconds per repetition   † Optional set   ‡ Start with the body-weight version, and when you can do 12 reps with each leg, add a barbell or dumbbells

INTERMEDIATE LEVEL

This is called a split routine, meaning you divide your muscle groups and work them on separate days. In this case, you'll do three different workouts. Workout A hits chest and upper back. Workout B goes after midsection and lower-body muscles. And Workout C focuses on shoulders, traps, and arms.

We recommend that you limit yourself to three workouts a week. These workouts give you a wide range of sets and reps. We recommend you do 2 warmup sets and 2 work sets of each exercise. Use perhaps one-third of your work-set weight on the first warmup set, and two-thirds on the second warmup. You can use a little more weight on the second work set than you used on the first.

INTERMEDIATE ALL-EQUIPMENT WORKOUT A: CHEST AND UPPER BACK

MUSCLES	EXERCISE	Sets	Target Reps	WEEK 1 Weight	Reps	WEEK 2 Weight	Reps	WEEK 3 Weight	Reps	WEEK 4 Weight	Reps
Chest, shoulders, triceps	Barbell bench press	Set 1	6–10								
		Set 2	6–10								
		Set 3*	6–10								
		Set 4*	6–10								
Upper back, biceps	Chinup or supinated lat pulldown	Set 1	6–10								
		Set 2	6–10								
		Set 3*	6–10								
		Set 4*	6–10								
Chest, shoulders, triceps	Dumbbell incline bench press	Set 1	6–10								
		Set 2	6–10								
		Set 3*	6–10								
		Set 4*	6–10								
Upper back	Seated row	Set 1	6–10								
		Set 2	6–10								
		Set 3*	6–10								
		Set 4*	6–10								

* Optional set

INTERMEDIATE ALL-EQUIPMENT WORKOUT B: MIDSECTION AND LOWER BODY

MUSCLES	EXERCISE	Sets	Target Reps	WEEK 1		WEEK 2		WEEK 3		WEEK 4	
				Weight	Reps	Weight	Reps	Weight	Reps	Weight	Reps
Abdominals	Kneeling cable crunch	Set 1	8–12								
		Set 2*	8–12								
Obliques	Dumbbell reverse woodchopper	Set 1	8–12†								
		Set 2*	8–12†								
Lower body (knee-dominant)	Barbell squat	Set 1	8–10								
		Set 2	8–10								
		Set 3*	8–10								
		Set 4*	8–10								
Lower body (hip-dominant)	Deadlift	Set 1	8–10								
		Set 2	8–10								
		Set 3*	8–10								
		Set 4*	8–10								
Lower-body (knee-dominant)	Dumbbell lunge	Set 1	8–10								
		Set 2	8–10								
		Set 3*	8–10								
		Set 4*	8–10								
Lower body (hip-dominant)	Romanian deadlift	Set 1	8–10								
		Set 2	8–10								
		Set 3*	8–10								
		Set 4*	8–10								

* Optional set   † Each side

INTERMEDIATE ALL-EQUIPMENT WORKOUT C: SHOULDERS, TRAPS, AND ARMS

MUSCLES	EXERCISE	Sets	Target Reps	WEEK 1		WEEK 2		WEEK 3		WEEK 4	
				Weight	Reps	Weight	Reps	Weight	Reps	Weight	Reps
Traps, shoulders	Barbell hang clean	Set 1	4–6								
		Set 2	4–6								
		Set 3*	4–6								
Shoulders, traps, triceps	Dumbbell rotation press	Set 1	6–10								
		Set 2	6–10								
		Set 3*	6–10								
Triceps	French press	Set 1	6–10								
		Set 2	6–10								
Biceps	Reverse curl	Set 1	6–10								
		Set 2	6–10								

* Optional set

ADVANCED LEVEL

This workout not only introduces some challenging new exercises but also pulls you back to full-body workouts. You'll work most of your major muscle groups in each of the three workouts. We recommend you do the intermediate routine before attempting this program, even if you're already an advanced lifter.

ADVANCED ALL-EQUIPMENT WORKOUT A

MUSCLES	EXERCISE	Sets	Target Reps	WEEK 1		WEEK 2		WEEK 3		WEEK 4	
				Weight	Reps	Weight	Reps	Weight	Reps	Weight	Reps
Lower body (hip-dominant), upper back	Power clean	Set 1	3–5								
		Set 2	3–5								
		Set 3	3–5								
		Set 4	3–5								
		Set 5	3–5								
Shoulders, triceps	Standing piston-style shoulder press	Set 1	3–5								
		Set 2	3–5								
		Set 3*	3–5								
Lower body (knee-dominant)	Front squat	Set 1	4–6								
		Set 2	4–6								
		Set 3*	4–6								
Lower body (hip-dominant)	Deadlift	Set 1	2–4†								
		Set 2	2–4†								
		Set 3	2–4†								
		Set 4	2–4†								
		Set 5	2–4†								
		Set 6	2–4†								
		Set 7*	2–4†								
		Set 8*	2–4†								
Abdominals	Barbell cable rollout	Set 1	5–10								
		Set 2	5–10								
		Set 3	5–10								

* Optional set   † Upon completion of each rep, set the weight on the floor, regrip the bar, and reset your body for the lift. In other words, each set is really a collection of 3 to 5 single deadlifts, rather than steady-speed repetitions, allowing you to use a heavier weight and still focus on form on each rep

ADVANCED ALL-EQUIPMENT WORKOUT B

MUSCLES	EXERCISE	Sets	Target Reps	WEEK 1		WEEK 2		WEEK 3		WEEK 4	
				Weight	Reps	Weight	Reps	Weight	Reps	Weight	Reps
Lower body (knee-dominant)	Back squat	Set 1	5								
		Set 2	5								
		Set 3	5								
		Set 4	5								
		Set 5	5								
Chest, shoulders, triceps	Barbell bench press	Set 1	3*								
		Set 2	3*								
		Set 3	3*								
		Set 4	3*								
		Set 5	3*								
Upper back, biceps	Pullup	Set 1	6–8								
		Set 2	6–8								
		Set 3	6–8								
Shoulders, external rotators	Standing sideways external rotation	Set 1	4–6								
		Set 2†	4–6								
Lower body (hip-dominant)	Good morning	Set 1	8–10								
		Set 2	8–10								
		Set 3†	8–10								
Obliques	Low woodchopper	Set 1	8–10‡								
		Set 2	8–10‡								
		Set 3†	8–10‡								

* Rack the weight after each rep, sit up, take a deep breath, and then completely reset your body and grip for the next rep. In other words, a "set" consists of 3 single reps, allowing you to use a heavier weight and focus on form each rep   † Optional set   ‡ Each side

ADVANCED ALL-EQUIPMENT WORKOUT C

MUSCLES	EXERCISE	Sets	Target Reps	WEEK 1		WEEK 2		WEEK 3		WEEK 4	
				Weight	Reps	Weight	Reps	Weight	Reps	Weight	Reps
Lower body (hip-dominant), upper back	Muscle snatch	Set 1	2–4*								
		Set 2	2–4*								
		Set 3	2–4*								
Upper back, chest, triceps	Incline cable pullover	Set 1	5–8								
		Set 2	5–8								
		Set 3†	5–8								
Triceps	Close-grip bench press	Set 1	6–8								
		Set 2	6–8								
		Set 3	6–8								
		Set 4†	6–8								
		Set 5†	6–8								
Triceps	Decline triceps extension (dumbbells or EZ-curl bar)	Set 1	4–6								
		Set 2	4–6								
		Set 3†	4–6								
Biceps	Prone 45-degree curl (dumbbells or EZ-curl bar)	Set 1	6–8								
		Set 2	6–8								
		Set 3†	6–8								
		Set 4†	6–8								
Calves	Standing calf raise	Set 1	6–10								
		Set 2	6–10								
		Set 3†	6–10								

* As with deadlifts in Workout A, set the weight on the floor upon completion of each rep, and reset your body and grip   † Optional set

RESOURCES

Fitness Factory Outlet
1900 South Des Plaines Avenue
Forest Park, IL 60130
(800) 383-9300
www.fitnessfactory.com

Hampton Fitness Products
1913 Portola Road
Ventura, CA 93003
(877) 339-9733
www.hamptonfit.com

Ironmaster
1005 Standard Street
Suite A
Reno, NV 89506
(800) 533-3339
www.ironmaster.com

Life Fitness
10601 West Belmont Avenue
Franklin Park, IL 60131
(888) FIT4LIFE
www.lifefitness.com

Performance Bicycle
1 Performace Way
Chapel Hill, NC 27514
(800) 727-2453
www.performancebike.com

Perform Better
11 Amflex Drive
Cranston, RI 02920
(800) 556-7464
www.performbetter.com

PowerBlock
1819 South Cedar Avenue
Owatonna, MN 55060
(800) 446-5215
www.powerblock.com

Power Systems Inc.
P. O. Box 31709
Knoxville, TN 37930
(800) 321-6975
www.power-systems.com

PreCor
P. O. Box 7202
Woodinville, WA 98072-4002
www.precor.com

ProSpot Fitness
1325 Oakbrook Drive
Suite E
Norcross, GA 30093
(800) 741-8794
www.prospotfitness.com

Smooth Fitness
717 Fellowship Road
Suite C
Mount Laurel, NJ 08054
(888) 211-1611
www.smoothfitness.com

StairMaster
12421 Willows Road, NE
Suite 100
Kirkland, WA 98034
(800) 635-2936
www.stairmaster.com

INDEX

Boldface page references indicate photographs. <u>Underscore</u> references indicate boxed text.